CURRENT AND FUTURE IMMUNOSUPPRESSIVE THERAPIES FOLLOWING TRANSPLANTATION

CURRENT AND FUTURE IMMUNOSUPPRESSIVE THERAPIES FOLLOWING TRANSPLANTATION

Edited by

Mohamed H. Sayegh

Harvard Medical School,
Boston, MA, U.S.A.

and

Giuseppe Remuzzi

Mario Negri Institute for Pharmacological Research,
Bergamo, Italy

Kluwer Academic Publishers

Dordrecht / Boston / London

A C.I.P. Catalogue record for this book is available from the Library of Congress.

ISBN 1-4020-0018-9

Published by Kluwer Academic Publishers,
P.O. Box 17, 3300 AA Dordrecht, The Netherlands.

Sold and distributed in North, Central and South America
by Kluwer Academic Publishers,
101 Philip Drive, Norwell, MA 02061, U.S.A.

In all other countries, sold and distributed
by Kluwer Academic Publishers,
P.O. Box 322, 3300 AH Dordrecht, The Netherlands.

Printed on acid-free paper

Printed in the Netherlands

TABLE OF CONTENTS

Contributors List   **xii**

I.   Introduction   **1**

1. The History of Immunosuppression for Organ   3
Transplantation
Johnny C. Hong and Barry D. Kahan

2. Clinical Trials in Transplant Immunosuppression: 19
What Have We Learned?
P. Schnuelle and F.J. van der Woude

II.   Pharmacological Immunosuppression   **41**

1. Pharmacologic Monitoring of Immunosuppressive   43
Drugs
F. Gaspari, N. Perico and G. Remuzzi

2. Use of Corticosteroids in Kidney Transplantation   61
Donald E. Hricik

3. Mycophenolate Mofetil and Azathioprine   85
John D. Pirsch and Elias David Neto

4. Cyclosporine Formulations   111
V. Ramanathan and Hal Helderman

5. Tacrolimus   123
Ron Shapiro

6. Sirolimus   143
Barry D. Kahan

7. New Agents on the Horizon   165
J. Klupp and Randall E. Morris

III.   Biologicals   185

1. Why Do We Need Induction Therapy?   187
    John Vella and John Neylan

2. Polyclonal Antilymphocyte Therapy   205
    Paul Morrissey and Anthony P. Monaco

3. Monoclonal Antibody Targeting of the T cell   221
    Receptor Complex
    Luciene Chatenoud

4. Monoclonal Antibody Targeting of IL-2R-   235
    Complex
    Flavio G. Vincenti

5. Monoclonal Antibody Targeting of Adhesion   249
    Molecules
    Marcus H. Frank and David M. Briscoe

6. Costimulation Blocade   265
    Roy D Bloom and Laurence A. Turka

7. Immunomodulatory Function of MHC   279
    Peptides
    Barbara Murphy and Alan Krensky

8. Tolerance: Is It Time to Move to the Clinic?   293
    Markus H. Frank and Mohamed H. Sayegh

IV.   Gene Therapy   315

1. Molecular Medicine in Organ Transplantation: 317
    How and When?
    A. Benigni, N. Perico, and G. Remuzzi

2. Gene Therapy in Organ Transplantation: 335
    Applicabilities and Shortcomings
    John C. Magee, Randall S. Sung, and J. Bromberg

3. Immunomodulation Strategies in   357
    Xenotransplantation
    Ian P.J. Alwayn, Leo Bühler, Murali Basker,
    and David K.C. Cooper

CONTRIBUTORS LIST

Section I

1. Johnny C. Hong and Barry D. Kahan*
   The University of Texas Medical School, Department of Surgery, Division of Immunology and Organ Transplantation, 6431 Fannin, Suite 6.240, Houston, TX 77030, USA
2. P. Schnuelle, and F.J. van der Woude
   V. Medizinische Klinik, Universitätsklinik Mannheim GGmbH, Fakultät für Klinische Medizin der Universität Heidelberg, Theodor Kutzer Ufer 1-3, D-68167 Mannheim, Germany

Section II

1. Flavio Gaspari*, Norberto Perico and Giuseppe Remuzzi
   Department of Immunology and Clinics of Organ Transplantation, Ospedali Riuniti di Bergamo - Mario Negri Institute for Pharmacological Research, Via Gavazzeni 11, - 24125, Bergamo, Italy
2. Donald E. Hricik
   Department of Medicine, Case Western Reserve University; The Transplantation Service, Department of Medicine, University Hospitals of Cleveland, 11100 Euclid Avenue, Room 8124 Lakeside Building, Cleveland, Ohio 44106, USA
3. John D. Pirsch* and Elias David-Neto**
   Department of Surgery, H4/772 Clinical Science Center, 600 Highland Avenue Madison, WI 53792-7375, USA
   ***Renal Transplant Unit, University of Sao Paulo School of Medicine*
4. Venkataraman Ramanathan* and J. Harold Helderman**
   Vanderbilt Transplant Center, Vanderbilt University Medical Center, Nashville, Tennessee 37232-2372, USA
   ***Microbiology & Immunology, Division of Nephrology, Vanderbilt University Medical Center, S-3305 Medical Center North, Nashville, Tennessee 37232-2372, USA*

NOTE: When more than one author is listed, affiliation can be assumed to be associated with all authors listed, unless specifically listed otherwise.

5. Ron Shapiro
   Renal Transplantation, Thomas E. Starzl Transplantation Institute, University of Pittsburgh, 3601 Fifth Avenue, Pittsburgh, Pennsylvania 15213, USA

6. Barry D. Kahan
   The University of Texas Medical School, Department of Surgery, Division of Immunology and Organ Transplantation, 6431 Fannin, Suite 6.240, Houston, TX 77030, USA

7. Jochen Klupp and Randall E. Morris*
   * Department of Cardiothoracic Surgery, Stanford University School of Medicine, 300 Pasteur Drive, Stanford, CA 94305-3407, USA

Section III

1. John Vella* and John Neylan**
   * Department of Clinical Transplantation, Maine Medical Center(1), 22 Bramhall Street, Portland, Maine 04102, USA
   ** Emory University, Atlanta, Georgia 30322, USA

2. Paul Morrissey* and Anthony P. Monaco**
   * Division of Organ Transplantation, Department of Surgery, Rhode Island Hospital and Brown Medical School, Providence, Rhode Island 02912, USA
   **The Transplant Center, Department of Surgery, Beth Israel Deaconess Medical Center and Harvard Medical School, Boston, MA 02215, USA

3. Lucienne Chatenoud
   INSERM U25 - Hôpital Necker 161 Rue de Sèvres 75743 Paris Cedex 15, France

4. Flavio G. Vincenti
   Clinical Medicine, Kidney Transplant Service, University of California, San Francisco, 505 Parnassus Avenue, 884 M, San Francisco, California 94143-0116, USA

5. Marcus H. Frank* and David M. Briscoe
   *Laboratory of Immunogenetics and Transplantation, Renal Division, Brigham and Women's Hospital, Renal Division, Children's Hospital, Harvard Medical School, 75 Francis Street, Boston, MA 02115, USA

6. Roy D. Bloom and Laurence A. Turka*
   *Department of Medicine, University of Pennsylvania, 700 Clinical Research Building, 415 Curie Boulevard, Philadelphia, Pennsylvania 19104-6144, USA

7. Barbara Murphy and Alan Krensky
   Renal Division, Mount Sinai School of Medicine, New York and Department of Pediatrics, Stanford University School of Medicine, California 94306, USA

8. Markus H. Frank and Mohamed H. Sayegh*
    ** Laboratory of Immunogenetics and
    Transplantation, Renal Division, Brigham and
    Women's Hospital, Renal Division, Children's
    Hospital, Harvard Medical School, 75 Francis Street,
    Boston, MA 02115, USA*

Section IV

1. Ariela Benigni*, Norberto Perico, and Giuseppe Remuzzi
    ** Department of Immunology and Clinics of Organ
    Transplantation, Ospedali Riuniti di Bergamo - Mario
    Negri Institute for Pharmacological Research, Via
    Gavazzeni, 11 24125 Bergamo, Italy*
2. John C. Magee, Randall S. Sung, and Jonathan S. Bromberg
    *University of Michigan Health Systems, 1500 E.
    Medical Center Drive, Ann Arbor, Michigan 48109,
    USA and Mount Sinai Medical Center, Miami Beach,
    Florida, USA*
3. Ian P.J. Alwayn, Leo Bühler, Murali Basker, *David K.C.
    Cooper
    *Transplantation Biology Research Center,
    Massachusetts, General Hospital / Harvard Medical
    School, Boston, USA
    *Transplantation Biology Research Center,
    Massachusetts General Hospital, GH-East, Building
    149, 13th Street, Boston, MA 02129, USA*

PART ONE: INTRODUCTION

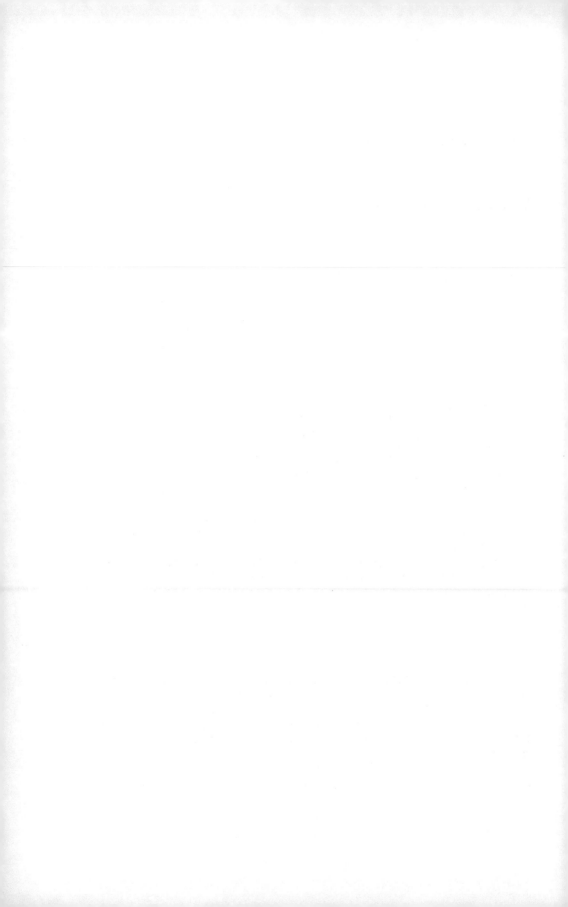

THE HISTORY OF IMMUNOSUPPRESSION FOR ORGAN TRANSPLANTATION[1]

Johnny C. Hong and Barry D. Kahan

[1]This work was supported by a grant from the National Institute of Diabetes and Digestive and Kidney Diseases (NIDDK 38016-12)

Conceptualization of Transplantation

Legends of both Eastern and Western cultures include tales of organ transplantation. Around 1200 B.C., the Hindu icon Ganesha, the god of wisdom and vanquisher of obstacles, was created by Shiva, who xenografted the head of an elephant onto the body of the child [1]. In the Iliad, Homer describes the Chimaera, a fabulous creature that is part lion, part goat, and part serpent. The writings of Lieh Tzu in 300 B.C. report the use of a "wonderful drug" by the noted Chinese physician Pien Ch'iao to promote the survival of heart allografts exchanged between two patients [2]. In the third century A.D., the twin brothers, Cosmas and Damian, used a cadaveric donor limb from an Ethiopian Moor gladiator to replace the gangrenous, cancerous leg of Justinian, the sacristan of their church in Rome [3].

Experimental to Clinical Transplantation

The technical advances for transplantation were made early in the second millennium. In 1902, Emerich Ulmann reported the heterotropic autotransplantation of a dog kidney using magnesium tube stents and ligatures to construct vascular anastomoses to the carotid artery and the internal jugular vein [4]. That same year Alexis Carrel, the noted French surgeon, reported a revolutionary technique of vascular suture—namely, triangulation with fine silk material [5]. In 1906, Mathieu Jaboulay, Carrel's teacher, performed technically successful

Mohamed Sayegh and Giuseppe Remuzzi (editors), Current and Future
Immunosuppressive Therapies Following Transplantation, 3-17.
© *2001 Kluwer Academic Publishers. Printed in the Netherlands.*

xenotransplantations using pig, and thereafter goat, kidneys to the artery and the vein in the arm of two patients [6]; however, the grafts only survived a few days. In 1909, Ernst Unger [7] concluded that there was a biochemical barrier to transplantation after he engrafted a monkey kidney into the thigh of a young girl dying of renal failure and the graft failed to produce urine.

On 3 April 1933, Soviet surgeon Yu Yu Voronoy [8] performed the first human kidney allograft on a 26-year-old female suffering from acute renal failure caused by mercuric chloride poisoning. Voronoy transplanted the right kidney of a 60-year-old head injury victim, six hours after the man's death, to the right femoral vessels of the recipient under local anesthesia. The ureter was drained through a cleft in the skin of the thigh. There was good perfusion via the vascular anastomoses; indeed, a drop of urine was produced, and the patient survived for two days. Voronoy reported five additional unsuccessful kidney transplants between 1933 to 1949, leading him to conclude that the procedure was technically feasible, but that rejection represented the real barrier. This view was reinforced by Hume's observation that canine renal allografts transplanted into the thigh afforded life-sustaining function.

Between 1950 and 1953, human kidney transplants were performed in both Paris [9-11] and Boston [12] without adjunctive immuno-suppression. Although most of these kidneys failed immediately, one recipient displayed life-sustaining renal function for several months. Kuss et al [9, 13] later revised the procedure—he performed anastomoses using the extra-peritoneal iliac, rather than the femoral, vessels of the recipient. The renal artery was anastomosed end-to-end to the hypogastric artery, and the renal vein was anastomosed end-to-side to the common iliac vein. The ureter was either implanted into the bladder or sutured to the ureter of the recipient. Based upon the report of Barrett-Brown that identical twins accept skin grafts (1935), Merrill et al [14] reported, in 1956, long-term success with excellent long-term function of renal grafts exchanged between monozygotic twins.

The Evolution of Transplant Immunology

In the 18th Century, the Scottish surgeon John Hunter, father of experimental surgery, argued against the earlier theory of Tagliacozzi on biochemical individuality as a barrier to allotransplantation [15]. Tagliacozzi wrote, "the singular character of the individual entirely dis-suades us from attempting this work on another person. For such is the force and power of individuality, that if any one should believe that he could accelerate and increase the beauty of union, nay more, achieve even the least part of the operation, we consider him plainly super-stitious and badly grounded in physical sciences" [15]. Two centuries later, Hunter made remarkable claims of successful transplantation of the spurs or the testicles of a cock into the abdomen of a hen, and of a human tooth into the comb of a cock. He attributed these successes to "the disposition of all living substances to unite when brought in contact with one another, although they are of different structure and even though the circulation is carried in one of them" [16,17].

During the first half of the twentieth century, two opposing postulates sought to explain host resistance to foreign transplants. Paul Herlich [18] postulated, in his "athrepsia" theory, that rejection was mediated by a *local* incompatibility of the protein templates of the donor and the host, a theory that was supported by Loeb [19]. In contrast, Jensen [20] postulated that foreign grafts were destroyed by a *systemic* active immunity, a theory that was confirmed by the experiments of both Bashford et al [21] and Russell et al [22]. Da Fano, in 1910 [23], and Woglom, in 1933 [24], suggested that lymphocytes and antibodies, respectively, mediate the *systemic* active immunity. The dispute between the *local* and the *systemic* postulates was resolved by the works of P.B. Medawar on skin allografts in humans [25] and rabbits [26]. The experiments conclusively documented that transplantation induces a *systemic*, donor-specific memory response of active immunization [27].

In 1962, Miller described the critical role of the thymus in the maturation of T cells, vectors of cell-mediated resistance [28]. Removal of the thymus from newborn animals prevented the development of cellular immunity, and from adult animals, lymphocyte repopulation after irradiation [29, 30]. In 1975, Lafferty and Cunningham [31] proffered the "two-signal hypothesis," which stated that, for T cells that receive a first antigen signal to display full activation, they also must receive costimulatory signals. Indeed, Bretscher and Cohn [32] found that T cell-generated humoral signals were critical for the subsequent maturation of the immune army, including the production of alloantibodies. Thus, interference with the humoral mediators of this cooperation prevents the alloimmune response.

The Development of Immunosuppressive Therapy

The antiproliferative paradigm: Lymphocyte proliferation is one of the most characteristic findings in the lymphoid structures of hosts displaying alloimmune responses. Initially, Benjamin and Sluka [33] observed that total-body irradiation interrupted cell proliferation and prevented rabbits from producing antibodies directed toward bovine serum. Murphy [34] confirmed that the radiosensitivity of lymphoid tissues mitigated the development of resistance toward tumor allografts, an observation that was later confirmed by Taliaferro et al [35], and applied to animal transplantation models by both Mannick et al [36] and by Rapaport et al [37]. Hamburger et al [38] and Murray et al [39] performed human kidney allografts after conditioning patients with sublethal total-body irradiation. Despite a few successes [38, 40,

41], this approach was abandoned owing to its irreversible effects and high mortality rates. Levin et al [42] used a variant of the procedure—total lymphoid irradiation, which focuses the treatment on lymph nodes to spare radiation exposure of marrow in long bones—to produce a transient immunosuppression—namely, a six-week window of protection prior to transplant that permitted successful engraftment with only modest chemical treatment. However, because the protocol is cumbersome, total lymphoid irradiation has been deemed impractical for routine application in cadaveric donor transplantation.

The first phase of the pharmacologic approach to immunosuppression began in 1914 when investigators used chemical compounds to block rejection. Murphy [34], followed two years later by Hektoen [43], documented the lymphocytotoxic effects of the simple organic compounds, benzene and toluene. In 1952, Baker et al noted that the combination of nitrogen mustards (methyl-bis [β-chloroethyl] amine hydrochloride), corticosteroids, and splenectomy prolonged the survival of mongrel canine allografts [44]. However, owing to the severe toxicities of these agents, the modern era of pharmacological immunosuppression did not begin until the introduction of the antiproliferative drug, 6-Mercaptopurine (6-MP; Purinethol, Glaxo Wellcome, Inc., Research Triangle Park, NC), which was originally developed for the treatment of cancer [45].

In 1959, Schwartz and Dameshek [46] demonstrated that 6-MP prevented rabbits from producing antibody against bovine serum albumin. The following year, both Calne [47] and Zukoski et al [48] reported that 6-MP prolonged allograft survival in dogs. Also in 1960, Murray et al reported that only one out of 12 patients treated with whole-body irradiation (WBI) survived, whereas five of six patients treated with either 6-MP or its imidazole derivative azathioprine (BW57-322, AZA, Imuran®, Glaxo Wellcome, Inc., Research Triangle Park, NC) showed graft function with one recipient surviving beyond four months [39]. Two years later, Calne reported that the use of AZA consistently prolonged canine renal transplant survival, caused less bone marrow suppression, and displayed better oral bioavailability than 6-MP [49]. In 1964, Calne reported three clinical cases of renal homotransplantation treated with 6-MP—two grafts were taken from cadaveric donors and one from a paternal living-related donor. The two patients who received kidneys from cadaveric donors died from uremia and infection within the first few days postoperatively, while the one who received a kidney from a living-related donor survived for seven weeks [50]. A number of investigators later documented the beneficial effects of the AZA/prednisone (Pred) combination regimen in man [51,52]. From 1966 to 1983, the AZA/Pred regimen was considered the "conventional" immunosuppressive protocol (Figure 1).

However, the AZA/Pred regimen was clouded both by a low therapeutic index and by major dose-related side effects—bone marrow aplasia, gastrointestinal visceral perforations, and overwhelming sepsis,

Established Immunosuppressive Agents

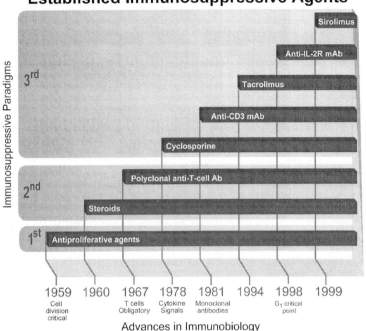

Figure 1. Major milestones in the history of immunosuppression.

primarily as a consequence of the high steroid doses nec-essary to control the frequent occurrence of acute rejection episodes. About 85 percent of renal allograft recipients on AZA/Pred regimens experienced acute rejection episodes, and only 50 percent of grafts survived a full year. Owing to the occasional occurrence of AZA-induced hepatitis, Starzl et al [53] recommended the use of cyclo-phosphamide (Cytoxan®, Bristol-Myers Squibb, New York, NY) as a maintenance immunosuppressive agent. Cyclophosphamide prevents replication by acting as an alkylating agent to cross-link DNA strands. However, the drug has been associated with refractory leukopenia, and in some patients, with leukemic transformation. At present, cyclophosphamide is used to control antibody-mediated responses, but only in a transient manner and at modest doses. The limitations of AZA and cyclophosphamide led to a search for a new nucleoside synthesis inhibitor.

Mycophenolic acid (MPA), produced by *Penicillium spp*, was discovered by Gosio in 1896 [54], purified by Alsberg and Black in 1913 [55], and shown to have antibacterial and antifungal activities in the late 1940s. Although widely used for autoimmune diseases, MPA was generally used in high doses and exhibited moderate toxicity. Mycophenolate mofetil (MMF, CellCept®, RS-61443, Roche Pharmaceuticals), a synthetic analog of MPA and the most recently approved antiproliferative agent, was designed to overcome these limitations.

The development of MMF was based on observations in children with genetic defects in purine metabolism. On one hand, children with inherited adenosine deaminase (ADA) deficiency display a selective decrease in T- and B-lymphocytes with normal numbers of neutro-phils, erythrocytes, and platelets, as well as normal brain function [56]. On the other hand, children with Lesh-Nyhan syndrome have es-sentially normal numbers of T- and B-lymphocytes, neutrophils, eryth-rocytes, and platelets, but exhibit mental deficiency [57]. This led to the hypothesis that *de novo* purine synthesis is more important for the proliferative responses of human T- and B-lymphocytes that are essential to antigenic stimulation, whereas the major salvage pathway primarily mediates neuronal activity, but not for T- and B-lymphocyte proliferation [58]. However, there is little doubt that both processes coexist in each target and that no nucleoside inhibitor shows an entirely specific pattern of immunosuppression without toxicity.

After Allison et al [57], and later Morris et al [59], showed that MMF prolonged allograft survival, Sollinger reported that ascending doses of MMF reduced the occurrence of acute rejection episodes in humans [60]. Although these observations were subsequently confirmed in randomized blinded trials [61-64], the hope that MMF might prevent chronic rejection was never realized [65], leaving the issue of the appropriate length of treatment to achieve prophylaxis of acute rejection episodes without the not uncommon complications of MMF therapy—severe cytomegalovirus disease (CMV) or lymphoprolif-erative transformation. In 1995, MMF was approved by the United States Food and Drug Administration for the prevention of acute rejection episodes in renal transplant patients. A recent major advance was the development of the new ERL080A formulation (Novartis, Basel, Switzerland) [66] of MMF, which overcomes gastrointestinal intolerance, a complication that almost invariably prevents treatment with full therapeutic doses of MMF.

The T cell depletion paradigm: The T cell depletion paradigm marked the beginning of the second phase of the modern era of immunosuppression. Based on the observation that the participation of thymus-derived lymphocytes is critical for the development of both cellular and antibody-mediated alloimmune responses, T cell depletion was attempted by a physical means—thoracic duct drainage [67-70]. To achieve depletion without surgical intervention, Anderson et al [71] produced polyclonal antilymphocyte sera (and their immunoglobulin [Ig] fractions), marking a renewal of the work performed by Metchnikoff [72] seven decades earlier. After these findings were confirmed and extended in animal models by Russell and Monaco [73] and by Levey and Medawar [74], they were translated to clinical practice by Starzl et al [75] with subsequent refinements by Najarian et al [76]. Treatment with polyclonal antibodies was initially used to salvage grafts from rejection episodes refractory to high-dose steroids and, later, to prevent their occurrence in combinations for induction therapy. However, the intense T cell inhibition resulting from the use of powerful equine or rabbit polyclonal anti-human thymocyte antibodies increased the incidence and severity of opportunistic infections and posttransplant lymphoproliferative disease to levels greater than those observed during the AZA/Pred dual-drug regimen era. In addition, the polyclonal reagents contain a variety of xenoantibodies, some of which produced toxicities, including nephropathy, serum sickness, and enhanced destruction of platelets and granulocytes.

Based on the hypothesis that some of the toxicity produced by polyclonal antibodies was caused by cross-reactions with antigens distributed on platelets, monocytes and granulocytes, monoclonal anti-bodies (mAb) were produced that were selective for markers distinctive for human T-lymphocytes. From a panel of mAb that identified T cell subpopulations, Kung et al [77] described a murine IgG2a anti-CD3 mAb (Orthoclone®, OKT3, Ortho Pharmaceutical, Raritan, NJ) directed against the CD3ε component of the T cell receptor (TcR)-CD3 complex. This reagent was pioneered in clinical practice by Cosimi et al [78] for the reversal of acute rejection episodes. Unfortunately, OKT3 causes an initial activation of T cells, producing the cytokine release syndrome and production of human anti-mouse antibodies that attenuate the activity of monoclonal reagents. OKT3 mAb is currently used both for treatment of acute rejection and for induction immunosuppression.

Another line of investigation seeks to harness intense T cell depletion (or inactivation), with or without adoptive transfer of donor elements to achieve cellular chimerism, as a method to induce allograft tolerance. This strategy seeks to decrease T cell numbers so that there will be less chance of T cells meeting each other and thus allow the emergence of elements bearing the unique regulatory phenotype that promotes tolerance induction [79]. For example, Thomas et al [80] induced renal allograft tolerance in monkeys using a combination of anti-thymocyte globulin and donor bone marrow infusions [81]. More intense and selective deletion of antigen-reactive T cells has been proposed using anti-CD2, anti-CD3, or anti-CD52 reagents with or without conjugation to toxins, and in some cases in conjunction with radiation therapy. An alternate hypothesis to achieve tolerance proposes the use of as yet undefined agents that promote T cell apoptosis [82].

The cytokine paradigm: The cytokine paradigm, which includes four components—cyclosporine (CsA), tacrolimus (TRL, FK506, Prograf®, Fujisawa USA, Inc., Deerfield, Illinois), sirolimus (SRL, Rapamycin, Rapamune®, Wyeth-Ayerst, Princeton, NJ), and anti-CD25 mAb—marked the third phase of the pharmacologic era of immunosuppression. The cytokine paradigm heralded a revolution in immunosuppression—namely, the introduction of CsA, an agent that selectively dampens the production of pro-inflammatory cytokines that mediate T cell responses. Based upon a series of elegant preclinical observations, Jean-François Borel [83] concluded that CsA exerts a T cell-selective pharmacologic effect while sparing elements of nonspecific host resistance. Although Calne et al reported the earliest clinical experience with CsA [84], it was the randomized Canadian clinical trial [85] that made seminal observations of the benefits of a CsA/Pred double-drug regimen. Although CsA displays a low immunosuppressive hazard for infection and malignancy, the associated drug-induced renal dysfunction prevents the administration of sufficient doses of the drug to fully exploit its immunosuppressive potential in transplantation, even with the use of the new microemulsion formulation (Neoral®, Novartis, Basel, Switzerland).

To permit CsA dose reduction and thereby mitigate renal dysfunction, one approach sought to discover an agent that would act in synergistic fashion with CsA. First, the antiproliferative agents AZA and MMF were shown to act in additive, but not in synergistic, fashion. Second, TRL, which was discovered in culture filtrates of *Streptomyces tsukubaensis* by Goto et al [86], was initially claimed to potentiate CsA-based immunosuppression [87]. However, CsA and TRL were subsequently shown to be antagonistic with each other [88]. Indeed, they were later discovered to inhibit the same target, calcineurin [89]. TRL was subsequently shown in clinical trials [90, 91] to be an alternative to, rather than an adjunct to, CsA for baseline immunosuppression.

Third, SRL, a macrocyclic lactone product of *Streptomyces hygroscopicus* discovered in the soil of the Vai Atari region of Rapa Nui (Easter Island) [92, 93], exhibited synergistic interactions with CsA. Under the direction of Suren Sehgal, SRL was shown to suppress both auto- and alloimmune responses *in vitro* and *in vivo* [94, 95]. While SRL was only equipotent to CsA as baseline therapy [96], the combination of SRL and CsA displayed a marked reduction in the incidence of acute rejection episodes compared with CsA alone [97].

The rapamycin analog, 40-O-(2-hydroxyethyl)-rapamycin (SDZ-RAD, Novartis, East Hanover, NJ), displays a spectrum of adverse reactions [98], as well as immunosuppressive effects, similar to SRL. However, SDZ-RAD shows a greater hydrophilicity and a shorter half-life than SRL [98]—namely, the drug requires less time to attain steady state after administration or conversely, to dissipate its effects upon drug cessation.

Fourth, mAb directed against the CD25 polypeptide α–chain of the highly avid interleukin-2 receptor (IL-2R) α, β, and, γ complex. CD25 is one of the first markers to appear on T cells as they undergo the initial activation cascade from the G_0–G_1 phase. Humanized and chimeric mouse-human anti-CD25 mAb have been developed to avoid or limit the OKT3-related adverse cytokine release syndrome. Since these agents block the CD25 α-chain of the IL-2R, which is only expressed on activated T cells, the rest of the host immune repertoire remains intact. In addition, CD25 is an extrinsic membrane protein; thus, it does not trigger T cell activation and the consequent cytokine release syndrome. Furthermore, since the majority of the molecule is of human origin, it displays a prolonged serum half-life and only rarely elicits neutralizing antibodies. Basiliximab (Simulect®, Novartis, Basel, Switzerland) [99, 100] and daclizumab (Zenapax®, Hoffman–La Roche, Inc., Nutley, NJ) [101], two new IL-2R mAb reagents approved in 1998 for the prophylaxis of acute rejection episodes in renal transplantation, afford a modest reduction in the occurrence of acute rejection episodes.

A Glimpse of the Future

On the horizon, there are new therapeutic approaches to disrupt several paradigms of the host response to a transplant. One example is the adhesion/migration paradigm. Recognition of the impact of graft injury to both enhance cellular immunogenicity and promote the lymphocyte infiltration necessary for direct antigen recognition has exposed a new strategy for intervention. At present, a variety of mAb, antisense oligonucleotides, receptor conjugates, and structural analogs are under evaluation to interrupt adhesion events mediated by cell surface selectins, Ig-type adhesion molecules, integrins, or chemokine/cytokine mediators [102-105].

The costimulation paradigm: The ultimate goal of transplantation immunosuppression is to induce immunologic tolerance to donor alloantigens, obviating the need for chronic drug therapy. Anergy or functional inactivation of antigen-reactive cells may result when the antigenic stimulus (signal one) is delivered in the absence of professional costimulation delivered by specific cell surface markers or by humoral stimuli (signal two). In animal models, anergy has been obtained using either CTLA-4Ig or anti-B7 mAb to block B7 ligation with CD28, or, alternatively, using anti-CD40 ligand (CD154) mAb receptor conjugates to block CD154 reception of the CD40 stimulus from antigen-presenting cells [106]. Disruption of costimulation is most effective when both ligand pairs (B7/CD28 and CD40/CD154) are interrupted by antibodies or receptor conjugates [107].

The antigen paradigm: In the era of modern biotechnology, two strategies are being developed to induce immunologic tolerance to donor alloantigens [108]—The first uses designer peptides, the second uses genes that alter major histocompatibility complex antigens. Both strategies seek to use isolated alloantigens to induce regulatory cells that mediate unresponsiveness either by preventing the initial recognition stages or by disrupting the effector phases of rejection. Peptides derived from class I and/or II major histocompatibility complex proteins display immunomodulatory effects *in vitro* and *in vivo*, prolonging the survival of cardiac, kidney, and skin allografts in animal models [109]. Native peptides from histocompatibility molecules seem unlikely to be clinically useful because of their relatively modest tolerogenic activity and dependence on at least a brief course of adjunctive treatment with nonspecific immunosuppressive agents.

The first approach uses designer polypeptides (allochimeric molecules) [110]—namely, molecules that bear individual donor-type antigenic epitopes substituted in the corresponding positions on a host-type class I protein backbone. In a donor-recipient rat strain combination, which provokes rapid destruction of allografts, administration of allochimeric antigens alone, either by the portal venous or oral routes, induces tolerance. The allochimeric molecules seem to produce this effect by sending a tolerogenic signal, in the distinctive fashion of an altered peptide ligand, to the corresponding T cell receptor, driving the cell into a pathway that results in the appearance of regulatory T cells. The second approach is based on the introduction of genes that either modify the expression of major histocompatibility antigens or induce markers that trigger peripheral tolerance responses, possibly akin to allochimeric molecules.

Summary

Organ transplantation has captured the public imagination like no other recent development in surgery. The field has utilized multiple disciplines, including biology, immunology, and pharmacology, to improve our understanding of the responses of the human body to transplants. Although legends of transplantation may be found in classic Eastern and Western literature, the major clinical milestones in the field have occurred within only the past 50 years. These milestones include the first successful human kidney transplantation (followed by successful liver, heart, pancreas, and intestinal transplantations), the understanding of the molecular basis of transplant immunology, and the development of agents that have resulted in significant improvements in both graft and patient survival. Transplantation has moved from the era of nonselective antiproliferative treatments, through the era of selective T cell depression with specialized pharmaceuticals such as CsA and TRL, and into the new era of drug synergy, with the exploitation of the addition of SRL to a CsA-based regimen. Using innovative strategies developed in animal models, transplant tolerance, the ultimate goal of immunosuppressive therapy, now seems within our grasp.

Acknowledgments

The authors would like to thank Natasha Teixeira and Eric Beverly for their expert editorial assistance.

References

1. Kahan BD. Pharmacokinetics and pharmacodynamics of cyclosporine. Transplant. Proc. 1989; 21(3 Suppl 1): 9-15.
2. Kahan BD. Preface: Pien Ch'iao, the legendary exchange of hearts, traditional Chinese medicine, and the modern era of cyclosporine. Transplant. Proc. 1988; 20(2 Suppl 2): 3-12.
3. Kahan BD. Editorial: Cosmas and Damian in the 20th century? N. Engl. J. Med. 1981; 305: 280-281.
4. Ullmann E. Experimentelle nierentransplantation. Wien. Klin. Wochenschr. 1902.
5. Carrel A. La technique operatoire des anastomoses vascularis, et la transplantation des visceres. Lyon Med. 1902; 98: 859-880.
6. Jaboulay M. Greffe de reins sans pli du corde sur dures arterielles et veinuses. Lyon Med. 1906; 107: 575-576.
7. Unger E. Nierentransplantation. Berl. Klin. Wochenschr. 1909; 1: 1057.
8. Voronoy Y. Sobre el bloqueo del aparato reticuloendotelial del hombre en algunas formas de intoxicacion por el sublimado y sobre la transplantacion del rinon cadaverico como metodo de tratamiento de lo anuria consecutiva aquella intoxicacion. El Siglo Med. 1936; 97: 296.
9. Kuss R, Teinturier J, Milliez P. Quelques essais de greffe de rein chez l'homme. Mem. Acad. Chir. 1951; 77: 755-759.
10. Dubost C, et al. Resultants d'une tentative de greffe renale. Bull. Soc. Med. Hop. Paris 1951; 67: 1372.
11. Servelle M, et al. Greffe d'une reine de suppliere à une malade avec rein unique congenital, atteinte de nephrite chronique hypertensive azatemique. Bull. Soc. Med. Hop. Paris 1951; 67: 99.
12. Hume DM, Merrill JP, Miller BF et al. Experiences with renal homotransplantation in the human: Report of nine cases. J. Clin. Invest. 1955; 34: 327-382.
13. Kuss R, Legrain M, Mathe G et al. Homologous human kidney transplantation: Experience with six patients. Postgrad. Med. J. 1962; 38: 528.
14. Merrill JP, Murray JE, Harrison JH et al. Successful homotransplantation of the human kidney between identical twins. J.A.M.A. 1956; 160: 277-282.
15. Gnudi MT, Webster JP. The Life and Times of Gaspare Tagliacozzi. New York: Reichner; 1950.
16. Hunter J. Treatise on the Natural History and Diseases of the Human Teeth. London: J. Johnson; 1771.
17. Palmer J. *The Complete Works of John Hunter -- Volume 3, Part 3*. Philadelphia: Haswell, Barrington & Haswell; 1841:264.
18. Ehrlich P. Experimentelle karzinomstudien an mausen. Arb. Inst. Exp. Ther. Frankfut. 1906; 1: 77.
19. Loeb L. The biological basis of individuality. Thomas, Springfield, Thomas. 1945.
20. Jensen CO. Transplantation of mammary gland carcinoma in mice. Zentralbl. Bakteriol. 1903; 34: 28-34.
21. Bashford EF, et al. Resistance and susceptibility to inoculated cancer. Third Sci. Rep. Cancer Res. Fund. 1908: 359.
22. Russell B, et al. The manifestation of active resistance to growth of implanted cancer. Proc. R. Soc. Lond. 1908; 85: 201.
23. Da Fano C. Zellulare analyse der geschwulstimmunitatsreaktionen. Z. Immunitaetsforsch. 1910; 5: 1.
24. Woglom WH. Absorption of protective agent from rats resistant to transplantable sarcoma. Am. J. Cancer 1933; 17: 873.
25. Gibson T, Medawar PB. The fate of skin homografts in man. J. Anat. 1943; 77(4): 299-310.
26. Medawar PB. The behavior and fate of skin autografts and skin homografts in rabbits. J. Anat. 1944; 78: 176.

27. Medawar PB. Second study of behavior and fate of skin autografts and skin homografts in rabbits. J. Anat. 1945; 79: 157.
28. Miller JFAP. Role of the thymus in transplantation immunity. Ann. N. Y. Acad. Sci. 1962: 340-354.
29. Miller JFAP. Effect of a neonatal thymectomy on the immunological responsiveness of the mouse. Proc. R. Soc. Lond. B. Biol. Sci. 1962; 156: 415-428.
30. Miller JFAP, Doak SMA, Cross M et al. Role of the thymus in recovery of the immune mechanism in the irradiated adult mouse. Proc. Soc. Exp. Biol. Med. 1963; 112: 785-792.
31. Lafferty KJ, Cunningham AJ. A new analysis of allogeneic interactions. Aust. J. Exp. Biol. Med. Sci. 1975; 53(1): 27-42.
32. Bretscher P, Cohn M. A theory of self-nonself discrimination. Paralysis and induction involve the recognition of one and two determinants on an antigen, respectively. Science 1970; 169(950): 1042-1049.
33. Benjamin E, Sluka P. Antikorperbildung nach experimenteller Schadigung des hamatopoetischen systems durch rontgenstrahlen. Wien. Klin. Wochenschr. 1908; 21: 311.
34. Murphy JB. Heteroplastic tissue grafting effected through roentgen ray lymphoid destruction. J.A.M.A. 1914; 62: 1459.
35. Taliaferro WH, Taliaferro LG. Effect of x-rays on immunity: A review. J. Immunol. 1951; 66: 181-212.
36. Mannick JA, Lochte Jr HL, Ashley CA et al. Autografts of bone marrow in dogs after lethal total-body radiation. Blood 1960; 15: 255-266.
37. Rapaport FT, Cannon FD, Blumenstock DA et al. Induction of unresponsiveness to canine renal allograft by total body irradiation and bone marrow transplantation. Nat. New Biol. 1972; 235(58): 191-192.
38. Hamburger J, Vayesse J, Crosnier J. Transplantation of kidney between nonhomozygotic twins after irradiation of the recipient. Presse Med. 1959; 67: 1771-1773.
39. Murray JE, Merrill JP, Dammin GJ et al. Study of transplantation immunity after total body irradiation: clinical and experimental investigation. Surgery 1960; 48(1): 272-284.
40. Kuss R, Legrain M, Mathe G et al. Premices d'une homotransplantation renale de souer à frere non jumeaux. Presse Med. 1960; 68: 755-760.
41. Merrill JP, Murray JE, Harrison H et al. Successful homotransplantation of the kidney between nonidentical twins. N. Engl. J. Med. 1960; 262: 1251.
42. Levin B, Hoppe RT, Collins G et al. Treatment of cadaveric renal transplant recipients with total lymphoid irradiation, antithymocyte globulin, and low-dose prednisone. Lancet 1985; 2(8468): 1321-1325.
43. Hektoen L. The effect of benzene on the production of antibodies. J. Infect. Dis. 1916; 19: 69.
44. Baker R, Gordon R, Huffer J et al. Experimental renal transplantation: I. Effect of nitrogen mustard, cortisone, and splenectomy. Arch. Surg. 1952; 65: 702-705.
45. Elion GB, Hitchings GH. *The Chemistry and Biology of Purines*. Boston: Little, Brown & Co.; 1957.
46. Schwartz RS, Dameshek W. Drug-induced immunological tolerance. Nature 1959; 183: 1682.
47. Calne RY. The rejection of renal homograft inhibition in dogs by 6-Mercaptopurine. Lancet 1960; 1: 417-418.
48. Zukoski CF, Lee HM, Hume DM. The effect of 6-mercaptopurine on renal homograft survival in the dog. Surg. Forum. 1960; 11: 470.
49. Calne RY, Alexandre GP, Murray JE. A study of the effects of drugs in prolonged survival of homologous renal transplantation in dogs. Ann. N. Y. Acad. Sci. 1962; 99: 743.

50. Hopewell J, Calne RY, Beswick I. Three clinical cases of renal transplantation. Brit. Med. J. 1964; 1: 411-413.
51. Goodwin WE, Kaufman JJ, Mims MM et al. Human renal transplantation. I. clinical experiences with 6 cases of renal homotransplantation. J. Urol. 1963; 89: 13.
52. Starzl TE, Marchioro TL, Huntley RT et al. Experimental and clinical homotransplantation of the liver. Ann. N. Y. Acad. Sci. 1964; 120: 739-765.
53. Starzl TE, Halgrimson CG, Penn I et al. Cyclophosphamide and human organ transplantation. Lancet 1971; 2(7715): 70-74.
54. Gosio B. Ricerche batteriologich e chimiche sulle alterazoni del mais. Rivista D'Igiene e Sanita Pubblica Ann. 1896; 7: 825.
55. Alsberg C, Black OF. Contribution to the study of maize deterioration. Bureau Plant Industry Bulletin, USDA 1913; 270: 7-48.
56. Giblett ER, Anderson JE, Cohen F et al. Adenosine-deaminase deficiency in two patients with severely impaired cellular immunity. Lancet 1972; 2(7786): 1067-1069.
57. Allison AC, Hovi T, Watts RW et al. Immunological observations on patients with Lesch-Nyhan syndrome, and on the role of de-novo purine synthesis in lymphocyte transformation. Lancet 1975; 2(7946): 1179-1183.
58. Eugui EM, Allison AC. Immunosuppressive activity of mycophenolate mofetil. Ann. N. Y. Acad. Sci. 1993; 685: 309-329.
59. Morris RE, Wang J, Blum JR et al. Immunosuppressive effects of the morpholinoethyl ester of mycophenolic acid (RS-61443) in rat and nonhuman primate recipients of heart allografts. Transplant. Proc. 1991; 23(2 Suppl 2): 19-25.
60. Sollinger HW. Mycophenolate mofetil for the prevention of acute rejection in primary cadaveric renal allograft recipients. U.S. Renal Transplant Mycophenolate Mofetil Study Group. Transplantation 1995; 60(3): 225-232.
61. Sollinger HW, Deierhoi MH, Belzer FO et al. RS-61443 -- a phase I clinical trial and pilot rescue study. Transplantation 1992; 53(2): 428-432.
62. Deierhoi MH, Sollinger HW, Diethelm AG et al. One-year follow-up results of a phase I trial of mycophenolate mofetil (RS61443) in cadaveric renal transplantation. Transplant. Proc. 1993; 25(1 Pt 1): 693-694.
63. Sollinger HW, Belzer FO, Deierhoi MH et al. RS-61443 (mycophenolate mofetil). A multicenter study for refractory kidney transplant rejection. Ann. Surg. 1992; 216(4): 513-519.
64. Laskow DA, Deierhoi MH, Hudson SL et al. The incidence of subsequent acute rejection following the treatment of refractory renal allograft rejection with mycophenolate mofetil (RS61443). Transplantation 1994; 57(4): 640-643.
65. Halloran P, Mathew T, Tomlanovich S et al. Mycophenolate mofetil in renal allograft recipients: a pooled efficacy analysis of three randomized, double-blind, clinical studies in the prevention of rejection. The International Mycophenolate Mofetil Renal Transplant Study Groups. Transplantation 1997; 63(1): 39-47.
66. Schmouder R, Arns W, Merkel F et al. Pharmacokinetics of ERL080A: a new enteric coated formulation of mycophenolic acid-sodium. 18th Annual Meeting of the American Society of Transplantation 1999; Abstract 787.
67. Gowans JL. The recirculation of lymphocytes from blood to lymph in the rat. J. Physiol. (Lond.) 1959; 146: 54.
68. Woodruff MFA, Anderson NF. Effect of lymphocyte depletion by thoracic duct fistula and administration of antilymphocyte serum on the survival of skin homographs in rats. Nature 1963; 200: 702.
69. Frankson C, Bloomstrand R. Drainage of the thoracic lymph duct during homologous kidney transplantation in man. Scand. J. Urol. Nephrol. 1967; 1: 123.
70. Fish JC, Sarles HE, Remmers Jr AR. Thoracic duct fistulas in man. Surg. Gynecol. Obstet. 1970; 131(5): 869-872.

71. Anderson NF, James K, Woodruff MF. Effect of antilymphocytic antibody and antibody fragments on skin-homograft survival and the blood-lymphocyte count in rats. Lancet 1967; 1(7500): 1126-1128.
72. Metchnikoff E. Etudes sur la resorption des cellules. Ann. Inst. Pasteur 1899; 13: 737.
73. Russell PS, Monaco AP. Heterologous antilymphocyte sera and some of their effects. Transplantation 1967; 5(4): 1086-1099.
74. Levey RH, Medawar PB. Some experiments on the action of anti lymphoid antisera. Ann. N. Y. Acad. Sci. 1966; 129: 164.
75. Starzl TE, Marchioro TL, Porter KA et al. The use of heterologous antilymphoid agents in canine renal and liver homotransplantation and in human renal homotransplantation. Surg. Gynecol. Obstet. 1967; 124(2): 301-308.
76. Najarian JS, Simmons RL, Gewurz H et al. Antihuman lymphoblast globulin. Fed. Proc. 1970; 29(1): 197-201.
77. Kung P, Goldstein G, Reinherz EL et al. Monoclonal antibodies defining distinctive human T cell surface antigens. Science 1979; 206(4416): 347-349.
78. Cosimi AB, Colvin RB, Burton RC et al. Use of monoclonal antibodies to T cell subsets for immunologic monitoring and treatment in recipients of renal allografts. N. Engl. J. Med. 1981; 305(6): 308-314.
79. Thomas FT, Ricordi C, Contreras JL et al. Reversal of naturally occurring diabetes in primates by unmodified islet xenografts without chronic immunosuppression. Transplantation 1999; 67(6): 846-854.
80. Thomas JM, Carver FM, Foil MB et al. Renal allograft tolerance induced with ATG and donor bone marrow in outbred rhesus monkeys. Transplantation 1983; 36(1): 104-106.
81. Thomas J, Carver M, Cunningham P et al. Promotion of incompatible allograft acceptance in rhesus monkeys given posttransplant antithymocyte globulin and donor bone marrow. I. In vivo parameters and immunohistologic evidence suggesting microchimerism. Transplantation 1987; 43(3): 332-338.
82. Van Parijs L, Abbas AK. Homeostasis and self-tolerance in the immune system: turning lymphocytes off. Science 1998; 280(5361): 243-248.
83. Borel JF, Feurer C, Gubler HU et al. Biological effects of cyclosporin A: A new antilymphocytic agent. Agents Actions 1976; 6(4): 468-475.
84. Calne RY, White DJ, Thiru S et al. Cyclosporin A in patients receiving renal allografts from cadaver donors. Lancet 1978; 2(8104-5): 1323-1327.
85. The Canadian Multicentre Transplant Study Group. A randomized clinical trial of cyclosporine in cadaveric renal transplantation. Analysis at three years. N. Engl. J. Med. 1986; 314(19): 1219-1225.
86. Goto T, Kino T, Hatanaka H et al. Discovery of FK506, a novel immunosuppressant isolated form *Streptomyces tsukubaensis*. Transplant. Proc. 1987; 19(5 Suppl 6): 4-8.
87. Zeevi A, Duquesnoy R, Eiras G et al. Immunosuppressive effect of FK-506 on in vitro lymphocyte alloactivation: synergism with cyclosporine A. Transplant. Proc. 1987; 19(5 Suppl 6): 40-44.
88. Vathsala A, Goto S, Yoshimura N et al. The immunosuppressive antagonism of low doses of FK506 and cyclosporine. Transplantation 1991; 52(1): 121-128.
89. Schreiber SL, Crabtree GR. The mechanism of action of cyclosporin A and FK506. Immunol. Today 1992; 13(4): 136-142.
90. Pirsch JD, Miller J, Deierhoi MH et al. A comparison of tacrolimus (FK506) and cyclosporine for immunosuppression after cadaveric renal transplantation. Transplantation 1997; 63(7): 977-983.
91. Yang HC, Holman MJ, Langhoff E et al. Tacrolimus/"low-dose" mycophenolate mofetil versus microemulsion cyclosporine/"low-dose" mycophenolate mofetil after kidney transplantation -- 1-year follow-up of a prospective, randomized clinical trial. Transplant. Proc. 1999; 31(1-2): 1121-1124.

92. Vezina C, Kudelski A, Sehgal SN. Rapamycin (AY-22,989), a new antifungal antibiotic: I. Taxonomy of the producing streptomycete and isolation of the active principle. J. Antibiot. (Tokyo) 1975; 28(10): 721-726.
93. Sehgal SN, Baker H, Vezina C. Rapamycin (AY-22,989), a new antifungal antibiotic: II. Fermentation, isolation and characterization. J. Antibiot. (Tokyo) 1975; 28(10): 727-732.
94. Morris RE, Meiser BM. Identification of a new pharmacologic action for an old compound. Med. Sci. Res. 1989; 17: 877-878.
95. Calne RY, Collier DS, Lim S et al. Rapamycin for immunosuppression in organ allografting. Lancet 1989; 2(8656): 227.
96. Groth CG, Backman L, Morales JM et al. Sirolimus (rapamycin)-based therapy in human renal transplantation: similar efficacy and different toxicity compared with cyclosporine. Transplantation 1999; 67(7): 1036-1042.
97. Kahan BD, Podbielski J, Napoli KL et al. Immunosuppressive effects and safety of a sirolimus/cyclosporine combination regimen for renal transplantation. Transplantation 1998; 66(8): 1040-1046.
98. Kahan BD, Wong RL, Carter C et al. A phase I study of a four-week course of the rapamycin analogue SDZ-RAD (RAD) in quiescent cyclosporine-prednisone-treated renal transplant recipients. Transplantation 1999; 68(8): 1100-1106.
99. Kahan BD, Rajagopalan PR, Hall ML et al. Reduction of the occurrence of acute cellular rejection among renal allograft recipients treated with basiliximab, a chimeric anti-interleukin-2-receptor monoclonal antibody. Transplantation 1999; 67(1): 276-284.
100. Nashan B, Moore R, Amlot P et al. Randomised trial of basiliximab versus placebo for control of acute cellular rejection in renal allograft recipients. Lancet 1997; 350(9086): 1193-1198.
101. Vincenti F, Kirkman R, Light S et al. Interleukin-2-receptor blockade with daclizumab to prevent acute rejection in renal transplantation. N. Engl. J. Med. 1998; 338(3): 161-165.
102. Dulkanchainun TS, Goss JA, Imagawa DK et al. Reduction of hepatic ischemia/reperfusion injury by a soluble P-selectin glycoprotein ligand-1. Ann. Surg. 1998; 227(6): 832-840.
103. Palma-Vargas JM, Toledo-Pereyra L, Dean RE et al. Small-molecule selectin inhibitor protects against liver inflammatory response after ischemia and reperfusion. J. Am. Coll. Surg. 1997; 185: 365-372.
104. Schmid RA, Yamashita M, Boasquevisque CH et al. Carbohydrate selectin inhibitor CY-1503 reduces neutrophil migration and reperfusion injury in canine pulmonary allografts. J. Heart Lung Transplant. 1997; 16(10): 1054-1061.
105. Snapp KR, Ding H, Atkins K et al. A novel P-selectin glycoprotein ligand-1 monoclonal antibody recognizes an epitope within the tyrosine sulfate motif of human PSGL-1 and blocks recognition of both P- and L- selectin. Blood 1998; 91(1): 154-164.
106. Gimmi CD, Freeman GJ, Gribben JG et al. Human T cell clonal anergy is induced by antigen presentation in the absence of B7 costimulation. Proc. Natl. Acad. Sci. U. S. A. 1993; 90(14): 6586-6590.
107. Kirk AD, Harlan DM, Armstrong NN et al. CTLA4-Ig and anti-CD40 ligand prevent renal allograft rejection in primates. Proc. Natl. Acad. Sci. U. S. A. 1997; 94(16): 8789-8794.
108. Wood KJ. Transplantation tolerance. Curr. Opin. Immunol. 1991; 3(5): 710-714.
109. Magee CC, Sayegh MH. Peptide-mediated immunosuppression. Curr. Opin. Immunol. 1997; 9(5): 669-675.
110. Wang M, Stepkowski SM, Yu J et al. Localization of cryptic tolerogenic epitopes in the alpha1-helical region of the RT1.A^u alloantigen. Transplantation 1997; 63(10): 1373-1379.

CLINICAL TRIALS IN TRANSPLANT IMMUNOSUPPRESSION: WHAT HAVE WE LEARNED?

P. Schnuelle and F.J. van der Woude

Introduction

Evidence-based medicine relies on clinical trials, which are mandatory prior to the introduction of novel therapeutic strategies into clinical practice. The experimental design most appropriate for the comparison of therapeutic intervention is the randomized controlled clinical trial. These trials are designed to assess the efficacy of treatment in quantitative terms which are frequency of defined events (primary end-points) and time course of disease. Randomization minimizes selection bias and prevents bias in the comparison between study groups due to regression toward the mean. However, there is no guarantee that bias is entirely eliminated even in a prospective study with double blinding.

External validity is very important in the interpretation of any controlled clinical trial. Subjects willing to participate in a controlled clinical trial fulfill certain inclusion criteria, others are usually excluded according to protocol restrictions. Therefore, it should be clear whom the study population represents and if the findings of the study can be generalized to other patient categories.

Changes in therapy or dropouts are special problems concerning the internal validity of a clinical trial; for instance, study subjects who continue not to respond to the experimental therapy may request for a prohibited medication or may want to be switched to another study group, which must be permitted because of ethical reasons. Early withdrawal from the study may be unavoidable in cases of unpleasant side effects even when the study medication is effective. Monitoring of

Mohamed Sayegh and Giuseppe Remuzzi (editors), Current and Future Immunosuppressive Therapies Following Transplantation, 19-40.
© *2001 Kluwer Academic Publishers. Printed in the Netherlands.*

unexpected side effects is of major importance featuring the safety analysis of any therapeutic intervention. Nevertheless, the clinical investigator should be aware of the fact that the prospective clinical trial is more suitable to study intended events rather than unintended ones like major side-effects.

The best strategy to deal with early study termination or switching between study groups is to analyze the data on intention-to-treat-basis even though the efficacy analysis might be offended due to a rising number of dropouts. The intention-to-treat-approach means that each subject is considered as if he or she had remained in the original treatment group. Thus, any negative outcome will be assigned to the initial therapy.

Pooled analysis of several single studies is increasingly used in efficacy research. The procedure may provide a more accurate estimate of the quantitative and qualitative benefits of a particular treatment, especially if the trials in themselves do not reach statistical power to detect a difference between the alternative interventions. However, there is some bias imminent that needs to be addressed; the question of study selection and comparability of the trials taken for a pooled analysis is the most troublesome issue. For purposes of quantitative assessment, only studies with identical endpoints and at least similarity in design and methods meet the criteria to be included. This may however be difficult to achieve.

Apart from these basic methodological limitations, the randomized controlled clinical trial represents the gold standard in efficacy research. This chapter focuses on the most outstanding clinical trials in the field of solid organ transplantation and will provide some guidelines for the clinician who faces an increasing number of new generation immuno-suppressants during the last decade (**Table 1**).

Cyclosporin / Neoral

The introduction of cyclosporin into clinical practice has stimulated transplantation world wide resulting in a 10-15% increase of 1 year graft survival after renal cadaveric transplantation as compared to conventional immunosuppression [1,2]. This is why various clinical study protocols which have been designed for the assessment of new generation immunosuppressants are based on a combination with cyclosporin for the verum groups or refer to a cyclosporin containing immunosuppressive regimen for the controls. However, cyclosporin is associated with several adverse side-effects such as hypertension, hyperlipidemia and nephropathy, and little has been gained with regard to the most important problem: the prevention of chronic allograft vasculopathy. Histological changes of chronic rejection appearing in obliterative vasculopathy and tubulointer-stitial fibrosis are difficult to

Table 1: Evolution of immunosuppressive agents in clinical transplantation: mechanisms of action, indication, and drug specific adverse side profiles

Drug	Year	Mechanism of action	Prevention of rejection	Treat-ment	Adverse side effects
Azathio-prine	1961/62	Antimetabolite of nucleic acid synthesis	+	-	Myelotoxicity Alopecia
Cyclo-sporin	1983	Inhibition of calcineurin mediated IL-2 expression by T-lymphocytes	+	-	Hypertension Nephrotoxicity Hyperlipidemia Gum hyperplasia Hirsutism
Tacro-limus	1993/94	Inhibition of calcineurin mediated IL-2 expression by T-lymphocytes	+	+	Diabetes mellitus Nephrotoxicity Neurotoxicity
Myco-pheno-late Mofetil	1995/96	Selective inhibition of purine de-novo synthesis pathway	+	(+)	Diarrhea Abdominal pain Leucopenia Anemia Thrombocytopenia
Siro-limus	1999	Inhibition of the IL-2 driven signal transduction pathway	+	-	Hyperlipidemia Leucopenia Thrombocytopenia

differentiate from cyclosporin nephro-toxicity in advanced cases [3,4]. Monitoring of trough levels is therefore routinely performed to achieve an optimum balance between adequate immunosuppression and toxic side-effects. Registry data indicate that graft survival is correlated with the maintenance dosage of cyclosporin during long-term follow-up [5].

Thus, besides various non-immunological factors which are thought to play a key-role in the pathogenesis of chronic rejection, inadequacy of immunosuppression obviously has a detrimental effect on graft survival. The occurrence of chronic cyclosporine nephrotoxicity may be less dose-dependent than attributable to an elevated individual susceptibility to the drug. This is in line with the observation that genetic differences exist in the quantitative expression of the cytokine transforming growth factor beta [6] after administration of cyclosporin

[7]. Halving target levels of cyclosporin in stable renal transplant recipients one year after transplantation was associated with less incidence of cancer but enhanced frequency of acute rejection episodes, which has been demonstrated by a prospective trial. Nevertheless, graft function and graft survival at 66 months of follow-up were not affected [8].

The administration of the new cyclosporin microemulsion neoral resulted in a 20% reduction of acute rejection episodes in the early phase after transplantation, due to a significantly higher bioavailability of the drug as compared to the standard oil-based formulation [9]. Furthermore, a larger concentration-controlled prospective study including 1097 stable renal transplant patients has clearly demonstrated that safety and tolerability remained similar despite a more efficient immunosuppression, and renal function parameters were not compromised due to the increased drug exposure during the follow-up period of 18 months [10,11]. But it is still a matter of debate if all patients who are stable on standard cyclosporin need to be switched to the microemulsion formulation.

Ongoing concerns about chronic cyclosporin nephrotoxicity prompted a large number of clinical trials in which attempts have been performed to withdraw cyclosporin after a given time post-transplant. Major differences in the designs, duration of follow-up, and outcomes make it difficult however to draw a final conclusion from these investigations. Several studies have reported improvements in renal function, lipid profile and hypertension [12-14] others have failed to confirm these findings [15,16] owing to the fact that the reduction in cyclosporin toxicity was offset by the occurrence of acute rejection [17]. A systematic meta-analysis involving 10 randomized [12-15,17-22] and 7 non-randomized clinical trials [23-29] has concluded that short-term graft or patient survival are not affected despite an increased incidence of acute rejection episodes following elective cyclosporine withdrawal after renal transplantation. Furthermore, none of the outcomes was influenced by the timing or manner of cyclosporin taper [30]. However, it remains unclear from the pooled analysis whether the higher incidence of acute rejection associated with cyclosporin withdrawal leads to an increased incidence of chronic rejection during the ongoing follow-up. At least one randomized trial has demonstrated improved renal function parameters at 5 years and a trend towards a reduced cardiovascular mortality after 8 years post-transplant in patients who had been withdrawn from cyclosporin [31].

Tacrolimus (FK506)

Tacrolimus, a macrolide molecule isolated from Streptomyces tsubucaensis is, like cyclosporin, an inhibitor of interleukin-2 expression by T-lymphocytes. Data from clinical studies indicate that tacrolimus is more potent than cyclosporin and to some extent, exhibits a different pattern of adverse side-effects. Tacrolimus has been compared with cyclosporin for primary immunosuppression in liver transplantation in two randomized controlled multicenter trials involving a total of 1074 patients [32,33]. In both trials, there was no difference in patient and graft survival between the two treatment groups at one year. Consistently higher rates of acute rejection episodes, in part steroid-resistant and refractory, were observed in the cyclosporin groups, despite a significantly lower usage of corticosteroids in the tacrolimus arm of the European study [32]. Nephrotoxicity, neurological complications and disturbances of glucose metabolism accounted for the most serious side-effects, requiring discontinuation of tacrolimus more frequently in the U.S. study [33]. The tolerability of tacrolimus appeared to be dosage related and improved after dose reduction. It can be concluded that tacrolimus is well established for primary immunosuppression in hepatic transplantation today. Furthermore, conversion from cyclosporin to tacrolimus has been shown an effective rescue therapy in liver allografts with chronic rejection [34]. Ongoing trials are comparing tacrolimus to neoral since standard cyclosporine may be more prone to inadequate reabsorption, especially in liver transplantation. Recently, a large multicenter study has been completed, clearly demonstrating the pharmacokinetic advantages of neoral translate into clinical superiority over conventional cyclosporin [35].

Based on the extending data supply from liver transplantation, tacrolimus has been used to attempt salvage of kidney allografts. The Pittsburgh Group was the first to report on a series of renal transplant patients with ongoing, biopsy-proven rejection, including vascular rejection, who were switched to tacrolimus for rescue therapy [36]. Meanwhile, the 5-year experience including a total of 169 renal transplant recipients is available and 85% had failed to respond to anti-lymphocyte globulins prior to conversion. A total of 125 patients (74%), among these, 13 out of 28 on dialysis, were salvaged successfully exhibiting a mean serum creatinine of 2.3 ± 1.1 mg/dl after an average follow-up of 30 months [37]. These results are in line with a multicenter study involving 73 kidney allograft recipients with steroid-resistant rejection. A 75% rate of graft survival could be achieved yielding a satisfactory renal function, a low incidence of recurrent rejection, and an acceptable profile of adverse side effects at 1 year of follow-up [38].

Two large multicenter studies comparing the 12-month efficacy and safety of a tacrolimus or cyclosporin based regimen in conjunction with azathioprine and low-dose corticosteroids for primary immunosuppression in kidney transplantation have been completed thus far [39,40]. Both trials were designed in a similar fashion concerning primary and secondary endpoints. However, patients in the U.S. study received an induction therapy and were given a higher average dose of tacrolimus during the study period. A consistently significant reduction of biopsy confirmed and steroid-resistant rejection episodes was evident for the tacrolimus treated groups in both trials. However, actuarial patient and graft survival at one year were not yet affected by this benefit. Neurological side-effects were more frequent in the tacrolimus groups, but were rarely severe enough to stop treatment. In the U.S study, a 19.9% incidence of post-transplant diabetes occurred in the tacrolimus arm as compared to 4% in the cyclosporin group, which was not observed at the same degree in the European study.

Although no difference was seen in 2-year protocol biopsies scored for acute and chronic histopathologic lesions according to the Banff classification [41] preliminary data from the U.S study indicate improved graft survival in tacrolimus treated patients at three years [42]. Extending experience with the drug is likely to further reduce complications which seem to be dose-dependent, and it remains to be seen whether the encouraging beneficial effects can be maintained during a longer period of follow-up.

Mycophenolate Mofetil

Mycophenolic acid, the active metabolite of mycophenolate mofetil (MMF), selectively inhibits lymphocyte proliferation by blocking the de-novo synthesis of guanosine nucleotides. The drug has been introduced into clinical transplantation as a replacement for azathioprine. Three randomized, double-blind multicenter parallel group trials have been conducted, which compared MMF at dosages of 2 or 3 g/day with either placebo or azathioprine (1-2mg/kg) as part of a combination therapy for the prevention of renal transplant rejection [43-45]. In summary, these trials confirm that MMF yields a 50% reduction in the incidence of (biopsy confirmed) acute rejec-tion during the first year after transplantation. Moreover, MMF compared favorably with either placebo or azathioprine in the severity of acute rejection as related to histopathologic grading, and to the need for antilymphocyte antibodies in the reversal of rejection. Nevertheless, even the pooled data analysis of the three studies failed to detect any beneficial effect on patient death and graft loss at one year [46]. Gastrointestinal complaints (abdominal pain, diarrhea, nausea, vomiting) and hematological disorders (leucopenia, anemia, thrombocytopenia) accounted for the most common adverse side-events resolving after drug discontinuation. There was a dose-dependent trend towards more opportunistic infections: tissue invasive CMV infection occurred more frequently in the MMF 3g/d group, but uniform CMV prophylaxis was not required. Extending clinical experience suggests that discontinuation of MMF during ganciclovir treatment is advisable since otherwise an adequate humoral immune response necessary to prevent a relapse of CMV disease may not occur. Because MMF does not induce hypertension, lipid metabolism abnormalities or nephrotoxic side-effects, one might expect improved survival of renal allografts during ongoing follow-up. Comparative studies have not yet demonstrated a long-term benefit so far, probably due to lack of statistical power [47]. On the other hand, there is preliminary evidence that long-term graft survival is substantially improved in certain subgroups of patients who have experienced delayed graft function [48]. In heart transplantation, data from a large double-blind, randomized multi-center trial comparing MMF (3g/d) with azathioprine (1,5-3mg/kg) in addition to cyclosporin and steroids indicate a significant reduction in the requirement of rejection therapy and in the 1-year mortality as well (6.2% vs. 11.4% in favor of MMF treatment), when the analysis was restricted to subjects on study medication. However, the ability to detect a statistically significant survival advantage was lost analyzing on intention-to-treat basis [49].

Large scaled randomized, multicenter trials involving MMF for primary prophylaxis of rejection in liver transplantation have not been published to date. MMF has been administered to render possible steroid taper either in combination with cyclosporine or tacrolimus after orthotopic liver tansplantation. A total of 97 patients was enrolled and the use of MMF with Neoral (n=49) or Tacrolimus (n=48) and an identical steroid was associated with a low incidence of rejection episodes (19.1%) and excellent graft and patient survival (96%) at 6 months [50]. Another open-label prospective protocol was conducted to compare the efficacy and toxicity of a double-drug therapy (tacrolimus and steroids) with a triple drug regimen including MMF at 1g b. i. d.. Two hundred liver transplant recipients were included and the interim analysis was reported after a mean follow-up of 12.7 months. During the study period, 28 of 99 patients (28.3%) in the double-drug group received MMF to reverse ongoing rejection, nephrotoxicity, and/or neurotoxicity, whereas 61 patients (60.4%) in the triple-drug group were withdrawn from MMF because of infection, myelosuppression, and/or gastrointestinal disturbances. By intention to treat, 1-year patient (85.1% vs. 83.1%) and graft survival (80.2% vs. 79.2%) were similar. Acute rejection episodes occurred more frequently in the double-drug group (41.4% vs. 31.7%), however the difference did not reach the level of statistical significance [51].

In kidney transplantation, MMF was noted to reverse rejection in approximately 70% of patients with refractory acute rejection which had been shown by a non-randomized pilot study some years prior to the approval of the drug for clinical transplantation [52]. MMF given at 3g/d in combination with high-dose intravenous steroids was further tested prospectively for the treatment of first acute cellular rejection in kidney transplantation and compared favorably to azathioprine and steroid bolus showing a significant reduction of any treatment failure and requirement for antilymphocyte therapy, respectively. Graft failure and patient death at one year, defined as the combined primary end-point, was 8.9% in the MMF treated and 14.8% in the control group, but more patients on MMF discontinued the study medication owing to adverse side effects [53].

Following the drug's mechanism of action it was hoped that MMF would prevent or delay progression of chronic allograft nephropathy. Preliminary clinical data derived from single center studies appear to confirm this hypothesis [54,55]. Further investigation is required, however, to clarify if transient improvements of renal function parameters definitely translate into improved long-term survival.

Sirolimus (Rapamycin)

Rapamycin, a macrolide produced by Streptomyces hygroscopicus, is structurally related to tacrolimus but does not affect lymphokine synthesis. The mechanism of action relies on the inhibition of the interleukin-2 mediated signal transduction pathway thus targeting at a later stage in the cascade of lymphocyte proliferation. The drug was thought therefore to be synergistic in addition with calcineurin inhibitors. Rapamycin administered in conjunction with cyclosporin resulted in enhanced immunosuppression in 49 mismatched living-donor renal transplant recipients when compared with a historical cohort of 65 demographically similar, consecutive patients on a concentration controlled cyclosporin / prednisone regimen. A substantial reduction in the overall incidence of acute rejection from 32% to 7.5% was evident, whereas rates of patient and graft survival as well as morbid complications did not differ between the treatment groups at 18-47 month follow-up period [56]. Rapamycin displays a different profile of adverse side effects but is equivalent to cyclosporin in the prevention of acute rejection which was demonstrated by a recent comparative multicenter pilot study. 83 first cadaveric renal transplant recipients were randomized either to receive cyclosporin (n=42) or rapamycin (n=41) in combination with azathioprine and corticosteroids. Patient survival (100% vs. 98%), graft survival (98% vs. 90%), and occurrence of acute rejection (41% vs. 38%) did not differ significantly at one year comparing sirolimus and cyclosporin treated patients. Renal function parameters were favorable and there was less hypertension in patients on sirolimus. Adverse side-effects were mainly attributable to laboratory abnormalities like hyperlidemia and hematologic changes like leucopenia and thrombocytopenia, resolving within two months after lowering the target trough level [57].

Owing to the synergism with cyclosporin it is therefore likely that rapamycin will facilitate dose reductions of both calcineurin inhibitors and corticosteroids, thus reducing toxic side-effects in maintenance immunosuppression of the future [58].

Biologics and Induction

Xenogenic biologics, either monoclonal or polyclonal, as derived from sera of various immunized mammalian species, are widely used in clinical transplantation for prophylaxis and treatment of severe rejection (**Table 2**). Antibodies are also given to avoid cyclosporine therapy during the early postoperative period in trans-plant recipients deemed to be at high risk for delayed graft function. Initial graft function has been identified to predict a superior long-term outcome [59-61]. However, there is still no consensus in the field if delayed onset of the graft in the absence of rejection necessarily leads to reduced long-term survival probability [62,63].

OKT3, a murine monoclonol antibody directed against the T cell receptor/CD3 complex, has been proven to be superior to high-dose steroids in the reversal of acute rejection in renal transplant recipients, when compared in a randomized multicenter trial [64]. Side effects are related to the cytokine release syndrome characterized by fever, chills, vomiting, diarrhea, myalgia, bronchial spasmen and hypotension. Acute pulmonary edema must be avoided by correcting a preexisting fluid overload and close monitoring of the patient is advisable during the first three days of treatment. The use of OKT3 for induction has been evaluated by a multicenter study enrolling a total of 215 renal transplant recipients. Patients were randomized to receive either a 14-day course of OKT3 in conjunction with azathioprine, corticosteroids and sequential addition of cyclosporin on day 11, or a conventional cyclosporin-based triple drug therapy. OKT3 induction resulted in significantly lower incidence of acute rejection episodes and Kaplan-Meier estimates revealed a trend towards improved graft survival at two years, whereas patient survival was not affected [65].

OKT3 has also been compared prospectively to various polyclonal antilymphocyte preparations for induction therapy, and Minnesota anti-lymphocyte globulin (MALG) was shown to deliver equivalent immuno-suppression. There was no difference in actuarial patient and graft sur-vival at one and two years in 138 adult kidney and 35 kidney-pancreas recipients. The incidence of acute rejection and renal function were similar in both study arms. Tolerability of MALG was favorable to OKT3, which was however associated with less incidence of CMV [66]. Two additional randomized studies indicate some superiority of polyclonals for prophylactic use [67,68]. Both trials revealed less treatment failure according to a lower incidence of acute rejection and significantly im-proved graft survival was observed in patients who received ATG-F [68]. Recently, a randomized study has been completed comparing

Table 2: Survey of antibody preparations used in comparative clinical trials of transplantation

	Agent	Species	Molecular target	Induction therapy	Reversal of rejection	Adverse side effects
polyclonal	**MALG**	horse	multiple	+	+	serum sickness
	Atgam	horse	epitopes	+	+	leukopenia
	ATG-F	rabbit	on	+	+	thrombopenia
	Thymoglo-buline	rabbit	lymphoid cells	+	+	fever
monoclonal	**OKT3**	murine	T cell receptor-CD3 complex	+	+	cytokine release syndrome
	anti-LFA 1	murine	leukocyte function-associated antigen-1 (CD11a)	+	-	well tolerated
	Enlimomab	murine	adhesion molecule ICAM-1 (CD54), ligand of LFA-1	+	-	well tolerated
	33B3.1	rat	α-chain of interleukin-2 receptor	+	-	no major side effects
	anti-Tac	murine	α-chain of interleukin-2 receptor			no major side effects
	Basiliximab	chimeric: murine / humanized	α-chain of interleukin-2 receptor	+	-	no major side effects
	Daclizumab	fully humanized	α-chain of interleukin-2 receptor	+	-	no major side effects

the efficacy and safety of thymoglobulin (rabbit-derived polyclonal antibody) to ATGAM (horse-derived polyclonal antibody) for induction in adult renal transplant patients. Maintenance immunosuppression was based on a triple drug therapy with corticosteroids, neoral and azathioprine or MMF. Thymoglobin was shown to result in a lower incidence and severity of acute rejection, better tolerability and less CMV disease. Event free survival at on year was significantly enhanced ($94\pm4\%$ vs. $63\pm10\%$), and the rate of patients with functioning graft was superior (98% vs. 83%) [69].

Induction therapy is thought to ameliorate nephrotoxicity permitting delayed addition of cyclosporin in the early phase after transplantation. Whether this potential benefit is abrogated in the presence of calcium antagonists was tested by a clinical pilot study including 100 renal transplant recipients. Short-term outcome of immediate cyclosporin administration in combination with diltiazem was compared to sequential cyclosporin following induction therapy with ATGAM: during the first 90 days graft failure and incidence of delayed graft function were similar and there was no difference in serum creatinine between the random groups [70].

Antilymphocyte induction therapy remains to be a troublesome issue and, since the majority of the U.S. transplantation centers routinely give induction whereas the Europeans do not, a striking difference in principal strategies on transplant immunosuppression exists. Registry data from the United Network of Organ Sharing indicate that the prophylactic use of antilymphocyte preparations in the early phase after cadaveric kidney transplantation results in improved graft outcomes. Using semiparametric logistic regression models, the relative risk of graft failure at 12 months was calculated to be 0.82 and 0.86 for Minnesota antilymphocyte globulin and OKT3, respectively [71]. These findings are in line with a meta-analysis on the impact of antilymphocyte induction therapy on renal allograft survival based on 7 randomized, controlled clinical trials. A significantly beneficial effect on two year graft survival was cal-culated according to an odds ratio of 0.69 [95%CI 0.45-0.97] [72].

OKT3 with sequential cyclosporine is efficient to improve long-term graft survival substantially in certain patient categories at high immunological risk like pediatric and black recipients and presensitized patients [73,74]. However, the use of antilymphocyte antibodies has been shown to be associated with increased incidence of lymphoma in kidney and heart transplant recipients [75,76], and there is evidence that the risk of malignant disorders during long-term follow-up is related to the power and dosage of immunosuppression [8]. Induction therapy is therefore discussed controversially and opinions differ whether the benefit on early outcome counterbalances the risk of cancer development during long duration follow-up. It is also questionable if the advantage on transplant survival will be maintained in the view of growing clinical expertise with new generation immunsuppressants that may facilitate a more specific immunosuppression in the future.

Monoclonal antibodies directed against leukocyte function-associated antigen-1 (LFA-1) were compared to rabbit ATG in a randomized multi-center trial with patients after their first renal transplantation. Anti LFA-1 was well tolerated, and seemed to be less protective against very early acute rejection, but the difference did not reach statistical significance. There was suggestion however for some beneficial effects on delayed graft function (19% vs. 35% for rATG) [77]. A recently completed multicenter trial using a mouse monoclonal antibody against ICAM-1 (enlimomab), which resembles the molecular counterpart to LFA-1 failed to detect any impact either on rate of acute rejection or immediate graft function [78].

Previous clinical trials with xenogenic monoclonal antibodies targeting the p55 chain of the human IL-2 receptor (33B3.1 / anti-Tac) indicated equivalent immunosuppressive capacity in comparison to a rabbit-derived polyclonal antilymphocyte preparation, or even superiority when compared to a cyclosporin based triple drug regimen without induction [79,80]. Surprisingly, the increase of immunosuppressive efficiency did consistently not translate in a rise of infectious complications. Advances in molecular engineering have enabled the preparation of either chimeric or fully humanized antibodies, which can be administered for prolonged periods without eliciting a clinically relevant host immune response. Meanwhile, two large multicenter phase III studies have been completed highlighting the clinical efficacy and safety of the novel humanized monoclonal antibodies, basiliximab and daclizumab, which are directed against the alpha chain of the interleukin-2 receptor molecule of activated T-lymphocytes [81,82]. Both trials were designed in a similar fashion, but basiliximab and daclizumab were dosed by different schedules either in conjunction with a cyclosporin containing dual-drug, or a triple-drug regimen with addition of azathioprine. The same medication served for baseline immunosuppression in the corresponding control groups. Concerning the primary endpoints, the prophylactic use of both basiliximab and daclizumab, resulted in a consistently lower incidence of biopsy confirmed acute rejection and steroid-resistant rejection. Acute rejection at 6 months was reduced from 52.2% to 34.2% in conjunction with cyclosporin and steroids, and from 35% to 22% in conjunction with triple drug therapy, respectively. There was no difference in patient and graft survival at 12 months. Tolerability was excellent with no evidence of cytokine release syndrome. Despite of improved effectiveness, no increase in infections or malignant disorders was observed during the study period. Data from a recently published U.S. multicenter study have provided similar results [83] and there is evidence from a subgroup analysis that the beneficial effects of interleukin-2 receptor blockade with basiliximab is extended to recipients of living related kidneys with at least a one-haplotype mismatch [84].

Maintenance Immunosuppression and Steroid Withdrawal

Corticosteroids are commonly used as a component of immunosuppressive therapy in transplantation and steroid-related side-effects are thought to add considerably to post-transplant morbidity and mortality [85,86]. These side-effects refer to hypertension, post-transplant diabetes, hyperlipidemia, osteoporosis, and cataracts. In pediatric transplantation, maintenance of steroids retains growth retardation, even though the renal allograft is well functioning. Epidemiological data suggest improved long-term patient and graft survival in renal transplant recipients who were withdrawn from steroids [87]. Results from controlled prospective trials indicate that steroid withdrawal from a cyclosporin based immunosuppressive regimen is feasible in approximately 50% of patients when performed early within 6 months [88-90] and between 67-87% when steroids were discontinued at a later stage beyond one year post-transplant [91,92]. A persisting risk of acute rejection episode was obvious which did not affect patient and graft survival in short-term [93]. Withdrawal of steroids was associated with proven benefits on hypertension, hyperglycemia, hypercholesterolemia and weight abnormalities. However, a progressive rise in serum creatinine occurred in a substantial number of patients [91]. The Canadian Multicentre Study including a total of 523 patients who were randomized after 3 months to receive either placebo or low-dose alternate day prednisone, revealed a less favorable graft survival on steroid-free immunosuppression at five years (73% vs. 85%). These findings raise concern on detrimental effects on graft function which become apparent only after a longer follow-up period. Therefore, it was concluded that steroid withdrawal should be approached with caution [94].

Recently, the 12-month results of a double blind randomized multicenter study have been published comparing two corticosteroid regimens in combination with MMF and cyclosporine. Steroids were tapered from 30mg to 10mg and from 15mg to 0 during the first 3 months respectively. The primary endpoint (biopsy proven rejection) was met at a very low incidence in both study arms (15% vs. 25%) and graft function was not deteriorated at one year [95]. Another large scaled multicenter trial on steroid taper at 3 months [96] enrolling 266 renal transplant patients on a triple drug therapy including MMF revealed a higher cumulative incidence of acute rejection episodes in the withdrawal arm (30.8% vs. 9.8% at one year post-transplant). However, the majority of patients remained free of acute and chronic rejection. There was no difference in patient and graft survival. Patients off steroids had lower cholesterol levels (p=0.005) and were less likely to use blood pressure lowering drugs (p=0.001). In liver transplantation, the additional administration of MMF to tacrolimus and prednisone was associated with a trend to a lower incidence of rejection, reduced nephrotoxicity, and a lesser amount of maintenance steroids, which has been shown by a randomized clinical study [51]. MMF in combination with either tacrolimus or cyclosporin has been demonstrated to permit prednisone cessation even at 14 days post-transplant which was associated with a moderate rejection rate only, but no immunologic graft loss. Early steroid withdrawal resulted in less metabolic complications like post-transplant diabetes, hypercholesterolemia, and hypertension as compared to a historical group of 100 liver transplant recipients on cyclosporin and prednisone [97]. Furthermore, there is evidence that steroid cessation can be safely accomplished after combined pancreas kidney transplantation which was demonstrated by the Pittsburgh Group in a series of 124 patients maintained on tacrolimus-based immunosuppression. Steroid withdrawal was achieved in 47% of patients after a mean duration of 15.2 months post-transplant. No rise in the incidence of rejection was observed, and both patient and graft survival rates at 4 years were superior in the steroid withdrawal group [98]. Further investigation on steroid cessation is in progress in patients who are treated with neoral, or tacrolimus, or mycophenolate mofetil, or sirolimus, or a combination of these. At least in kidney transplantation, preliminary results suggest that complete steroid withdrawal will be feasible under a combination therapy with cyclosporin and sirolimus [58].

Conclusions

The large comparative multicenter trials have clearly shown efficacy of the new generation immunosuppressants on prevention and, in part, on reversal of acute rejection. To some extent, these trials reveal considerable differences in the safety profile among the various agents. It is remarkable that the new generation of humanized IL-2 antibodies offers the unique property of immunosuppressive efficiency without any known side-effect. Long-term data on this issue are lacking however. Minimizing the exposure to drug-related adverse side-effects has the potential to improve morbidity and mortality of transplant patients during ongoing follow-up. A randomized trial on early cyclosporin withdrawal in stable renal transplant patients with uneventful course after transplantation, has shown feasibility and long-term benefits owing to better renal function, less proteinuria and more importantly, reduction in cardiovascular mortality [31]. On the other hand, the controversy on steroid-withdrawal with the intention to control late cardiovascular risks, points out that the advantage of less drug-related side-effects may be counterbalanced by an increased incidence of chronic rejection. An increasing number of reports from uncontrolled studies which have incorporated the novel immunosupressants tacrolimus, mycophenolate mofetil, or sirolimus in combination therapy, created hopes for reaching superiority in treatment efficacy, thereby allowing to taper more inadvertent components to reduce long-term complications. However, from a scientific point of view, these studies remain hypothesis generating and require further confirmation by controlled clinical trials, which have to be designed and powered properly for assessment during long-term follow-up. Furthermore, since more clinically approved agents become available, it needs to be evaluated which drug fits best for which indication or patient category eliciting a more individualized immunosuppressive therapy in the future. Another important question is, if the novel therapeutic strategies are capable to offer a more selective, rather than a more powerful immunosuppression. A more potent immunosuppression is likely to cause an unacceptable excess of malignant disorders in long-term [99]. It remains to be seen if enhanced early efficacy in the prevention of rejection is equivalent to clinical superiority during ongoing follow-up resulting in prolongation of graft function. Recent data from the United Network of Organ Sharing provide evidence that there has been a substantial increase in the projected graft half-life after kidney transplantation, between 1988 and 1996 [100]. The current clinical trials on transplant immunosuppression raise optimism that epidemiological data from the large transplant registries will continue to show improvement of graft survival beyond one year post-transplant.

References

1. Opelz G. Collaborative transplant study – 10 year report. Transplant Proc 1992; 24: 2342-2355
2. Hata Y, Ozawa M, Takemoto S, Cecka J. HLA matching. In: Cecka J, Terasaki P, eds. Clinical transplants. Los Angeles: UCLA Tissue Typing Laboratory, 1996: 381-396
3. Mihastsch MJ, Ryffel B, Gudat F. The differential diagnosis between rejection and cyclosporine toxicity. Kidney Int 1995, 48 (Suppl 52): S63-S69
4. Bennet W, Dem Mattos A, Meyer M, Andoh T, Barry J. Chronic cyclosporin nephropathy: The Achilles' heel of immunosuppressive therapy. Kidney Int 1996; 50: 1089-1100
5. Opelz G. Relation between maintenance dose of cyclosporine and long-term kidney-graft survival: collaborative transplant study. Transplant Proc 1998; 30: 1716-1717
6. Hutchinson IV, Pravica V, Perrey C, Sinnott P. Cytokine gene polymorphisms and relevance to forms of rejection. Transplant Proc 1999; 31: 734-736
7. Shin G, Khanna A, Ding R, Sharma VK, Lagman M, Li B, Sunthanthiran M. In vivo expression of transforming growth factor-beta 1 in humans: stimulation by cyclosporine. Transplantation 1998; 65: 313-318
8. Dantal J, Hourmant M, Cantarovitch D, Giral M, Blancho G, Dreno B, Soulillou JP. Effect of long-term immunosuppression in kidney-graft recipients on cancer incidence: randomised comparison of two cyclosporin regimens. Lancet 1998; 351: 623-628
9. Keown P. Niese D. Cyclosporine microemulsion increases drug exposure and reduces acute rejection without incremental toxicity in de novo renal transplantation. International Neoral Study Group. Kidney Int 1998; 54: 938-944
10. Keown P, Landsberg D, Halloran P, Shoker A, Rush D, Jeffrey J, Russell D, Stiller C, Muirhead N, Cole E, Paul L, Zaltzman J, Loertscher R, Daloze P, Dandavino R, Boucher A, Handa P, Lawen J, Belitsky P, Parfrey P. A randomized, prospective multicenter pharmacoepidemiologic study of cyclosporine microemulsion in stable renal graft recipients. Report of the Canadian Neoral Renal Transplantation Study Group. Transplantation 1996; 62: 1744-1752
11. Cole E, Keown P, Landsberg D, Halloran P, Shoker A, Rush D, Jeffrey J, Russell D, Stiller C, Muirhead N, Paul L, Zaltzman J, Loertscher R, Daloze P, Dandavino R, Boucher A, Handa P, Lawen J, Belitsky P, Parfrey P, Tan A, Hendricks L. Safety and tolerability of cyclosporine and cyclosporine microemulsion during 18 months of follow-up in stable renal transplant recipients: a report of the Canadian Neoral Renal Transplantation Study Group. Transplantation 1998; 65: 505-510
12. Hall BM, Tiller DJ, Hardie I, Mahony J, Mathew T, Thatcher G, Miach P, Thomson N, Sheil AG. Comparison of three immunosuppressive regimens in cadaver renal transplantation: long-term cyclosporine, short-term cyclosporine followed by azathioprine and prednisolone, and azathioprine and prednisolone without cyclosporine. N Engl J Med 1988; 318: 1499-1507
13. Kootte AM, Lensen LM, van Es LA, Paul LC. Controlled cyclosporine conversion at three months after renal transplantation. Long-term results. Transplantation 1988; 46: 677-680
14. Sweny P, Lui SF, Scoble JE, Varghese Z, Fernando ON, Moorhead JF. Conversion of stable renal allografts at one year from cyclosporin A to azathioprin: a randomized controlled study. Transpl Int 1990; 3: 19-22
15. Isoniemi H. Renal allograft immunosuppression. III. Triple therapy versus three different combinations of double drug treatment: two years results in kidney transplant patients. Transpl Int 1991; 4: 31-37

16. Heim-Duthoy KL, Chitwood KK, Tortorice KL, Massy ZA, Kasiske BL. Elective cyclosporine withdrawal 1 year after renal transplantation. Am J Kidney Dis 1994; 24: 846-853

17. Delmonico FL, Conti D, Auchincloss H Jr, Russell PS, Tolkoff-Rubin N, Fang LT, Cosimi AB. Long-term, low-dose cyclosporine treatment of renal allograft recipients. A randomized trial. Transplantation 1990; 49: 899-904

18. Hiesse C, Neyrat N, Deglise-Favre A, Lantz O, Bensadoun H, Bonigeit G, Charpentier B, Fries D. Randomized prospective trial of elective cyclosporine withdrawal from triple therapy at 6 months after cadaveric renal transplantation. Transplant Proc 1991; 23: 987-989

19. Spielberger M, Aigner F, Schmid T, Bösmüller C, Königsrainer A, Margreiter R. Long-term results of cadaveric renal transplantation after conversion from cyclosporine to azathioprine: a controlled randomized trial. Transplant Proc 1988; 20: 169-170

20. Büsing M, Hölzer H, Schareck WD, Mellert J, Greger B, Hopt UT, Lauchart W. Is long-term therapy without cyclosporin A (CsA) indispensable or dangerous? One-year results of a prospective randomized trial. Transplant Proc 1989; 21: 1601-1603

21. Sagalowski AI, Reisman ME, Dawidson I, Toto R, Peters PC, Helderman JH. Late cyclosporine conversion carried risk of irreversible rejection. Transplant Proc 1988; 20: 157-160

22. Land W, Castro LA, Hillebrand G, Günther K, Gokel JM. Conversion rejection consequences by changing the immunosuppressive therapy from cyclosporine to azathioprine after kidney transplantation. Transplant Proc 1983: 15:2857-2861

23. Woodle ES, Heffron TG, Stuart JK, Thistlethwaite JR Jr, Stuart FP. Effect of discontinuing or restricting cyclosporine on late renal allograft rejection and function. Transplant Proc 1989; 21: 1641-1642

24. Venning MC, Lennard TWJ, Stevens ME, Proud G, Ward MK, Elliott RW, Taylor RM, Wilkinson R. Cyclosporin A treatment with successful selective conversion after six months in 70 renal allograft recipients. Transplant Proc 1989; 21: 1633-1634

25. Veitch PS, Taylor JD, Feehally J, Walls J, Bell PRF. Elective conversion from cyclosporine to azathioprine: long-term follow-up. Transplant Proc 1987; 19: 2017

26. Oka T, Omori Y, Aikawa I, Yasumura T, Yoshimura N, Yoshida T. Early conversion from cyclosporine to combination therapy with azathioprine in living related kidney transplantation. Transplant Proc 1989; 21: 1628-1630

27. Maddux MS, Veremis SA, Bauma WD, Pollak R, Mozes MF. Conversion from cyclosporine to azathioprine after renal transplantation: long-term effects on renal function, rejection, and allograft survival. Transplant Proc 1988; 20: 152-154

28. Gonwa TA, Nghiem DD, Schulak JA, Corry RJ. Results of conversion from cyclosporine to azathioprine in cadaveric renal transplantation. Transplantation 1987; 43: 225-228

29. Kaiser BA, Lawless ST, Palmer JM, Dunn SP, Polinsky MS, Baluarte HJ. Safe conversion from cyclosporine to azathioprine with improved renal function in pediatric renal transplantation. Pediatr Nephrol 1989; 3: 401-405

30. Kasiske BL, Heim-Duthoy K, Ma JZ. Elective cyclosporine withdrawal after renal transplantation. JAMA 1993; 269: 395-400

31. Hollander AAMJ, van Saase JLMC, Kootte AMM, van Dorp WT, van Bockel HJ, van Es LA, van der Woude FJ. Beneficial effects of conversion from cyclosporin to azathioprine after kidney transplantation. Lancet 1995; 345: 610-614

32. European FK506 Multicentre Liver Study Group: Randomised trial comparing tacrolimus (FK506) and cyclosporin in prevention of liver allograft rejection. Lancet 1994; 344: 423-428

33. The U.S. Multicenter FK506 Liver Study Group: A comparison of tacrolimus (FK506) and cyclosporine for immunosuppression in liver transplantation. N Engl J Med 1994; 331: 1110-1115
34. Sher LS, Cosenza CA, Michel J, Makowka L, Miller CM, Schwartz ME, Busuttil R, McDiarmid S, Burdick JF, Klein AS, Esquivel C, Klintmalm G, Levy M, Roberts JP, Lake JR, Kalayoglu M, D'Alessandro AM, Gordon RD, Stieber AC, Shaw BW Jr, Thistlethwaite JR, Whittington P, Wiesner RH, Porayko M, Cosimi AB et al. Efficacy of tacrolimus as rescue therapy for chronic rejection in orthotopic liver transplantation: a report of the U.S. Multicenter Liver Study Group. Transplantation 1997; 64: 258-263
35. Otto MG, Mayer AD, Clavien PA, Cavallari A, Gunawardena KA, Mueller EA. Randomized trial of cyclosporine microemulsion (neoral) versus conventional cyclosporine in liver transplantation: MILTON study. Multicentre International Study in Liver Transplantation of Neoral. Transplantation 1998; 66: 1632-1640
36. Jordan ML, Shapiro R, Vivas CA, Scantlebury P, Rhandhawa P, Carrieri G, McCauley J, Demetris AJ, Tzakis A, Fung JJ, Simmons RL, Hakala TR, Starzl TE. FK506 "Rescue" for resistant rejection of renal allografts under primary cyclosporine immunosuppression. Transplantation 1994; 57: 860-865
37. Jordan ML, Naraghi R, Shapiro R, Smith D, Vivas CA, Scantlebury VP, Gritsch HA, McCauley J, Rhandhawa P, Demetris AJ, McMichael J, Fung JJ, Starzl TE. Tacrolimus rescue therapy for renal allograft rejection – five-year experience. Transplantation 1997; 63: 223-228
38. Woodle ES, Thistlethwaite JR, Gordon JH, Laskow D, Deierhoi MH, Burdick J, Pirsch JD, Sollinger H, Vincenti F, Burrows L, Schwartz B, Danovitch GM, Wilkinson AH, Shaffer D, Simpson MA, Freeman RB, Rohrer RJ, Mendez R, Aswad S, Munn SR, Wiesner RH, Delmonico FL, Neylan J, Whelchel J. A multicenter trial of FK506 (tacrolimus) therapy in refractory acute renal allograft rejection. A report of the Tacrolimus Kidney Transplantation Rescue Study Group. Transplantation 1996; 62: 594-599
39. Mayer AD, Dmitrewski J, Squifflet JP, Besse T, Grabensee B, Klein B, Eigler FW, Heemann U, Pichlmayr R, Behrend M, Vanrenterghem Y, Donck J, van Hooff J, Christiaans M, Morales JM, Andres A, Johnson RW, Short C, Buchholz B, Rehmert N, Land W, Schleibner S, Forsythe JL, Talbot D, Pohanka E et al. Multicenter randomized trial comparing tacrolimus (FK506) and cyclosporine in the prevention of renal allograft rejection: a report of the European Tacrolimus Multicenter Renal Study Group. Transplantation 1997; 64: 436-443
40. Pirsch JD, Miller J, Deierhoi MH, Vincenti F, Filo RS. A comparison of tacrolimus (FK506) and cyclosporine for immunosuppression after cadaveric renal transplantation. FK506 Kidney Transplant Study Group. Transplantation 1997; 63: 977-983
41. Solez K, Vincenti F, Filo RS. Histopathologic findings from 2-year protocol biopsies from a U.S. multicenter kidney transplant trial comparing tacrolimus versus cyclosporine: a report of the FK506 Kidney Transplant Study Group. Transplantation 1998; 66: 1736-1740
42. Jensik S. Tacrolimus (FK506) in kidney transplantation: three year survival results of the U.S. multicenter, randomized, comparative trial: FK506 Kidney Transplant Study Group. Transplant Proc 1998; 30: 1216-18
43. Pichlmayr R for the European Mycophenol Mofetil Cooperative Study Group: Placebo-controlled study of mycophenolate mofetil combined with cyclosporine and corticosteroids for prevention of acute rejection. Lancet 1995; 345: 1321-1325
44. Sollinger HW for the U.S. Renal Transplant Mycophenolate Mofetil Study Group: Mycphenolate mofetil for the prevention of acute rejection in primary cadaveric renal allograft recipients. Transplantation 1995; 60: 225-232

45. Keown PA for the Tricontinental Mycophenolat Mofetil Renal Transplantation Study Group: A blinded, randomized clinical trial of mycophenolate mofetil for the prevention of acute rejection in cadaveric renal transplantation. Transplantation 1996; 61: 1029-1037

46. Halloran P, Mathew T, Tomlanovich S, Groth C, Hooftman L, Barker C for the International Mycophenolate Mofetil Renal Transplant Study Groups. Mycophenolate mofetil in renal allograft recipients. A pooled efficacy analysis of three randomized, double-blind clinical studies in prevention of rejection. Transplantation 1997; 63: 39-47

47. Mathew T. A blinded, long-term, randomized, multicenter study of mycophenolate mofetil in cadaveric renal transplantation: results at three years: Tricontinental Mycophenolate Mofetil Renal Transplantation Study Group. Transplantation 1998; 65: 1450-1454

48. Cho S, Hodge E, Navarro M, and the International Mycophenolate Mofetil Renal Study Groups. Mycophenolate mofetil improves long-term graft survival following renal transplantation in patients experiencing delayed graft function. Transplant Proc 1999; 31: 322-323

49. Kobashigawa J, Miller L, Renlund D, Mentzer R, Alderman E, Bourge R, Costanzo M, Eisen H, Dureau G, Ratkovec R, Hummel M, Ipe D, Johnson J, Keogh A, Mamelok R, Mancini D, Smart F, Valantine H. A randomized active-controlled trial of mycophenolate mofetil in heart transplant recipients. Mycophenolate Mofetil Investigators. Transplantation 1998; 66:507-515

50. Fisher RA, Ham JM, Marcos A, Shiffman ML, Luketic VA, Kimball PM, Sanyal AJ, Wolfe L, Chodorov A, Posner MP. A prospective randomized trial of mycophenolate mofetil with neoral or tacrolimus after orthotopic liver transplantation. Transplantation 1998; 66: 1616-1621

51. Jain AB, Hamad I, Rakela J, Dodson F, Kramer D, Demetris J, McMichael J, Starzl TE, Fung JJ. A prospective randomized trial of tacrolimus and prednisone versus tacrolimus, prednisone, and mycophenolate mofetil in primary adult liver transplant recipients: an interim report. Transplantation 1998; 66: 1395-1398

52. Sollinger HW, Belzer FO, Deierhoi MH, Diethelm AG, Gonwa TA, Kauffman RS, Klintmalm GB, McDiarmid SV, Roberts J, Rosenthal JT et al. RS-61443 (mycophenolate mofetil). A multicenter study for refractory kidney transplant rejection. Ann Surg 1992; 216: 513-518

53. The Mycophenolate Mofetil Acute Renal Rejection Study Group. Mycophenolate mofetil for the treatment of first acute renal allograft rejection. Transplantation 1998; 65: 235-241

54. Weir MR, Anderson L, Fink JC, Gabregiorgish K, Schweitzer EJ, Hoehn-Saric E, Klassen DK, Cangro CB, Johnson LB, Kuo PC, Lim JY, Bartlett ST. A novel approach to the treatment of chronic allograft nephropathy. Transplantation 1997; 64: 1706-1710

55. Mourad G, Vela C, Ribstein J, Mimran A. Long-term improvement in renal function after cyclosporine reduction in renal transplant recipients with histologically proven chronic rejection. Transplantation 1998; 65: 661-667

56. Kahan BD, Podbielski J, Napoli KL, Katz SM, Meier-Kriesche HU, Van Buren CT. Immunosuppressive effects and safety of a sirolimus/cyclosorine combination regimen for renal transplantation. Transplantation 1998; 66: 1040-1046

57. Groth CG, Bäckman L, Morales JM, Calne R, Kreis H, Lang P, Touraine JL, Claesson K, Campistol JM, Durand D, Wramner L, Brattström C, Charpentier B for the Sirolimus European Renal Transplant Study Group. Sirolimus (rapamycin)-based therapy in human renal transplantation: similar efficacy and different toxicity compared with cyclosporine. Transplantation 1999; 67: 1036-1042

58. Kahan BD. Rapamycin: personal algorithms for use based on 250 treated renal allograft recipients. Transplant Proc 1998; 30: 2185-2188

59. Halloran PF, Aprile MA, Farewell V, Ludwin D, Smith EK, Tsai SY, Bear RA, Cole EH, Fenton SS, Cattran DC. Early function as the principal correlate of graft survival. Transplantation 1988; 46: 223-228

60. Ojo AO, Wolfe RA, Held PJ, Port FK, Schmouder RL. Delayed graft function: Risk factors and implications for renal allograft survival. Transplantation 1997; 63: 968-974

61. Tejani AH, Sullivan EK, Alexander SR, Fine RN, Harmon WE, Kohaut EC. Predictive factors for delayed graft function (DGF) and its impact on renal graft survival in children: a report of the North American Pediatric Renal Transplant Cooperative Study (NAPRTCS). Pediatr Transplant 1999; 3: 293-300

62. Lehtonen SR, Isoniemi HM, Salmela KT, Taskinen EI, von Willebrand EO, Ahonen JP. Long-term graft outcome is not necessarily affected by delayed onset of graft function and early acute rejection. Transplantation 1997; 64: 103-107

63. Marcen R, Orofino L, Pascual J, de la Cal MA, Teruel JL, Villafruela JJ, Rivera ME, Mampaso F, Burgos FJ, Ortuno J. Delayed graft function does not reduce the survival of renal transplant allografts. Transplantation 1998; 66: 461-466

64. Ortho Multicenter Transplant Study Group. A randomized clinical trial of OKT3 monoclonal antibody for acute rejection of cadaveric renal transplants. N Engl J Med 1985; 313: 337-342

65. Norman DJ, Kahana L, Stuart FP Jr, Thistlethwaite JR Jr, Shield CF, Monaco A, Dehlinger J, Wu SC, Van Horn A, Haverty TP. A randomized clinical trial of induction therapy with OKT3 in kidney transplantation. Transplantation 1993; 55: 44-50

66. Frey DJ, Matas AJ, Gillingham KJ, Canafax D, Payne WD, Dunn DL, Sutherland DE, Najarian JS. Sequential therapy – a prospective randomized trial of MALG versus OKT3 for prophylactic immunosuppression in cadaver renal allografts. Transplantation 1992; 54: 50-56

67. Hanto DW, Jendrisak MD, So SK, McCullough CS, Rush TM, Michalski SM, Phelan D, Mohanakumar T. Induction immunosuppression with antilymphocyte globulin or OKT3 in cadaver kidney transplantation. Results of a single institution prospective randomized trial. Transplantation 1994; 57: 377-384

68. Bock HA, Gallati H, Zurcher RM, Bachofen M, Mihatsch MJ, Landmann J, Thiel G. A randomized prospective trial of prophylactic immunosuppression with ATG-fresenius versus OKT3 after renal transplantation. Transplantation 1995; 59: 830-840

69. Brennan DC, Flavin K, Lowell JA, Howard TK, Shenoy S, Burgess S, Dolan S, Kano JM, Mahon M, Schnitzler MA, Woodward R, Irish W, Singer GG. A randomized, double-blinded comparison of thymoglobin versus atgam for induction immunosuppressive therapy in adult renal transplant recipients. Transplantation 1999; 67: 1011-1018

70. Kasiske BL, Johnson HJ, Goerdt PJ, Heim-Duthoy KL, Rao VK, Dahl DC, Ney AL, Andersen RC, Jacobs DM, Odland MD. A randomized trial comparing cyclosporine induction with sequential therapy in renal transplant recipients. Am J Kidney Dis 1997; 30: 539-645

71. Shield CF, Edwards EB, Davies DB, Daily OP. Antilymphocyte induction therapy in cadaver renal transplantation. A retrospective, multicenter United Network for Organ Sharing study. Transplantation 1997; 63: 1257-1263

72. Szczech LA, Berlin JA, Aradhye S, Grossman RA, Feldman HI. Effect of anti-lymphocyte induction therapy on renal allograft survival: A meta-analysis. J Am Soc Nephrol 1997; 8: 1771-1777

73. Opelz G. Efficacy of rejection prophylaxis with OKT3 in renal transplantation. Collaborative Transplant Study. Transplantation 1995; 60: 1220-1224

74. Abramowicz D, Norman DJ, Goldman M, De Pauw L, Kinnaert P, Kahana L, Thistlethwaite JR, Shield CF, Monaco AP, Vanherweghem JL, et al. OKT3 prophylaxis improves long-term renal graft survival in high-risk patients as

compared to cyclosporine: combined results from the prospective, randomized Belgian and US studies. Transplant Proc 1995; 27: 852-853

75. Swinnen LJ, Costanzo-Nordin MR, Fisher SG, O'Sullivan EJ, Johnson MR, Heroux AL, Dizikes GJ, Pifarre R, Fisher RI. Increased incidence of lymphoproliferative disorder after immunosuppression with the monoclonal antibody OKT3 in cardiac-transplant recipients. N Engl J Med 1990; 323: 1723-1728

76. Opelz G, Henderson R. Incidence of non-Hodgkin lymphoma in kidney and heart transplant recipients. Lancet 1993; 342: 1514-1516

77. Hourmant M, Bedrossian J, Durand D, Lebranchu Y, Renoult E, Caudrelier P, Buffet R, Soulillou JP. A randomized multicenter trial comparing leukocyte function-associated antigen-1 monoclonal antibody with rabbit antithymocyte globulin as induction treatment in first kidney transplantations. Transplantation 1996; 62: 1565-1570

78. Salmela K, Wrammer R, Ekberg H, Hauser I, Bentdal O, Lins LE, Isoniemi H, Backman L, Persson N, Neumayer HH, Jorgensen PF, Spieker C, Hendry B, Nicholls A, Kirste G, Hasche G. A randomized multicenter trial of the anti-ICAM-1 monoclonal antibody (enlimomab) for the prevention of acute rejection and delayed onset of graft function in cadaveric renal transplantation: a report of the European Anti-ICAM-1 Renal Study Group. Transplantation 1999; 67: 729-736

79. Soulillou JP, Cantarovich D, Le Mauff B, Giral M, Robillard N, Hourmant M, Hirn M, Jacques Y. Randomized controlled trial of a monoclonal antibody against the interleukin-2 receptor (33B3.1) as compared with rabbit antithymocyte globulin for prophylaxis against rejection of renal allografts. N Engl J Med 1990; 322: 1175-1182

80. Kirkman RL, Shapiro ME, Carpenter CB, McKay DB, Milford EL, Ramos EL, Tilney NL, Waldmann TA, Zimmerman CE, Strom TB. A randomized prospective trial of anti-Tac monoclonal antibody in human renal transplantation. Transplantation 1991; 51: 107-113

81. Nashan B, Moore R, Amlot P, Schmidt AG, Abeywickrama K, Soulillou JP for the CHIB 201 International Study Group. Randomised trial of basiliximab versus placebo for control of acute cellular rejection in renal allograft recipients. Lancet 1997; 350: 1193-1198

82. Vincenti F, Kirkman R, Light S, Bumgardner G, Pescovitz M, Halloran P, Neylan J, Wilkinson A, Ekberg H, Gaston R, Backman L, Burdick J for the Daclizumab Triple Therapy Study Group. Interleukin-2-receptor blockade with daclizumab to prevent acute rejection in renal transplantation. N Engl J Med 1998; 338: 161-165

83. Kahan BD, Rajagopalan PR, Hall M for the United States Simulect Renal Study Group. Reduction of the occurrence of acute cellular rejection among renal allograft recipients treated with basiliximab, a chimeric anti-interleukin-2-receptor monoclonal antibody. Transplantation 1999; 67: 276-284

84. Mulloy LL, Wright F, Hall ML, Moore M. Simulect (basiliximab) reduces acute cellular rejection in renal allografts from cadaveric and living donors. Transplant Proc 1999; 31: 1210-1213

85. Veenstra DL, Best JH, Hornberger J, Sullivan SD, Hricik DE. Incidence and long-term cost of steroid-related side effects after renal transplantation. Am J Kidney Dis 1999; 33: 829-839

86. Kasiske B, Guijarro C, Massy Z, Wiederkehr M, Ma J. Cardiovascular diseases after renal transplantation. J Am Soc Nephrol 1996; 7: 971-977

87. Opelz G. Effect of the maintenance immunosuppressive drug regimen on kidney transplant outcome. Transplantation 1994; 58: 443-446

88. Maiorca R, Cristinelli L, Brunori G et al. Prospective controlled trial of steroid withdrawal after six months in renal transplant patients treated with cyclosporine. Transplant Proc 1988; 20: 121-125

89. Schulak JA, Mayers JT, Moritz CE, Hricik DE. A prospective randomized trial of prednisolone versus no prednisolone maintenance therapy in cyclosporine-treated and azathioprine-treated renal transplant patients. Transplantation 1990; 49: 327-332

90. Gulanikar AC, Belitsky P, MacDonald AS, Cohen A, Bitter-Suermann H. Randomized controlled trial of steroids versus no steroids in stable cyclosporine treated renal graft recipients. Transplant Proc 1991; 23: 990-991

91. Ratcliffe PJ, Dudley CR, Higgins RM, Firth JD, Smith B, Morris PJ. Randomised controlled trial of steroid withdrawal in renal transplant recipients receiving triple immunosuppression. Lancet 1996; 348: 643-648

92. Hollander HA, Hene RJ, Hermans J, van Es LA, van der Woude FJ. Late prednisone withdrawal in cyclosporine-treated kidney transplant patients: a randomized study. J Am Soc Nephrol 1997; 8: 294-301

93. Hricik DE, O'Toole MA, Schulak JA, Herson J. Steroid-free immunosuppression in cyclosporine-treated transplant recipients: a meta-analysis. J Am Soc Nephrol 1993; 4: 1300-1305

94. Sinclair NRS, for the Canadian Multicentre Transplant Study Group. Low-dose steroid therapy in cyclosporine treated renal transplant recipients with well functioning grafts. Can Med Assoc J 1992; 147: 645-657

95. Lebranchu Y for the M 55002 Study Group. Comparison of two corticosteroid regimens in combination with cellcept and cyclosporine A for prevention of acute allograft rejection: 12 month results of a double-blind, randomized multi-center study. Transplant Proc 1999; 31: 249-250

96. Ahsan N, Hricik D, Matas A, Rose S, Tomlanovich S, Wilkinson A, Ewell M, McIntosh M, Stablein D, Hodge E. Prednisone withdrawal in kidney transplant recipients on cyclosporine and mycophenolate mofetil—a prospective randomized study. Steroid Withdrawal Study Group. Transplantation 1999; 68: 1865-1874

97. Stegall MD, Wachs ME, Everson G, Steinberg T, Bilir B, Shrestha R, Karrer F, Kam I. Prednisone withdrawal 14 days after liver transplantation with mycophenolate: a prospective trial of cyclosporine and tacrolimus. Transplantation 1997; 64: 1755-1760

98. Jordan ML, Chakrabarti P, Luke P, Shapiro R, Vivas CA, Scantlebury VP, Fung JJ, Starzl TE, Corry RJ. Results of pancreas transplantation after steroid withdrawal under tacrolimus immunosuppression. Transplantation 2000; 69: 265-271

99. Denton MD, Magee CC, Sayegh MH. Immunosuppressive strategies in transplantation. Lancet 1999; 353: 1083-1091

100. Hariharan S, Johnson CP, Bresnahan BA, Taranto SE, McIntosh MJ, Stablein D. Improved graft survival after renal transplantation in the United States, 1988 to 1966. N Engl J Med 2000; 342: 605-612

PART TWO: PHARMACOLOGICAL IMMUNOSUPPRESSION

PHARMACOLOGIC MONITORING OF IMMUNOSUPPRESSIVE DRUGS

Flavio Gaspari, Norberto Perico & Giuseppe Remuzzi

Introduction

Organ transplantation as a treatment modality for patients with end-stage organ diseases of kidney, heart, liver, and pancreas has achieved impressive results in the past 2 decades thanks to better understanding of basic immunobiology and more advanced measures for medical and surgical management. Although immunosuppressive therapies to overcome host reaction to allografts have been employed since the early days of clinical transplantation, immunosuppressive agents and treatment protocols are constantly evolving. Since the 1978 introduction of cyclosporine (CsA) [1] there has been some doubt about its value as the single most important agent in the armamentarium of maintenance immunosuppression for organ transplantation. Triple-drug therapy with CsA, corticosteroid and azathioprine is now the most frequently used regimen for cadaver kidney recipients. However, the continuing search for more selective and specific agents has become, in the past decade, one of the priorities for transplant medicine. Some of these compounds are now entering routine clinical practice: among them are tacrolimus, mycophenolate mofetil (MMF) and sirolimus.

Current antirejection drugs, however, invariably reduce systemic immunity non-selectively which translates in more risk of infections and cancer. Several approaches can be used to assess the appropriateness of the dosing regimen for an immunosuppressive drug. One involves the assessment of clinical response. This approach has serious limitations because signs of rejection or toxicity may be difficult to recognize clinically. Another involves assessment of the pharmacokinetic

Mohamed Sayegh and Giuseppe Remuzzi (editors), Current and Future
Immunosuppressive Therapies Following Transplantation,43-59.
© 2001 Kluwer Academic Publishers. Printed in the Netherlands.

properties of the drug and relates parameters such as trough concentration or area under the time-concentration curve (AUC) to immunosuppressive efficacy or toxicity. Also this strategy has some limitations. A novel method for optimizing drug dosing is the pharmacodynamic approach direct to monitor the biological response to a drug.

Here we will review the pharmacokinetic approaches currently employed in the routine clinical practice, examine their usefulness and limitation and evaluate the potential of pharmacodynamic strategy, alone or coupled with pharmacokinetics, to achieve the best monitoring of current and future immunosuppressive drugs.

The Pharmacokinetic Approach

Measuring the concentrations of drugs during clinical trials or routine patient follow-up may facilitate rapid determination of appropriate dosing regimens, objective measures of drug exposure, and drug interaction [2,3]. This applies particularly to immunosuppressive drugs most of them have a very narrow therapeutic index, so that optimal dosing in the individual patient can only be achieved by therapeutic drug monitoring as an essential component of the patient long-term management. Up-to-now in transplant medicine this has been the case of CsA and more recently of tacrolimus, whereas for azathioprine and steroids, which have been used extensively for more than 35 years in transplantation, and for the drugs more recently entering clinical practice such as mycophenolate mofetil (MMF) and sirolimus accurate pharmacokinetic monitoring has not occurred.

A Logistic-Regression Model to Optimize CsA Dosage Early Post-Kidney Transplant.

Measurement of whole-blood concentrations of CsA is a standard practice in virtually all transplant centers. Because of the considerable variability in the bioavailability, metabolism, and excretion of CsA in transplant patients and because the drug's narrow therapeutic index, dosage individualization based on blood CsA concentration as a guide is required to reduce the risk for either underdosage or toxicity [4].

Current methods include measurements of trough whole blood CsA concentration by sampling immediately before the next dose is given [5]. However, target values for CsA trough concentrations at different time points early after transplant have not been defined in sufficient detail, primarily because of the lack of a model correlating them with probability of rejection or toxicity. Recently, we developed a logistic regression model and applied it to data collected retrospectively from two post-operative periods, day 0 to 9 and day 10 to 30 in 135 consecutive cadaver renal transplant recipients on triple immunosuppressive therapy (CsA, azathioprine, steroid) for a total of 1851 determinations [6].

Only minimum and maximum trough concentrations were considered from each period. Whole blood trough concentration of 330 to 430 ng/ml from day 0 to 9 and of 260 to 390 ng/ml for day 10 to 30 predicted an incidence of acute rejection of 22% and 12%, respectively. The model predicts no further improvement of antirejection activity for trough levels of CsA higher than indicated above. Moreover, within these therapeutic intervals, the model predicts a rather low frequency of toxic reactions mainly characterized by a mild but reversible increase in serum aminotransferase. These findings are in line with a recent observation [7] in 92 consecutive renal allograft recipients receiving triple therapy and studied for episodes of renal dysfunction with respect to whole blood CsA concentrations within the first 100 days after transplantation. Specificity was good for the prediction of CsA nephrotoxicity by high (>400 ng/ml) CsA trough concentrations and of acute rejection by low (>150 ng/ml) concentrations, although the sensitivity was relatively low. It should be, however, considered that the theoretical finding of this model should be validated by means of a prospective trial to verify whether the therapeutic intervals proposed here indeed offer the predicted degree of protection. This is actually more required today given the fact that the traditional Sandimmun formulation, with which the above data have been generated, has now been substituted worldwide with the new oral formulation Sandimmun Neoral.

Measurement of CsA Area Under the Curve Using an Abbreviated Sampling Strategy To Monitor Long-Term Drug Exposure in Kidney Transplantation.

Therapeutic monitoring of trough blood CsA concentration has been widely adopted to adjust CsA dose in individual subjects. However, trough level monitoring is not of universal help, as documented by findings that some patients may experience rejection in the presence of adequate or even high blood CsA levels, whereas others may develop toxicity even when blood trough values are low [4]. More informative than trough CsA concentration is the area under the concentration time curve (AUC), calculated from the individual complete pharmacokinetic profile [8]. Although AUC is an accurate index of patient's exposure to the drug, this approach is quite expensive and time-consuming, and increases discomfort for the patients, making it seldom feasible in routine outpatient clinic monitoring. Thus abbreviated CsA AUC profiles have been proposed, but data with the traditional formulation of Sandimmun were inconsistent due to the lack of correlation between the predicted and measured CsA AUC when a limited sample strategy was used, as it was recently reported [9].

Recently a new oral formulation of CsA (CsA microemulsion, CsA-ME) has become available in clinical practice. CsA-ME displays more consistent pharmacokinetic properties than the original formulation, and may, therefore, allow successful implementation of abbreviated AUC strategy [10], thus providing a better monitoring of the actual exposure of patients to CsA and enhancing the therapeutic index of the drug. Stepwise multiple regression analysis of CsA blood levels recorded after CsA-ME administration to 20 renal transplant patients showed the best results in AUC prediction with three sampling points (1.5, 8, 11 hours after CsA-ME dosing; r=0.992 with an associated error in AUC prediction ranging from -8.0 to 8.8%) (**Table 1**). Because blood sampling at 8 and 11 hours is not feasible in routine clinical practice, sample points from 0 to 3 hours after CsA-ME dosing, that is, up to the time of maximum mean blood CsA concentration plus 2 standard deviations, were considered. The best results were obtained with a three-point strategy (0, 1 and 3 hour afters CsA-ME dosing; error in prediction -9.0 to 7.2%), which gave an excellent correlation between measured and predicted AUC (r=0.989). A similar analysis after Sandimmun given to the same patients always resulted in poor AUC prediction with a wide associated error. Other studies have favored a two-time sample strategy after drug dosing (2, 6 hours or 0, 2 hours) [11,12]. We analyzed our data according to the model equation proposed by Amante and coworkers [11] for 2 and 6 hours time point sampling to predict AUC. Using this model equation, however, the AUC prediction was not as good, and the correlation coefficient was numerically lower as compared to the three-point sampling at 0, 1 and 3 hours after CsA-ME dosing. The discrepancy may be the consequence of the analysis performed in different sets of data or related to differences in the analytical method employed for CsA blood determination. Moreover, the greater pharmacokinetic consistency of the CsA-ME and the characteristic of the pharmacokinetic profile obtained with this microemulsion formulation, which invariably results in CsA blood level at 10 hours after dosing comparable to trough

Table 1. Abbreviated CsA AUC as an alternative to complete pharmacokinetic profile. Comparison of measured versus predicted CsA AUC values in 20 kidney transplant recipients on maintenance Neoral dose: multiple and stepwise regression analysis.

Number of sampling	Time points of sampling	Correlation coefficient (r)
5	1, 1.5, 8, 10, 11	0.995
3	1.5, 8, 11	0.992
3	1, 3, 5	0.994
3	0, 1, 3	0.989
2	2, 6	0.949
2	0, 2	0.931
1	10	0.947

concentration, would overwhelm the concern of the possible bias of trough point blood sampling, related to the possible variability in the timing of self-administration of CsA-ME by patients, as previously suggested [13]. We have also analyzed our CsAconcentration data using the model equation of the 0 and 2 hour sampling point [13]. Although in this case the correlation coefficient between measured and predicted AUC was very similar to that obtained with 0, 1, 3 hour points after CsA-ME dosing (r=0.89), the associated error in AUC prediction was wider (from -31.5% to 50%) (**Figure 1**). When one compares two methods for evaluating AUC, the agreement between the two is usually estimated by calculating the correlation coefficient (r). However, r does not measure the agreement but only the strenght of a relationship between two variables. Actually, the correlation depends on the range of values considered for the analysis, and data with quite high cor-relation may be in poor agreement [14]. Thus, given the large limit of agreement, expressed by the wide error in prediction of the 0 and 2 hour point strategy, this abbreviated estimation of AUC seems less realiable than the three-point sampling approach. The possibility of estimating the CsA AUC within a reasonable percentage of error (less than 10%) by using only three very early blood samples after CsA-ME dosing indicates that, with this novel formulation, drug therapy and patient exposure to the drug could be monitored accurately with minimum effort.

How Is a Limited Sampling Strategy Applied to New Immuno-suppressants in Routine Clinical Practice?

The case of tacrolimus. Tacrolimus is a macrolide immunosuppressive agent, 100 times more potent than CsA *in vitro* [15-17], and according to some reports, its use is associated with a lower incidence of acute rejection as compared to Sandimmun [18-22]. Although the structure and origin of tacrolimus are different from CsA, pharmacokinetics and pharmacodynamics are remarkably similar [15-17]. Indeed the pharm-acokinetics of tacrolimus are highly variable between individuals and are affected by many factors, including alterations in absorption, liver func-tion, patient's age, or time of administration [17,23,24]. As with CsA, a major side effect of tacrolimus is dose-dependent nephrotoxicity, al-though other side effects such as neurotoxicity, gastrointestinal dis-turbances, or diabetogenicity appear to be more common than CsA [19,25]. Preventing serious graft rejection or toxicity rests on trough concentration monitoring with a recommended therapeutic range of 5 to 15 ng/ml whole blood tacrolimus concentrations [26]. However, the difficulty in establishing useful relationship between trough concen-trations and clinical events exists [27,28]. Although trough concentra-tions of tacrolimus appears to reasonably predict clinical events inclu-ding graft rejection or toxicity [27], various studies have questioned the usefulness of trough levels in differentiating graft rejection from

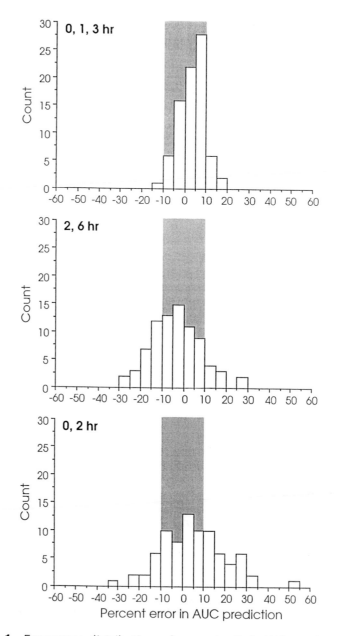

Figure 1. Frequency distribution of error in CsA AUC prediction in 81 stable kidney transplant patients. Shaded area represents the interval of acceptance error (-10% to 10%). Top, middle and lower panel report analysis using equation for 0, 1, 3 hr; 0, 6 hr and 0, 2 hr sampling points, respectively. (Modified from [13]).

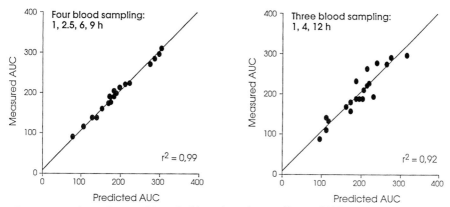

Figure 2. The relationship of abbreviated tacrolimus AUC from four sampling times (1, 2.5, 6, and 9 hours) and three sampling times (1, 4, and 12 hours) and the measured area under the curve from 0 to 12 hours in liver transplant recipients at steady state. (Modified from [24]).

tacrolimus toxicity [28-31]. Because pharmacokinetic and pharmaco-dynamic characteristics of CsA and tacrolimus are similar, AUC monitoring has recently been attempted [16,17]. In an effort to minimize the disadvantages of frequent blood samples, some recent studies have examined abbreviated pharmacokinetic profiles or limited sampling strategies for tacrolimus monitoring, but data are scanty. In a pilot study in 12 stable patients with liver transplant at steady state given tacrolimus as a part of their antirejection therapy, a stepwise multiple regression analysis showed that the abbreviated AUC at 1, 2.5, 6 and 9 hours after drug dosing could predict the total AUC with a high degree of confidence ($r^2=0.99$). Similarly, blood levels at 1, 4, and 12 hours as an abbreviated AUC were as good as a full pharmacokinetic study ($r^2=0.92$) (**Figure 2**). But both strategies may not be convenient for an outpatient visit since 9h or 12h whole blood sampling remain time consuming and therefore impractical for routine clinical monitoring. Alternatively, the tacrolimus concentration at 4 hours either morning or evening concentration, correlated reasonably well with AUC ($r^2=0.73$) and can predict 73% of drug exposure with a single concentration.

These preliminary data seem indicate that, at least in liver transplant recipients an abbreviated AUC monitoring for tacrolimus is feasible, but can not be applicable to outclinic patients. Studies are required to extend this observation to kidney transplant recipients. Moreover, it remains to be established the relationship between abbreviated AUC profile or the 4-hour tacrolimus concentrations and the clinical outcome.

The case of mycophenolate mofetil. MMF is an immunosuppressive agent approved for the prophylaxis of acute graft rejection in renal transplantation. In that indication is given at a dose of 1 gr twice daily, as adjunctive therapy with CsA and corticosteroids. Although this is the

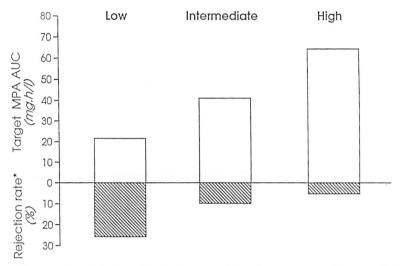

Figure 3. Relationship between risk of acute rejection and the time-concentration curve for mycophenolic acid in kidney transplant recipients. *: Biopsy-proven rejection. Low, Intermediate and High represent target AUC for the analysis. (Modified from [35]).

standard dose regimen of MMF currently employed, one may wonder whether a uniform-dose strategy for MMF is appropriate to provide adequate immunosuppression in kidney transplant patients. This rests on the fact that as in the case for CsA and tacrolimus, there is great interpatient pharmacokinetic variability for mycophenolic acid (MPA), the active metabolite. Indeed although the bioavailability of MPA is reportedly high (94%) in healthy subjects and renal transplant patients [32], the 12-h dose interval MPA AUC shows a >10-fold range for renal transplant patients on a fixed MMF dose of 2 gr/day [32]. Correction of the AUC values for patients weight did not lessen the magnitude of AUC range for the fixed MMF dose. Moreover in earlier studies involving renal transplant patients receiving MMF, CsA and steroids it was shown that there was a correlation between the complete MPA AUC 12h and the risk for acute rejection such that as the MPA AUC 12h increased, the risk for acute rejection decreased [32-34] (**Figure 3**). This observation was evaluated in a prospective randomized concentration controlled trial which confirmed the relationship between risk for rejection and the MPA AUC 12h [34,35]. This suggests that individualization of MMF dose and thus monitoring AUC 0-12h is of value in the follow-up of patients being on immunosuppression with MMF. As for all other drugs, full MPA AUC is laborious, requires multiple blood sampling and is costly. Therefore, a limited sampling approach in which two or three points are determined would be useful. This has been recently assessed in 36 pediatric kidney transplant recipients on a combined immunosuppression of CsA, steroids and MMF [36]. A two-point model utilizing only the predose and 2h postdose MPA concentrations (0, 2h) was found to be less satisfactory (r^2=0.64) than three-point models for adequately estimating AUC 0-12h. Using the three time points predose (i.e. time 0), 75 minutes and 6 hours postdose, a model equation could be formulated that gave a close correlation (r^2=0.88) between the abbreviated and the full MPA AUC. Because, a 6-hour blood sample after dosing may be considered unacceptable in some centers, particularly for ambulatory patients, a three-point limited sampling strategy based on the first 2 hours after the MMF dose was also considered. A reasonable correlation (r^2=0.74) was found between estimated and actual AUC with a model based on the time points 0 minutes, 40 minutes and 2 hours, but a greater discrepancy as compared with the model based on the three time point up to 6 hours. Others have made use of a 2-hours abbreviated MPA AUC (0, 4 h postdose timed plasma samples) in adult renal transplant patients and showed to correlate well with the full 12-hour AUC, which appears a much more appropriate sampling strategy in the patient care setting [37]. Hopefully these findings will provide the basis for routine monitoring of MPA in transplanted patients. The clinical validity of these limited sampling approaches needs, however, validation in prospective studies.

The case of sirolimus. Sirolimus is a potent immunosuppressive macrolide under development for maintenance therapy in organ transplantation. Some data suggest that a uniform dose of sirolimus may provide adequate immunosuppression for virtually all renal transplant patients [38]. However, a mean 40% inter- and intraindividual coefficient of variation in sirolimus oral bioavailability poses doubt for this strategy. Thus even standard sirolimus doses may need to be adjusted by estimating drug exposure accurately. Nevertheless, some evidence suggests that trough concentration monitoring may not be sufficient for sirolimus in all patients [39]. Indeed, despite the high correlation coefficient between the trough blood concentration and the AUC value, the former shows a 30% prediction error to estimate AUC. On the other hand, since a full pharmacokinetic profile of sirolimus is cumbersome and costly, abbreviated sampling protocols using whole-blood aliquots has been attempted also for this new immunosuppressive agent. In 27 renal transplant recipients given sirolimus once daily, the drug AUC values were well predicted on the basis of data from one early (C2) and one late (C14) sample (r^2= 0.99) [39]. However, a strategy that involves a late sample compromises the clinical utility of the limited sampling approach. Using a stepwise regression analysis, a correlation coefficient >0.90 between abbreviated sample strategy and full AUC was observed for samples obtained at 2 and 6 h; 2, 4, and 6 h; and 0, 2, 4, and 6 hours after dosing [39]. Good coefficient of determination were observed for the samples collected at all time points except for the trough sample, but only two sets of samples, namely those obtained at 0, 2, 4, and 6 h and those obtained at 0, 2, and 6 h, were clinically acceptable. Indeed they yielded 85% of the AUC estimates within a ±15% prediction error range compared with the corresponding full AUC [39]. Because the mean prediction error and standard deviation for both models are almost identical, the latter model with fewer time points is preferable. However, it has been recommended to use full pharmacokinetic profiles during the first post-transplant month to estimate drug exposure accurately and assess the maximal tolerated exposure. Thereafter, abbreviated profiles on a bimonthly base may be useful for at least 1 year [40]. The therapeutic window for sirolimus concentrations has yet to be defined. Evidence is available that the hyperlipidemic and pancytopenic toxic effects of siro-limus are concentration-dependent and correlate with trough values. Thus monitoring sirolimus AUC as a measure of total drug exposure may allow to refine further the relationship between these toxic effects and blood concentrations and to elucidate the relationship between concentration and the immunosuppressive efficacy of the drug.

Pharmacodynamic Monitoring

The assessment of the pharmacokinetic properties of a drug, the most used approach for antirejection drug monitoring, has limitation in that the apparent concentrations of the drug measured may not accurately reflect the concentration of the pharmacologically active moieties, be-cause of cross-reactivity of inactive metabolites in the assay. In addi-tion therapeutic ranges for the drugs have been difficult to establish, given the dependency of such values on the type of transplant, the time post-transplant, and what regimen of immunosuppressive drugs is used in combination with the drug of interest [41,42]. In contrast to pharma-cokinetics, which measure effects of the body on a drug, pharmaco-dynamic assesses the effects of the drug on the body, thus providing numerous potential advantage for monitoring of immunosuppressive drugs. Indeed the pharmacodynamic approach measures not only the parent drug but the biologically relevant metabolites. Therapeutic ranges may be less dependent on comedication or on type or length of time since transplantation. Moreover other variables, such as cross-reactivity or interference from other drugs, may not be as significant as they are for traditional therapeutic drug monitoring.

Pharmacodynamic monitoring may be performed using a surrogate laboratory measure of immunosuppressive acivity, an approach attem-pted for CsA [43,44], azathioprine [45], MMF [46,47], and sirolimus [48]. Thus specific assays that measures the inhibitory effect of the drug of interest on its apparent enzyme target or on the generation of a relevant intermediary product, have been recently developed.

As for pharmacokinetics, most of the data concerning pharmaco-dynamic monitoring of immunosuppressive drug relate to CsA. Pharmacodynamic approaches for CsA monitoring have been based on the measurement of inhibition of the enzyme calcineurin, a serine-threonine phosphatase essential in calcium-dependent intracellular signal trans-duction [49,50] in peripheral blood lymphocytes (**Figure 4A**). The first clinical report of measurement of calcineurin activity to monitor CsA involved 62 adult bone marrow transplant patients [43]. In all instances calcineurin activity in patients receiving CsA was significantly less than that in normal subjects [43]. More recently, the degree of calcineurin blockade and cytokine expression (i.e. interleukin-2 and interferon-γ) was assessed in peripheral blood lymphocytes from stable CsA-treated renal-transplant recipients [44]. CsA *in vitro* inhibited completely both calcineurin activity and cytokine induction with an IC50 of 10 to 20 µg/l [44]. In CsA-treated patients with therapeutic trough concentrations of CsA, calcineurin activity was 50% less than in controls [44]. The dif-ferential sensitivity of calcineurin inhibition *in vivo* versus *in vitro* most probably results for the difference between the free fraction of CsA in biological fluids and that in culture medium. Studies have also shown a significant negative correlation of calcineurin activity with CsA trough concentrations [44,51], but the correlation coefficient value was not so straightforward (**Figure 4B**). More recently, to clarify the relationship between the daily exposure of patients to CsA and changes in the enzyme activity of calcineurin, we correlated the pharmacokinetic

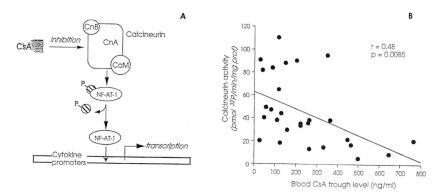

Figure 4.

A. Mechanism of action of cyclosporine in T-lymphocytes. The CsA-cyclophyllin complex selectively inhibits calcineurin, a serine-threonine phosphatase with an essential role in calcium-dependent signal transduction ultimately leading to cytokine gene transcription and T cell proliferation. CnB/CnA: subunits of calcineurin enzyme; CaM calmodulin; NF-AT-1: nuclear factor activation T cell; P: phosphorus.

B. Regression analysis of baseline calcineurin activity in peripheral blood mononuclear cells from kidney transplant patients given different CsA doses plotted against trough CsA level. (Modified from [51]).

profile of CsA in 30 renal transplant patients given different CsA dosing (<4, 4-6, >6-8, >8 mg/Kg) with the profile of calcineurin activity at different intervals after dosing. For each of the above CsA doses an inverse relationship was found between CsA concentrations and calcineurin activity throughout the dosing interval [51]. Although encouraging as pharmacodynamic CsA monitoring approach, we are still in early stages of development of a reliable and reproducible method for measurement of calcineurin activity *in vitro*. Indeed recovery of samples requires careful handling, and there may be significant variability introduced by sampling procedures. Thus developments are underway in calcineurin assay methodology so that the whole blood matrix has been proposed as alternative to peripheral blood mononuclear cells, in order to overcome the high variability of results with the latter approach, which is related to procedure of leukocyte separation [52]. More importantly, further studies are required to determine whether calcineurin activity or drug concentrations better correlate with clinical responses.

Tacrolimus also mediates its immunosuppressive activity in a manner similar to CsA, through inhibition of calcineurin activity. Therefore pharmacodynamic monitoring of this drug would be also possible. However, detailed studies on pharmacodynamic monitoring of tacrolimus have not been reported.

Measurement of inosine monophosphate dehydrogenase in the whole blood, an enzyme involved in the de novo biosynthesis of purine nucleotides [53,54], has been recently reported as means to assess immunosuppression induced by MPA and ultimately as a pharmacodynamic monitoring of its prodrug MMF. Animal studies in both rabbits and dogs have shown an inverse relationship between inosine monophosphate dehydrogenase activity and drug concentration [46,47]. More recently a prospective study involving pharmacodynamic assessment of MPA-induced immunosuppression has been performed in renal transplant recipients [55]. Similarly to animals, in these patients an inverse relationship was found between MPA concentrations and inosine monophosphate dehydrogenase activity in whole blood. The peak concentration of MPA, achieved 1h-postdose, inhibited 40% of inosine monophosphate dehydrogenase activity. As the MPA concentration is decreased through the dosing interval, the inosine monophosphate dehydrogenase activity was gradually restored. In a recent study, a relationship between inhibition of inosine monophosphate dehydrogenase activity, MPA concentrations, and acute rejection episodes was investigated in 25 renal transplant patients during the first 3 months post-transplant. Both the MPA concentrations and the inosine monophosphate dehydrogenase enzyme activity demonstrated considerable intra- and interpatient variability. At the time of rejection, no inhibition of inosine monophosphate dehydrogenase activity was observed, despite adequate drug concentrations. Moreover, many patients who had no inhibition of inosine monophosphate dehydrogenase activity at certain times through the monitoring period did nor experience rejection episodes. The cause for the considerable variability of the inosine monophosphate dehydrogenase activity in renal transplant patients remains ill defined. Future studies, beside addressing this issue, should focus on whether measurement of inosine monophosphate dehydrogenase activity or MPA concentrations better correlates with immunosuppressive efficacy and graft outcome.

As surrogate for estimating the pharmacodynamic effect of sirolimus, measurement of p70^{S6} kinase, a critical enzyme for microsomal protein synthesis necessary for cell cycle progression through the G1 phase [56] has been proposed. Almost all of the activity of this enzyme in whole blood resides in lymphocytes. Because this test is relatively cumbersome, its routine clinical application seems remote. However, it may provide useful indices to establish limits between drug concentrations and immunosuppressive effects, and thereby yield reliable insights into sirolimus dosage.

Conclusion

The assessment of an individual state of immunosuppression remains an unfulfilled important goal in transplant medicine. Pharmacodynamic monitoring has the potential to augment pharmacokinetic and trough level monitoring to optimize the dosing regimen of immunosuppressive drugs. Many of the assays, however, are time-consuming and not amenable for use in routine clinical laboratories. Thus, the challenge is for investigators to develop robust pharmacodynamic assays to facilitate further evaluation of this approach. Moreover clinical trials are required to investigate the relationship of pharmacokinetic and pharmacodynamic monitoring to clinical events. The ultimate goal is to establish the ideal approach for monitoring of patients receiving immunosuppressive drugs to optimize the quality of care given to them.

References

1. Kahan BD: Cyclosporine. N Engl J Med 321:1725-1738, 1989
2. Peck CC, Barr WH, Benet LZ, Collins J, Desjardins RE, Furst DE, Harter JG, Levy G, Ludden T, Rodman JH: Opportunities for integration of pharmacokinetics, pharmacodinamics, and toxokinetics in rational drug development. Clin Pharmacol Ther 51:465-473, 1992
3. Shaw LM, Bonner HS, Fields L, Lieberman R: The use of concentration measurements of parent drug and metabolites during drug trials. Ther Drug Monit 15:483-487, 1993
4. Kahan BD, Grevel J: Optimization of cyclosporine therapy in renal transplantation by a pharmacokinetic strategy. Transplantation 46:631-644, 1988
5. Lindholm AS, Kahan BD: Influence of cyclosporine pharmacokinetics, trough concentrations, and AUC monitoring on outcome after kidney transplantation. Clin Pharmacol Ther 54:205-218, 1993
6. Perna A, Gotti E, De Bernardis E, Perico N, Remuzzi G: A logistic-regression model provides novel guidelines to maximize the anti-acute rejection properties of cyclosporine with a minimum of toxicity. J Am Soc Nephrol 7:786-791, 1996
7. Nankivell B, Hibbins M, Chapman J: Diagnostic utility of whole blood cyclosporine measurements in renal transplantation using triple therapy. Transplantation 58:989-996, 1994
8. Grevel J, Welsh MS, Kahan BD: Cyclosporine monitoring in renal trasplantation: area under the curve is superior to trough level monitoring. Ther Drug Monit 11:246-248, 1989
9. Gaspari F, Ruggenenti P, Torre L, Bertocchi C, Remuzzi G, Perico N: Failure to predict cyclosporine area under the curve using a limited sampling strategy. Kidney Int 44:436-439, 1993
10. Gaspari F, Anedda MF, Signorini O, Remuzzi G, Perico N: Prediction of cyclosporine area under the curve using a three-point sampling strategy after Neoral administration. J Am Soc Nephrol 8:647-652, 1997
11. Amante AJ, Kahan BD: Abbreviated AUC strategy for monitoring cyclosporine microemulsion therapy in the immediate posttransplant period . Transplant Proc 28:2162-2163, 1996
12. Keown P, Landsberg D, Halloran P, Shoker A, Rush D, Jeffrey J, Russel D, Stiller C, Muirhead N, Cole E, Paul L, Zaltzman J, Loertscher R, Daloze P, Dandavino R, Boucher A, Handa P, Lawen J, Belitsky P, Parfrey P: A randomized, prospective multicenter pharmacoepidemiologic study of cyclosporine microemulsion in stable renal graft recipients. Transplantation 62:1744-1752, 1996
13. Gaspari F, Perico N, Signorini O, Caruso R, Remuzzi G: Abbreviated kinetic profiles in area-under-the-curve monitoring of cyclosporine therapy. Kidney Int 54:2146-2150, 1998
14. Bland JM, Altman DG: Statistical methods for assessing agreement between two methods of clinical measurement. Lancet 1:307-310, 1986
15. Hooke MA: Tacrolimus, a new immunosuppressant - a review of the literature. Ann Pharmacother 28:501-511, 1994
16. Kelly PA, Burkart GJ, Venkataramanan R: Tacrolimus: a new immunosuppressant. Am J Health-Syst Pharm 52:1521-1535, 1995
17. Jusko WJ, Pickozewski W, Klintman GB, Shaefer MS, Hebert MF, Piergies AA, Lee CC, Schechter P, Mekki QA: Pharmacokinetics of tacrolimus in liver transplant patients. Clin Pharmacol Ther 57:281-290, 1995
18. Fung J, Abu-Elmagd K, Jain A, Gordon A, Tzakis A, Todo S, Takaia S, Alessiani M, Demetris A, Bronster O, Martin M, Mieles L, Selby R, Reyes J, Doyle H, Stieber A, Casavilla A, Starzl T: A randomized trial of primary liver transplantation under

immunosuppression with FK 506 vs cyclosporine. Transplant Proc 23:2977-2983, 1991

19. U.S.Multicenter FK 506 Liver Study Group : A comparison of tacrolimus (FK 506) and cyclosporine for immunosuppression in liver transplantation. N Engl J Med 331:1110-1115, 1994

20. Laskow DA, Vincenti F, Neylan JF, Mendez R, Matas AJ: An open-label, concentration-ranging trial of FK 506 in primary kidney transplantation. Transplantation 62:900-905, 1996

21. Mayer AD, Dmitrewski J, Squifflet JP, Besse T, Grabensee B, Klein B, Eigler FW, Heemann U, Pichlmayr R, Beherend M, Vanrenterghem Y, Donk J, Van Hoof J, Christiaans M, Morales JM, Andres A, Johnson RWG, Short C, Buchholz B, Rehemert N, Land W, Schleibner S, Forsythe JLR, Talbot D, Neumayer HH, Hauser I, Ericzon B, Brattström C, Claesson K, Mülbacher F, Pohanka E: Multicenter randomized trial comparing tacrolimus (FK 506) and cyclosporine in the prevention of renal allograft rejection. Transplantation 64:436-442, 1997

22. Pirsch JD, Miller J, Deierhoi MH, Vincenti F, Filo RS: A comparison of tacrolimus (FK 506) abd cyclosporine for immunosuppression after cadaveric renal transplantation. FK506 Kidney Transplant Study Group. Transplantation 63:977-983, 1997

23. Ku Y, Min DI: An abbreviated Area-under-the-curve monitoring for tacro-limus in patients with liver transplants. Ther Drug Monit 20: 219-223, 1998

24. Min DI, Chen H, Lee M, Ashton K, Martin M: Time-dependent disposition of tacrolimus and endothelin-1 in liver transplant.. Pharmacotherapy 17:457-463, 1997

25. European FK 506 multicenter liver study group : Randomized trial comparing tacrolimus (FK 506) and cyclosporin in prevention of liver allograft rejection. Lancet 344:423-428, 1994

26. Jusko WJ, Thomson AW, Fung J, McMaster P, Wong SH, Zylber-Katz E, Christians U, Winkler M, Fitzsimmons WE, Lieberman R: Consensus document: therapeutic monitoring of tacrolimus (FK 506). Ther Drug Monit 17:606-614, 1995

27. Kershenr RP, Fitzsimmons WE: Relationship of FK 506 whole blood concentrations and efficacy and toxicity after liver anf kidney transplantation. Transplantation 62:920-926, 1996

28. Takahara S, Kokado Y, Kameoka H, Takano Y, Jiang H, Moutbarrik A, Ishibashi M, Okuyama A, Sonoda T: Monitoring of FK 506 blood levels in kidney transplant recipients. Transplant Proc 26:2106-2108, 1994

29. Winkler M, Ringe B, Rodeck B, Melter M, Stoll K, Baumann J, Wonigeit K, Pichlmayr R: The use of palsma levels for FK 506 dosing in liver-graft patients. Transpl Int 7:329-333, 1994

30. Bäckman L, Nicar M, Levey M, Distant D, Eisenstein C, Renard T, Goldstein R, Husberg B, Gonwa T, Klintman G: FK 506 trough levels in whole blood and plasma in liver transplant recipients: correlation with toxicity. Transplant Proc 26:1804, 1994

31. Erden E, Warty V, Magnone M, Shapiro R, Demetris J, Randhawa P: Plasma FK 506 levels in patients with histopatologically documented renal allograft rejection (letter). Transplantation 58:397, 1994

32. Bullingham RES, Nicholls AJ, Hale M: Pharmacokinetics of mycophenolate mofetil (RS61443): a short review. Transplant Proc 28:925-929, 1996

33. Takahashi K, Ochiai T, Ukida K, Yasamura T, Ishibashi M, Suzuki S, Otsubo O, Isono K, Takagi H, Oka T, Okuyama A, Sonoda T, Amamiya H, Ota K: Pilot study of mycophenolate mofetil (RS-61443) in the prevention of acute rejection following renal transplantation in japanese patients. Transplant Proc 27:1421-1424, 1995

34. Vanrenterghem Y,for the Mycophenolate Mofetil RCCT Trial Group: In: edited by Int'l Congress of Nephrology, Sydney, Australia, 1997, p. 1015
35. Hale MD, Nicholls AJ, Bullingham RES, Hené R, Hoitsma A, Squifflet JP, Weimar W, Vanrenterghem Y, Van de Woude FJ, Verpooten GA: The pharmacokinetic-pharmacodinamic relationship for mycophenolate mofetil in renal transplantation. Clin Pharmacol Ther 64:672-683, 1998
36. Schütz E, Armstrong VW, Shipkova M, Weber L, Niedmann PD, Lammersdorf T, Wiesel M, Mandelbaum A, Zimmerhackl LB, Mehls O, Tönshoff B, Oellerich M, and Members of the German Study Group on MMF in Pediatric Renal Transplant Recipients: Limited sampling strategy for the determination of mycophenolic acid area under the curve in pediatric kidney recipients. Transplant Proc 30:1182-1184, 1998
37. Hale M: The population approach: measuring variability in response, concentration and dose. In: Cost B1 Medicine, European Commission, edited by Aarons L, Balant LP, Danhof Met al, Luxembourg, 1997, p. 229
38. Kahan BD: Sirolimus: a new agent for clinical renal transplantation. Transplant Proc 29:48-50, 1997
39. Kaplan B, Meier-Kriesche HU, Napoli K, Kahan BD: A limited sampling strategy for estimating sirolimus area-under-the-concentration curve. Clin Chem 43:539-540, 1997
40. Kahan BD, Napoli K: Role of therapeutic drug monitoring of rapamycin. Transplant Proc 30:2189-2191, 1998
41. Oellerich M, Armstrong VW, Kahan BD, Shaw L, Yatscoff R, Lindholm A, Halloran P, Gallicano K, Wonigeit K: Lake Louise consensus conference on cyclosporine monitoring in organ transplantation: report of the consensus panel. Ther Drug Monit 17:642-654, 1995
42. Sketris I,, Yatscoff RW, Keown P, Canafax DM, First MR, Holt DW, Schroeder TJ, Wright M: Optimizing the use of cyclosporine in renal transplantation. Clin Biochem 28:195-211, 1995
43. Pai SY, Fruman DA, Leong T, Neuberg D, Rosano TG, McGarigle C, Antin JH, Bierer BE: Inhibition of calcineurin phosphatase activity in adult bone marrow transplant patients treated with cyclosporine A. Blood 84:3974-3979, 1994
44. Batiuk TD, Pazdeva F, Halloran PF: Calcineurin activity is only partially inhibited in leukocites of cyclosporine-treated patients. Transplantation 59:1400-1404, 1995
45. Mircheva J, Legendre C, Soria-Royer C, Thervet E, Beaune P, Kreis H: Monitoring of azathioprine-induced immunosuppression with htiopurine methyltransferase activity in kidney transplant recipients. Transplantation 60:639-642, 1995
46. Langman LJ, Shapiro AJ, Lakey RT, LeGatt DF, Kneteman NM, Yatscoff RW: Pharmacodynamic assessement of mycophenolic acid-induced immunosuppression by measurement of inosine monophosphate dehydrogenase activity in a canine model. Transplantation 61:87-92, 1996
47. Langman LJ, LeGatt DF, Yatscoff RW: Pharmacodynamic assessement of mycophenolic acid-induced immunosuppression by measuring IMP dehydrogenase activity. Clin Chem 41:295-299, 1995
48. Gallant HL, Yatscoff RW: P70 S6 kinase assay: a pharmacodynamic monotoring strategy for rapamycin; assay development. Transplant Proc 28:3058-3061, 1996
49. Clipstone NA, Crabtree GR: Identification of calcineurin as a key signalling enzyme in T-lymphocyte activation. Nature 357:695-697, 1992
50. Schreiber SL, Crabtree GR: The mechanism of action of cyclosporin A and FK 506. Immunol Today 13:136-142, 1992
51. Piccincini G, Gaspari F, Signorini O, Remuzzi G, Perico N: Recovery of blood mononuclear cell calcineurin activity segregates two populations of renal

transplant patients with different sensitivities to cyclosporine inhibition. Transplantation 61:1526-1531, 1996

52. Caruso R, Piccinini G, Bonazzola S, Cattaneo D, Gaspari F, Perico N, Remuzzi G: Whole blood calcineurin (CN) activity to monitor cyclosporine (CsA)-immune effect. (Abstract). J Am Soc Nephrol in press:1999

53. Eugui EM, Mirkovich A, Allison A: Lymphocyte-selective antiproliferative and immunosuppressive effects of mycophenolic acid in mice. Scand J Immunol 33:175-183, 1991

54. Eugui EM, Almquist S, Mullen G, Allison A: Lymphocyte-selective cytostatic and immunosuppressive effects of mycophenolic acid *in vitro*: role of deoxyguanosine nucleotide depletion. Scand J Immunol 33:161-173, 1991

55. Yatscoff RW, Aspeslet LJ, Gallant HL: Pharmacodynamic monitoring of immunosuppressive drugs. Clin Chem 44:428-432, 1998

56. Brown EJ, Albers MW, Shin TB, Ichikawa K, Keith CT, Lane WS, Schreiber SL: A mammalian protein targeted by G1-arresting rapamycin-receptor complex. Nature 369:756-758, 1994

USE OF CORTICOSTEROIDS IN KIDNEY TRANSPLANTION

Donald E. Hricik

Historical Background

Corticosteroids have played a key role in the evolution of successful organ transplantation. Azathioprine was actually the first immunosuppressive agent used for human kidney transplant recipients in the late 1950s. However, in 1951, Billingham et al demonstrated that steroids prevented rejection and prolonged the survival of skin grafts in rabbits [1]. The effectiveness of large doses of corticosteroids in suppressing and reversing human renal allograft rejection was first reported in the early 1960s [2,3]. Thereafter, combination of azathioprine and steroids became the conventional maintenance immunosuppression regimen in organ transplantation and remained so for almost two decades.

During the early years of kidney transplantation, it became clear that chronic corticosteroid therapy was responsible for a great deal of post-transplantation morbidity. Well-recognized long-term side effects of steroid therapy include increased susceptibility to infection, weight gain with cushingoid changes, cataracts, glucose intolerance, myopathy, sodium retention manifested by edema and hypertension, hyperlipidemia, and a number of skeletal effects including osteopenia, aseptic necrosis, and impaired growth. Even before the availability of cyclosporine (CsA) in the early 1980s, a trend had begun toward lowering steroid doses used both for maintenance immunosuppression [4-6] and for treatment of acute rejection [7,8] in order to minimize side effects. The "low-dose" steroid regimens described in the 1970s were initiated at a time when our understanding of the immunosuppressive mechanisms of corticosteroids was rudimentary. CsA proved to

Mohamed Sayegh and Giuseppe Remuzzi (editors), Current and Future
Immunosuppressive Therapies Following Transplantation, 61-84.
© 2001 Kluwer Academic Publishers. Printed in the Netherlands.

be even further steroid sparing and its introduction was accompanied by continued interest in steroid sparing regimens. However, interest in *steroid-free* immunosuppression in patients receiving CsA-based therapy waxed and waned between the mid-1980s and the mid-1990s. Declining interest in steroid-free protocols during that era was based on 1) a clear risk of acute and chronic allograft rejection associated with steroid withdrawal and 2) an inability to identify patients at risk for rejection on the basis of immunologic or clinical criteria.

In the past fifteen years, there has been an expansion in our knowledge of the cellular and subcellular mechanisms of corticosteroid immunosuppression. Despite their toxicities, corticosteroids are still prescribed in combination with other immunosuppressants for the vast majority of organ transplant recipients. In addition, corticosteroids remain the agents most commonly used for initial treatment of acute allograft rejection. Since 1994, the introduction of several new induction and maintenance immunosuppressive agents has renewed interest in steroid-free immunosuppression. The remainder of this review will focus on current understanding of the mechanisms by which corticosteroids suppress rejection, on the pharmacology of corticosteroids, and on current patterns of steroid usage in immunosuppression regimens prescribed for renal transplant recipients, with an emphasis on the results of recent trials of steroid withdrawal.

Mechanisms of Action

Corticosteroids exert two principal effects on the immune system. First, they transiently alter the distribution of circulating lymphocytes. Within four to eight hours of administration, CD4+ T lymphocytes are sequestered in the reticuloendothelial system, thereby reducing egress to inflammatory sites [9]. Secondly, corticosteroids inhibit the proliferation and function of lymphocytes by blocking the expression of various lymphokines and cytokines.

Owing to their hydrophobic nature, glucocorticoids easily diffuse into cells and bind to cytoplasmic receptors [10,11] that exist in association with a heat shock protein (see **Figure 1**). Binding of the corticosteroid molecule results in dissociation of heat shock protein from the complex and translocation of the steroid-receptor complex into the nucleus, where it binds to a number of DNA sites collectively referred to as glucocorticoid response elements (GRE). Binding of the steroid-receptor complex to GRE may inhibit transcription of cytokine genes either 1) by acting on distant genes to induce expression of transcription inhibitory factors, or 2) by acting on adjacent genes [12,13]. However, a number of genes involved in inflammation have no identifiable GRE in their promoter regions, suggesting that other mechanisms may mediate the antiinflammatory and immunosuppressive effects of steroids.

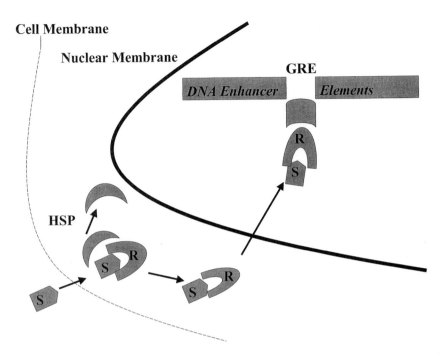

Figure 1. Corticosteroids (S) exert their immunosuppressive effects by blocking the expression of various cytokine genes. The steroid molecule enters the cytoplasm in association with a heat shock protein (HSP). Binding of this complex to the cytoplasmic glucocorticoid receptor (R) leads to dissociation of the HSP. The steroid-receptor complex then enters the nucleus and binds to one of a number of glucocorticoid response elements (GRE), ultimately inhibiting the transcription of mRNA for proinflammatory cytokines.

Recent evidence suggests that corticosteroids inhibit the action of transcription factors such as activating protein-1 (AP-1) and nuclear factor-κB (NF-κB)[14,15]. There may be direct protein-protein interactions between activated glucocorticoid receptors and these transcription factors. In the case of NF-κB, activated glucocorticoid receptors may bind to activated NF-κB and prevent it from binding to κB sites on proinflammatory genes [16,17] (see **Figure 2**). Corticosteroids also increase transcription of the gene for IκBα which binds to activated NF-κB. The IκBα protein probably causes dissociation of NFκB from target genes, resulting in its movement back to the cytoplasm [18].

The major consequence of these intracellular effects of corticosteroids is an inhibition of the production of interleukin-1 (IL-1) and IL-6 by antigen-presenting cells such as macrophages and monocytes [19-21]. Because IL-1 is a primary co-stimulus for helper T cell activation and IL-6 is a major inducer of B cell activation, corticosteroid administration has the potential to inhibit both the cellular and hormonal

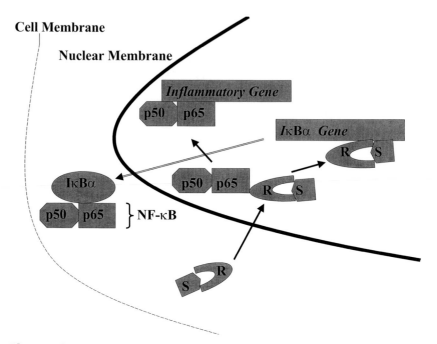

Figure 2. Schematic diagram of the effects of glucocorticoids on the activation of NF-κB. NF-κB is a heterodimer that consists of two proteins, a p50 subunit and a p65 subunit. In unstimulated cells, NF-κB is bound in the cytoplasm to IκBα which prevents it from entering the nucleus. The glucocorticoid (S) receptor (R) complex exerts at least two effects: 1) it prevents binding of active NK-κB to promoter regions of proinflammatory genes, and 2) it activates transcription of IκBα that promotes movement of NF-κB out of the nucleus.

arms of the immune response. Steroids also inhibit expression of other proinflammatory cytokines, including IL-3 [22], interferon-γ [23,24], and tumor necrosis factor [25]. Finally, recent studies indicate that corticosteroids inhibit the expression of IL-2, a potent growth factor for lymphocytes, by impeding the effects of DNA binding proteins that normally stimulate IL-2 gene transcription [13,26].

Corticosteroid inhibition of the expression of cytokines is reversible. However, *in vitro* studies suggest that abrupt withdrawal of corticosteroids is associated with a vigorous rebound in T cell activation. This phenomenon may be related to steroid-induced upregulation of various cytokine receptors on the surface of lymphocytes. It is known, for example, that corticosteroids increase the density of receptors for IL-1 [27], IL-6 [28], and interferon-γ [29]. As a clinical corollary, corticosteroid dose reduction or withdrawal should probably be performed slowly in transplant recipients to avoid a surge in T cell activation that could lead to rejection.

Pharmacologic Considerations

The commonly prescribed corticosteroids differ with respect to potency and duration of action [30] (see **Table 1**). Prednisone, prednisolone, and methylprednisolone exhibit intermediate durations of action and are the agents most commonly used for the prevention and treatment of allograft rejection. Prednisone must be converted to prednisolone by the liver enzyme 11-ß-hydroxydehydrogenase. In most patients, however, the systemic bioavailability of prednisone, prednisolone, and methyl-prednisolone is comparable and no clinically significant differences in immunosuppressive efficacy or toxicity have been discerned among these agents. Prednisone is probably the oral steroid preparation most commonly prescribed for transplant recipients. However, some centers prefer prednisolone for maintenance immunosuppression in order to minimize concerns about the effects of alterations in liver function on steroid metabolism over time.

 In vitro data indicate that corticosteroid blockade of T cell activation and cytokine expression is concentration dependent, with a 50% effective concentration of 1-10 nM for dexamethasone [31]. Blockade of IL-1 by dexamethasone is also concentration dependent. Dexamethasone concentrations ranging from 10 to 100 nM completely block the transcription of IL-1 mRNA after *in vitro* stimulation with toxic shock supernatant, whereas greater than 500 nM is necessary to completely block IL-1 expression by prestimulated cells [19]. Thus, *in vitro*, low doses of corticosteroids are sufficient to block cytokine transcription in activated cells, while high doses are necessary to block cytokine production in activated cells. As a clinical corollary, low doses of steroids appear to be adequate for the prevention of acute allograft rejection, while high doses are required to treat an active episode of acute rejection.

Table 1. Relative potencies and duration of action of commonly prescribed corticosteroids

Drug	Equivalent Anti-inflammatory Dose (mg)	Duration of Action (hr)	Relative Anti-inflammatory Potency	Relative Mineralo-corticoid Potency
Hydrocortisone	20	8 – 12	1	1
Cortisone	25	8 – 12	0.8	0.8
Prednisolone	5	12 – 36	4	0.8
Methylprednisolone	5	12 – 36	5	0.5
Dexamethasone	0.75	36 –72	25	0

Corticosteroids most often are prescribed according to fixed and empiric dose-tapering schedules. The observation that some transplant recipients exhibit more steroid-related toxicities than others receiving comparable doses suggests, however, that there may be substantial interindividual variations in the pharmacokinetics and pharmacodynamics of corticosteroids in such patients. Tornatore et al have identified a number of clinical factors accounting for interindividual differences in the metabolism of methylprednisolone in transplant recipients [32-35]. Clearance of this corticosteroid varies with time after transplantation, being 2-fold more rapid in the first few weeks after transplantation than several months later [32]. Compared to men, post-menopausal women exhibit a significantly slower clearance [33]. Finally, African-American patients exhibit a significantly slower clearance of methylprednisolone than Caucasian counterparts [34,35]. Interindividual variation in steroid metabolism is also supported by the observation that the hypothalamic-pituitary-adrenal axis is not consistently suppressed in renal transplant recipients receiving "standard" doses of corticosteroids [36]. Collectively, these findings suggest that fixed dose-tapering regimens provide inconsistent corticosteroid exposure to transplant recipients and may account for wide variations in both toxicity and efficacy. Additional studies are required, however, to determine whether the routine use of pharmacokinetic analyses as a guide to corticosteroid dosing can substantially alter patient outcomes.

Clinical Use of Corticosteroids in Renal Transplantation

Use of Corticosteroids for the Treatment of Acute Rejection

Even before their routine use in maintenance immunosuppression regimens, corticosteroids were found to be effective in reversing acute allograft rejection. In the early 1960s, typical regimens for treatment of acute rejection included the administration of prednisone or prednisolone in oral doses ranging from 150 to 600 mg for up to 3 weeks. Bell et al [37] first demonstrated the efficacy of administering a single large dose of intravenous methylprednisolone in reversing acute renal allograft rejection. Thereafter, others confirmed the benefit of administering intravenous bolus ("pulse") doses of prednisone or prednisolone for several days. Bolus administration of steroids intravenously results in a very rapid lympholytic effect that persists for up to two days. In addition, the short serum half-life of the intravenously administered drug serves to minimize side effects when compared to the use of longer-acting oral preparations.

Despite the theoretical advantages of intravenous pulse steroid therapy, comparative trials have failed to demonstrate an advantage of intravenous methylprednisolone over oral steroids with regard to reversal of acute renal allograft rejection [38-41]. Data accumulated from studies performed prior to the availability of CsA indicate that 60 to 76% of rejection episodes were reversed with intravenous methylprednisolone compared to 56 to 72% of episodes reversed by treatment with oral steroids [39-41]. In two studies, oral doses were associated with a higher frequency of adverse effects such as gastrointestinal bleeding, infection, and diabetes mellitus [39,40]; however, the higher frequency of side effects was probably more closely related to the duration of therapy than to the total dose administered.

The optimal dose of corticosteroids for the treatment of acute rejection also remains a matter of controversy. In the 1960s and 1970s, doses used for pulse therapy ranged from 1 gm of prednisolone daily for three days [37] to 2 gm of methylprednisolone daily for ten days [42]. In 1974, Webel et al [43] studied the effects of a single intravenous bolus of methylprednisolone on lymphocytes stimulated by allogeneic cells and found no significant difference in the magnitude of the response to 80 mg, 250 mg, 500 mg, or 1 gm. Fan et al [44] similarly compared intravenous methylprednisolone doses of 50 mg and 1 gm administered on three consecutive days and found that each dose produced a similar suppression of lymphocyte responsiveness to a variety of mitogens. These studies suggested that the corticosteroid doses used for the treatment of acute rejection in the mid-1970s may have been excessive. However, current steroid dosing schedules used for the treatment of acute rejection vary widely and continue to be chosen empirically. Randomized trials comparing low dose (3 mg/kg or 250 mg) and high-dose (30 mg/kg or 1 gm) intravenous methylprednisolone have shown no significant differences in the rate of reversing acute renal allograft rejection [7,45]. In one study, however, patients receiving the higher dose tended to have greater reductions in serum creatinine concentrations while those receiving the lower dose tended to have fewer infections [45].

A number of polyclonal or monoclonal antilymphocyte antibodies have proven to be effective in reversing acute renal allograft rejection. Many centers continue to use high-dose steroid therapy as first-line treatment for acute allograft rejection, reserving antibody therapy for patients with steroid-resistant rejection. However, several studies suggest that the use of antilymphocyte antibodies for first-line treatment of rejection may be associated with better outcomes. Investigations performed in the late 1970s and early 1980s suggested that use of polyclonal antilymphocyte antibodies for first-line treatment of rejection resulted in higher graft survival rates 1 to 4 years following the rejection episode than did the use of high-dose steroids [46-48]. In a randomized prospective trial comparing use of the monoclonal antibody OKT3 to intravenous methylprednisolone for the treatment of acute renal allograft rejection, OKT3 reversed significantly more rejection episodes than did steroids (94% versus 75%, respectively)[49]. One-year allograft survival was also significantly better with OKT3 (62% versus 45%, respectively). A retrospective study of kidney transplant recipients receiving either OKT3 or oral prednisone for first-line therapy of acute rejection showed a significantly superior 2-year actuarial graft survival among patients treated with OKT3 (87%) compared with patients receiving steroids (54%)[50]. Many centers remain reluctant to use antilymphocyte antibodies routinely for first-line treatment of rejection based on concerns about cost and overimmunosuppression. An alternative strategy individualizes first-line therapy according to the severity of rejection assessed by renal biopsy, such that steroids are administered to patients with histologically mild rejection and antilymphocyte antibodies to those with moderate or severe rejection. Single center experiences suggest that such an approach may improve outcomes compared to the empiric approach of using high-dose steroid therapy as first-line therapy in all patients [51].

The Use of Corticosteroids for the Prevention of Rejection

Low- versus high-dose regimens. In the 1960s and early 1970s, most transplant centers used relatively high doses of corticosteroids, usually in conjunction with azathioprine, for prophylaxis of acute rejection in renal transplant recipients. Daily doses as high as 200 mg of oral prednisone or 1 gm of intravenous methylprednisolone were used for induction of immunosuppression and then tapered over three to four months to maintenance doses of 0.25 – 0.5 mg/kg/day of prednisone or 0.4 – 1.5 mg/kg/day of methylprednisolone [37,38,42,52]. McGeown et al first reported that low-dose steroid therapy (i.e., 20 mg of prednisone daily) instituted immediately after transplantation was associated with patient and allograft survival rates comparable to those of historical controls [53]. Some centers reported higher rates of acute rejection in patients receiving low-dose steroid therapy [54,55], particularly in patients receiving suboptimal doses of azathioprine [56]. However, these early studies generally showed that relatively low doses of corticosteroids were associated with a lower incidence of side effects without jeopardizing allograft survival. Buckels et al reported a significantly lower mortality rate in patients receiving low doses of steroids [6].

Alternate-day corticosteroid regimens. Alternate-day steroid therapy, usually accomplished by slowly tapering steroid doses in patients previously maintained on daily doses, represented the next historical step in efforts to minimize steroid-related side effects after renal transplantation. In two large randomized controlled trials, alternate-day steroid therapy was as effective in maintaining allograft function as daily dosing [57,58]. In one study of 91 cadaveric renal transplant recipients, 5-year actuarial patient survival was 97% and 83%, and allograft survival was 85% and 67% in the alternate-day and daily-dose treatment groups, respectively [58]. In another study of 38 patients maintained on alternate-day therapy, the frequency of acute rejection episodes and serum creatinine concentrations were similar to those of 38 patients maintained on daily steroids [57].

Some [4,59,60] but not all [58] studies suggest that alternate-day steroid therapy reduces the incidence of side effects such as infectious complications, gastrointestinal bleeding, cataracts, obesity, and post-transplant diabetes mellitus. Dumler et al [57] reported that a 2.6% incidence of aseptic necrosis of the hip in patients maintained on alternate-day therapy, significantly lower than the 18.6% incidence in patients maintained on daily therapy. Curtis et al [61] reported that 75% of 74 patients were normotensive after receiving alternate-day therapy for an average of 3.9 years. Conflicting data have been obtained on the effect of alternate-day therapy on post-transplant hyperlipidemia. In two prospective, controlled trials [62,63], conversion from daily to alternate-day therapy resulted in a significant reduction of total cholesterol and/or triglyceride levels. However, a similar study limited to children did not confirm this benefit [64]. Results of several prospective [59,60,65] and retrospective [66] studies indicate that alternate-day therapy is associated with accelerated growth in pediatric renal transplant recipients with good renal allograft function, although increased growth may not be appreciated until more than one year following conversion to the alternate-day regimen.

Steroid-Free Immunosuppression

The introduction of CsA in the early 1980s revolutionized the field of organ transplantation and permitted effective immunosuppression with even lower doses of corticosteroids than used previously. However, the observations that corticosteroids and CsA independently promote the development of hypertension [67-69], hyperlipidemia [70,71] and glucose intolerance [72,73] probably account for the fact that the decline in steroid-induced morbidity has not been proportional to the reduction in steroid dosage that most centers incorporated into their CsA-based immunosuppression protocols. The independent influence of steroids and CsA on cardiovascular risk factors is particularly concerning because cardiovascular disease emerged as the major cause of late post-transplant morbidity and mortality in the decade following the introduction of CsA [74,75]. Complete withdrawal of steroid therapy was attempted only rarely in the pre-CsA era [76-79] and the best outcomes were observed in recipients of renal allografts from HLA-identical donors [79]. The availability of CsA rekindled an interest in steroid-free immunosuppression for kidney transplant recipients, either by avoidance of steroids from the time of transplantation or by withdrawal of steroid therapy at some arbitrary time after transplantation.

Experience with Steroid-free Immunosuppression in the CsA-Azathioprine Era

Corticosteroid avoidance. The early experience with CsA monotherapy demonstrated that renal transplantation could be performed successfully in some patients without the use of corticosteroids. However, between 15 and 79% of patients initially treated with cyclosporine alone ultimately required the addition of steroids, usually because of acute allograft rejection [80-86]. Relatively short-term follow-up studies of patients entered into randomized trials failed to show any advantage in patient or graft survival when CsA monotherapy was compared to the combination of CsA and steroids [81-83]. However, a recent 6-year follow-up analysis of patients enrolled in such a study in Italy [87] indicated that renal allograft survival was significantly lower in patients initially randomized to CsA without steroids (see below). Steroid avoidance also has been attempted in patients maintained on CsA and azathioprine from the time of transplantation. However, Bry et al. showed that approximately 50% of such patients ultimately require initiation of steroid therapy because of acute rejection [88].

Steroid Withdrawal. The more popular approach to achieving steroid-free immunosuppression in renal transplant recipients has consisted of withdrawing maintenance corticosteroids slowly at some arbitrary time after transplantation. The widely varying success of steroid withdrawal in patients receiving CsA-based immunosuppression probably reflects differences in patient selection, the timing of steroid withdrawal after the transplant operation, the rapidity of the steroid taper, the intensity of residual immunosuppression, duration of follow-up, and the criteria for defining successful withdrawal or for renewing steroids in patients previously withdrawn from these agents. During the decade following the introduction of CsA, a large body of data was generated regarding the benefits of steroid withdrawal and on the subsequent risk of acute and chronic rejection.

A number of studies have shown that corticosteroid avoidance [89,90] or withdrawal of steroid therapy [91,92] results in accelerated growth in children following transplantation. Although corticosteroids undoubtedly contribute to post-transplant osteopenia, it has been more difficult to determine whether steroid withdrawal has any discernible benefit on bone density. Wolpaw et al were unable to demonstrate a statistically significant difference in vertebral bone density when patients maintained on corticosteroid therapy were compared with those successfully withdrawn from steroids for at least 6 months, although there was a trend toward higher bone densities in the steroid-free group [93].

Studies in adult and pediatric renal transplant recipients indicate that withdrawal of steroid therapy is accompanied by significant declines in systolic and diastolic blood pressure as well as a decrease in the number of administered antihypertensive medications [94-97]. In one study, approximately 15% of previously hypertensive transplant recipients successfully withdrawn from corticosteroids were able to discontinue all antihypertensive medications [97]. Withdrawal of steroids from CsA-treated renal transplant recipients results in a 10 to 20% reduction in total plasma cholesterol, low-density lipoprotein and triglyceride concentrations [95,96,98-100]. The decrease in total cholesterol levels is even more dramatic in children successfully withdrawn from steroids [94]. However, the decrease in low-density lipoprotein cholesterol concentration is accompanied by a proportional decrease in the concentration of high-density lipoproteins such that the ratio of total to high-density lipoprotein cholesterol remains unchanged [100]. Thus, it remains unclear whether withdrawal of steroids will reduce cardiovascular morbidity related to post-transplant hyperlipidemia. In CsA-treated renal transplant recipients with pre-existing diabetes mellitus, steroid withdrawal is accompanied by reduced insulin requirements [94]. In patients with acquired post-transplant diabetes mellitus, a majority of patients can be withdrawn from insulin or oral hypoglycemic agents within months following successful steroid withdrawal [101]. However, Fabrega et al have noted long-term deterioration in glycemic control in many of their patients with post-transplant diabetes after withdrawal of steroids [102,103].

The benefits of steroid withdrawal must be weighed against the risks of precipitating allograft rejection. It has been difficult to assess the risks because much of the published experience with steroid-free immunosuppression consists of results of uncontrolled trials. Moreover, even controlled studies of steroid withdrawal in CsA-treated patients vary greatly with respect to factors that may influence the risk of allograft rejection. In fact, the definition of "success" and "failure" in steroid withdrawal protocols has varied from one center to another. Allograft rejection is undoubtedly the most common reason for renewing corticosteroid therapy after attempted withdrawal, but the severity, frequency, and reversibility of rejection episodes that trigger renewal of steroids are rarely delineated in published studies. In some centers, protocol failures include patients in whom steroids are renewed because of adrenal insufficiency, leukopenia, recurrent renal disease, or for the treatment of comorbid conditions. However, allograft rejection remains the most serious concern in judging the safety of steroid withdrawal protocols.

In patients maintained on either CsA and azathioprine or CsA alone, the reported incidence of acute renal allograft rejection associated with corticosteroid withdrawal has ranged from 3 to 81% [104-112]. A meta-analysis of 7 randomized, prospective controlled trials [83-86,104,105,113] compared the outcomes of 681 steroid-free patients with those of 592 patients maintained on steroids [114]. The collective incidence of acute rejection was 48% in the steroid-free group compared with 30% in patients maintained on steroids (p=0.012). There were no statistically significant differences in patient or allograft survival. However, 4 of the 7 studies incorporated into this analysis were steroid avoidance studies and, in 2 of the 3 steroid withdrawal studies, prednisone was withdrawn less than 3 months following transplantation. In an uncontrolled study limited to living related renal transplant recipients, Stratta et al similarly reported that 21 of 46 patients (46%) withdrawn from steroids within one month of transplantation sustained acute rejection episodes that prompted renewal of steroid therapy [115]. Thus, results of both controlled and uncontrolled trials and of a meta-analysis suggest that steroid avoidance or early discontinuation of steroids (less than 3 months after transplantation) is associated with a high incidence of rejection. A list of randomized prospective trials of steroid withdrawal in patients maintained on CsA-based therapy (updated since the above-mentioned meta-analysis) is shown in **Table 2**.

Results from uncontrolled trials suggested that the risk of precipitating acute rejection might be reduced in patients subjected to later steroid withdrawal (more than 6 months after transplantation) [116,117]. Asidefrom timing, few clinical variables reliably predict the outcome of attempted steroid withdrawal. It is generally acknowledged that steroid withdrawal in children is associated with higher rates of acute rejection compared to adults. Although this review focuses on kidney transplant recipients, it should be noted that the risk of acute rejection associated with steroid withdrawal may be different with other solid organ transplants. In liver transplant recipients, acute rejection rates are low enough that some centers have routinely withdrawn steroids from stable patients. In renal allograft recipients, data from single centers indicate higher rates of rejection in patients with elevated serum creatinine concentrations prior to steroid withdrawal, donor-recipient racial mismatches, and suboptimal doses of CsA [116-118].

However, none of these variables has proven to be sensitive enough to provide meaningful predictive value. In addition, no satisfactory means of immunologic monitoring have been established to date to guide the withdrawal of steroids or other immunosuppressants.

Several long-term follow-up studies of renal transplant recipients withdrawn from steroids and maintained on CsA-based regimens indicate that steroid withdrawal increases the risk of chronic allograft dysfunction, irrespective of the timing of steroid withdrawal [107, 119,120]. A placebo-controlled trial organized by the Canadian Multicenter Transplant Study Group concluded that withdrawal of corticosteroids results in deterioration of renal function that could be appreciated only after 5 years of follow-up [107]. Similarly, Tarantino et al compared the long-term outcomes of patients randomized to CsA monotherapy or triple drug therapy [119]. After 6 years, they observed an allograft survival rate of 67% for patients assigned to CsA

Table 2. Randomized controlled trials of corticosteroid withdrawal in renal transplant patients receiving azathioprine and/or cyclosporine

Study [ref #]	Group	n	Timing of steroid Withdrawal (months post-transplant)	Residual therapy	Duration of follow-up (years)	Acute rejection (%)	1-year graft survival (%)
Schulak et al [104]	Control	35	NA	CsA, STE, AZA	1	54	83
	Study	32	< 1	CsA, AZA		81	87
Maiorca et al [105]	Control	31	NA	CsA, STE	4	13	81
	Study	35	6	CsA		46	84
Sinclair et al [109]	Control	263	NA	CsA, STE	5	NR	85
	Study	260	3	CsA		NR	73
Ratcliffe et al [120]	Control	51	NA	CsA, STE, AZA	1	0	NR
	Study	49	12-36	CsA, AZA		0	NR
Hilbrands et al [108]	Conrol	63	NA	AZA, STE	5	25	NR
	Study	64	3	CsA		30	NR
Hollander et al [121]	Control	42	NA	CsA,STE	1	2	NR
	Study	42	>12	CsA		26	NR

n = number of patients; CsA = cyclosporine; STE = corticosteroids;
AZA = azathioprine; NA= not applicable; NR = not reported

alone versus 86% for patients given triple therapy that included corticosteroids. At least two studies have shown that withdrawal of steroids is associated with higher rates of urine protein excretion, presumably reflecting "chronic rejection" [121,122]. In one study, however, the risk of proteinuria was limited to patients in whom steroids were renewed after sustaining multiple episodes of acute rejection associated with steroid withdrawal. Recent studies have described histological findings in patients withdrawn from cortico-steroids, and suggest higher rates of interstitial fibrosis [123], and sclerosing arteriopathy [124] when compared to steroid-treated controls. Although these observations suggest that withdrawal of steroids promotes chronic immune-mediated injury to the renal allograft in some patients, it remains possible that the absence of ster-oids also enhances the chronic nephrotoxicity of calcineurin inhibitors such as CsA or tacrolimus.

Results of these long-term follow-up studies contrast sharply with Opelz' retrospective analysis of more than 12,000 cadaveric renal transplant recipients from 188 centers that provided data to his registry

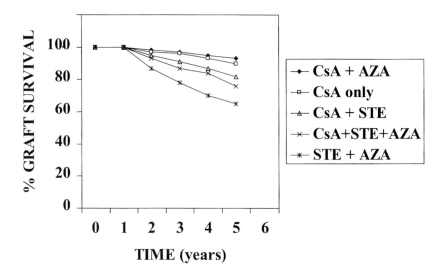

Figure 3. Long-term graft survival rates of first cadaver transplants according to the immunosuppressive regimen administered one year after transplantation. All patients were initially treated with cyclosporine (CsA), azathioprine (AZA), and steroids (STE). The number of patients followed (n) and the mean CsA dose at one year were: CsA + AZA (n=733; 4.60 mg/kg/day); CsA only (n=537; 4.70 mg/kg/day); CsA + STE (n=2829; 4.06 mg/kg/day); CsA+STE+AZA (n=8024; 3.92 mg/kg/day); STE + AZA (n=830). Modified with permission from Opelz [125].

[125]. Among patients who were initially treated with CsA, azathioprine, and corticosteroids, the 5-year allograft survival was significantly higher in a subgroup of patients who had been withdrawn from steroids during the first post-transplant year than in patients who remained on triple therapy (see **Figure 3**). Results of this analysis may have been influenced by bias in selection of patients for steroid withdrawal protocols. However, it is interesting that CsA doses administered to the patients withdrawn from steroids were significantly higher than those administered to patients who continued to receive steroids. Although the balance of evidence from long-term follow-up studies led to a decreased interest in the routine withdrawal of steroids from CsA-treated renal transplant recipients, results from Opelz' registry analysis certainly suggest that withdrawal of steroids might be accomplished more safely in renal transplant recipients maintained on potent residual immunosuppression.

Experience with Steroid Withdrawal in Patients Receiving Newer Immunosuppressants

Since 1994, the introduction and routine use of new CsA formulations, tacrolimus, mycophenolate mofetil, sirolimus, and a number of new monoclonal and polyclonal anti-lymphocyte antibodies has been accompanied by lower rates of acute allograft rejection in renal transplant recipients. Availability of these new immunosuppressants also has resurrected interest in the possibility of safely withdrawing corticosteroids with residual immunosuppression consisting of some combination of the newer agents. In addition to the results of uncontrolled and controlled studies summarized below, a number of prospective steroid withdrawal trials are ongoing with results expected in 2 to 4 years.

Tacrolimus. Although tacrolimus is widely regarded as a "steroid-sparing" immunosuppressant, there have been no randomized trials to determine whether the agent is superior to CsA in allowing withdrawal of corticosteroids. In a large, uncontrolled experience with tacrolimus at the University of Pittsburgh, 76% of adult patients have been successfully weaned from steroids at various times after transplantation and most often maintained on tacrolimus monotherapy [126]. Compared to patients maintained on steroids, those successfully weaned from steroids exhibit lower serum creatinine concentrations and a lower frequency of cumulative acute rejection episodes. However, these observations undoubtedly reflect bias in selecting ideal candidates for steroid withdrawal. In another uncontrolled study, Woodle et al have attempted to withdraw steroids one week after transplantation in patients maintained on relatively high doses of tacrolimus and mycophenolate mofetil [127]. The overall rate of acute rejection was 25% with a mean follow-up of 19 months. Notably, the incidence of acute rejection in African-American patients was 52%, significantly higher than that observed in Caucasians. Compared to Caucasians, African-Americans also exhibited lower 2-year graft survival rates (80% versus 54%) after attempted withdrawal of steroids. The overall rates of acute rejection are nonetheless lower than those reported in previous experiences with "early" steroid withdrawal [104,109,115], and form the basis for an ongoing prospective, double-blinded trial that will assess outcomes after early steroid withdrawal in patients treated with daclizumab, tacrolimus, and mycophenolate mofetil.

Mycophenolate mofetil/CsA. In an uncontrolled study of 26 patients maintained on mycophenolate mofetil and the Sandimmune® formulation of CsA, Grinyo et al [128] reported no episodes of acute rejection with a mean follow-up of 10 months in patients withdrawn from steroids 4 to 30 months after transplantation. Kupin et al reported relatively low rates of acute rejection after steroid withdrawal in living related kidney transplant recipients on mycophenolate mofetil and the Neoral® formulation of CsA compared to historical control group maintained on azathioprine and Sandimmune®[129].

A large, prospective randomized European multicenter study investigated the safety of steroid withdrawal in transplant recipients maintained on CsA and mycophenolate mofetil [130]. Patients were randomized to receive either a standard steroid regimen (n=248) or a low-dose steroid regimen (50% of the dose administered to the control group) followed by steroid withdrawal at 3 months post-transplant (n=252). The incidence of biopsy-proven rejection within the first year of follow-up was 25% in the low-dose/steroid withdrawal group versus 15% in the control group (p<0.01). Interestingly, most of the rejection episodes in the low-dose/withdrawal group occurred before steroids were actually discontinued. At 1 year post-transplant, patient and allo-graft survival rates were not significantly different (98 and 94% in the low-dose/withdrawal group versus 97 and 93% in the control group).

A US trial of steroid withdrawal in primary kidney transplant recipients maintained on mycophenolate mofetil and Neoral® was dis-continued prematurely by the study's data safety monitoring board because of a significantly higher rate of biopsy-proven acute rejection in the steroid withdrawal group [131]. In this prospective, double-blinded trial, patients free of acute rejection during the first 3 post-transplant months were randomly assigned to steroid withdrawal over a period of eight weeks (n=134) or continued therapy with steroids (n=132). In contrast to the European trial, steroid doses were similar in the two groups prior to randomization. The Kaplan-Meier estimate of the cumulative incidence of acute rejection within the first post-transplant year was 30.8% in the steroid withdrawal group and 9.8% in the steroid maintenance group. The risk of acute rejection was much higher in black patients (39.6%) than in nonblacks (16%) (p<0.001). However, when blacks were eliminated from the analysis, rejection rates remained significantly higher in nonblacks subjected to steroid withdrawal than in those maintained on corticosteroids. At 1 year post-transplant, patient and allograft survival rates were similar in each group; however, early discontinuation of the trial prevented the long-term follow-up needed to determine whether steroid withdrawal in-creases the risk of chronic allograft dysfunction in patients maintained on mycophenolate mofetil and CsA.

Sirolimus. Experience with steroid withdrawal in renal transplant recipients receiving sirolimus-based immunosuppression has been lim-ited. However, preliminary data from the University of Texas indicates that the combination of sirolimus and Neoral® may allow early elim-ination of corticosteroids with relatively low rates of acute allograft rejection [132]. Controlled, prospective, multicenter trials will test the safety of steroid withdrawal in patients receiving sirolimus-based therapy in the near future.

Summary

Corticosteroids have been a mainstay of immunosuppressive drug therapy in solid organ transplantation for more than 40 years.

Although our understanding of the immunosuppressive mechanisms of these agents has expanded greatly during that time, dosing of corticosteroids for organ transplant recipients has remained surprisingly empiric.   The well-recognized adverse effects of long-term steroid therapy have led to an understandable desire to develop steroid-sparing and steroid-free immunosuppressive regimens.   To date, virtually all controlled trials of steroid avoidance or steroid withdrawal have indicated that elimination of steroids increases the risk of acute and/or chronic rejection in a substantial minority of patients.   Data from studies performed in renal transplant recipients receiving CsA/azathioprine-based therapy indicate that long-term follow-up of at least 5 years is necessary to appreciate the negative effects of steroid withdrawal on graft function and survival.   Preliminary results from trials of steroid withdrawal in patients receiving some of the newer immunosuppressants suggest lower rates of acute rejection than in historical controls.   However, results of these and future trials should be interpreted cautiously until long-term follow-up is available.   Most studies suggest that African-American race increases the risk of acute and chronic rejection associated with steroid withdrawal.   Future trials of steroid-free immunosuppression should be particularly cognizant of the effects of race on outcome.

References

1. Billingham RE, Krohn PL, Medawar PB. Effect of cortisone on survival of skin homografts in rabbits. Br Med J 1951; 1: 4716.
2. Starzl TE, Marchioro TL, Waddel WR. The reversal of rejection in renal homografts with subsequent development of homograft tolerance. Surg Gynecol Obstet 1963; 117: 385-395.
3. Goodwin WE, Kaufman JJ, Mims MM, et al. Human renal transplantation. I. Clinical experiences with six cases of renal homotransplantation. J Urol 1963; 89: 13-17.
4. Siegel RR, Luke RG, Hellebusch AA. Reduction of toxicity of corticosteroid therapy after renal transplantation. Am J Med 1972; 53: 159-169.
5. Chan L, French ME, Beare J, Oliver DO, Morris PJ. Prospective trial of high-dose versus low-dose prednisolone in renal transplant patients. Transplant Proc 1980; 12: 323-326.
6. Buckels JA, Mackintosh P, Barnes AD. Controlled trial of low versus high dose oral steroid therapy in 100 cadaveric renal transplants. Proc EDTA 1981; 18: 394-399.
7. Park GD, Bartucci M, Smith MC. High- versus low-dose methylprednisolone for acute rejection episodes in renal transplantation. Nephron 1984; 36: 80-83.
8. Hricik DE, Almawi WY, Strom TB. Trends in the use of glucocorticoids in renal transplantation. Transplantation 1994; 57: 979-989.
9. Fauci AS. The effect of hydrocortisone on the kinetics of normal human lymphocytes. Blood 1975; 46: 235-240.
10. Hollenberg SM, Evans RM. Multiple and cooperative trans-activation domains of the human glucocorticoid receptor. Cell 1988; 55: 899-906.
11. Guigere V, Hollenberg SM, Rosenfeld MG, Evans RM. Functional domains of the human glucocorticoid receptor. Cell 1986; 46: 645-652.
12. Almawi WY, Hadro ET, Strom TB. Evidence that glucocorticosteroid-mediated immunosuppressive effects do not involve altering second messenger function. Transplantation 1991; 52: 133-140.
13. Vacca A, Felli MP, Farina AR, et al. Glucocorticoid receptor-mediated suppression of the interleukin 2 gene expression through impairment of the cooperativity between nuclear factor of activated T cells and AP-1 enhancer elements. J Exp Med 1992; 175: 637-646.
14. Barnes PJ, Adcock I. Anti-inflammatory actions of steroids: molecular mechanisms. Trends Pharmacol Sci 1993; 14: 436-441.
15. Barnes PJ, Karin M. Nuclear factor-κB – a pivotal transcription factor in chronic inflammatory diseases. N Engl J Med 1997; 336: 1066-1071.
16. Ray A, Prefontaine KE. Physical association and functional antagonism between the p65 subunit of transcription factor NF-κB and the glucocorticoid receptor. Proc Natl Acad Sci USA 1994; 91: 752-756.
17. Scheinman RI, Gualberto A, Jewell CM, Cidlowski JA, Baldwin AS. Characterization of mechanisms involved in transrepression of NF-κB by activated glucocorticoid receptors. Mol Cell Biol 1995; 15: 943-953.
18. Scheinman RI, Cogswell PC, Lofquist AK, Baldwin AS. Role of transcriptional activation of IκBα in mediation of immunosuppression by glucocorticoids. Science 1995; 270: 283-286.
19. Knudsen PJ, Dinarello CA, Strom TB. Glucocorticoids inhibit transcriptional and post-transcriptional expression of interleukin 1 in U937 cells. J Immunol 1987; 139: 4129-4134.
20. Kern JA, Lamb RJ, Reed JC, et al. Dexamethasone inhibition of interleukin 1 beta production by human monocytes: posttranscriptional mechanisms. J Clin Invest 1988; 81: 237-244.

21. Zanker B, Walz G, Wieder KJ, et al. Evidence that glucocorticoids block expression of the human interleukin-6 gene by accessory cells. Transplantation 1990; 49: 183-185.
22. CulpepperJA, Lee F. Regulation of IL-3 expression by glucocorticoids in cloned murine T lymphocytes. J Immunol 1985; 135: 3191-3197.
23. Gessani S, McCandless S, Baglioni C. The glucocorticoid dexamethasone inhibits synthesis of interferon by decreasing the level of its mRNA. J Biol Chem 1988; 263: 7454-7457.
24. Arya SK, Wong-Staal F, Gallo RC. Dexamethasone-mediated inhibition of human T cell growth factor and gamma interferon messenger RNA. J Immunology 1984; 133: 273-276.
25. Waage A, Baake O. Glucocorticoids suppress the production of tumour necrosis factor by lipopolysaccharide-stimulated human monocytes. Immunology 1988; 63: 299-302.
26. Granelli-Piperno A, Nolan P, Inaba K, et al. The effect of immunosuppressive agents on the induction of nuclear factors that bind to sites in the interlekin 2 promoter. J Exp Med 1990; 172: 1869-1872.
27. Shen V, Cheng SL, Kohler NG, et al. Characterization and hormonal modulation of IL-1 binding in neonatal mouse osteoblast-like cells. J Bone Miner Res 1990; 5: 507-515.
28. Schooltink H, Schmitz-Van der Leur H, Heinrich PC, et al. Upregulation of the interleukin-6-signal transducing protein (gp130) by interlekin-6 and dexamethasone in HepG2 cells. FBS Lett 1992; 297: 263-265.
29. Strickland RW, Wahl LM, Finbloom DS. Corticosteroids enhance the binding of recombinant interferon gamma to cultured monocytes. J Immunology 1986; 137: 1577-1580.
30. Haynes RC. Adrenocortical steroids and their synthetic analogs. In: Gilman AG, Rall TW, Nies AS, Taylor P, eds. The pharmacological basis of therapeutics. New York; Pergamon Press, 1990: 1431.
31. Snyers L, De Wit L, Content J. Glucocorticoid up-regulation of high-affinity interleukin 6 receptors on human epithelial cells. Proc Natl Acad Sci USA 1990; 87: 2838.
32. Tornatore KM, Reed KA, Venuto RC. Assessment of methylprednisolone pharmacokinetics and cortisol response during early and chronic postrenal-transplant periods. Transplantation 1995; 60: 1607-1611.
33. Cimminelli AM, Reed KA, Farooqui M, Venuto RC, Tornatore KM. Glucocorticoid pharmacokinetics in postmenopausal renal transplant recipients. Pharmacother (abstract) 1998
34. Tornatore KM, Biocevich D, Reed KA, Tousley K, Singh P, Venuto RC. Methylprednisolone pharmacokinetics, cortisol response, and adverse effects in black and white renal transplant recipients. Transplantation 1995; 59: 729-736.
35. Tornatore KM, Reed KA, Venuto RC. Racial differences in pharmacokinetics of methylprednisolone in black and white renal transplant recipients. Pharmacother 1993; 13: 481-486.
36. Tornatore KM, Reed K, Walshe JJ, Venuto RC. Cortisol pharmacodynamic response to long-term methylprednisolone in renal transplant recipients. Pharmacother 1994; 14: 111-118.
37. Bell PRF, Briggs JD, Calman KC, et al. Reversal of acute clinical and experimental organ rejection using large doses of intravenous prednisolone. Lancet 1971; 1: 876-880.
38. Alarcon-Zurita A, Ladefoged J. Treatment of acute allograft rejection with high doses of corticosteroids. Kidney Int 1976; 9:351354.
39. Mussche MM, Ringoir SMG, Lamiere NN. High intravenous doses of methylprednisolone for acute cadaveric renal allograft rejection. Nephron 1976; 16:287-291.

40. Gray D, Shepherd H, Daar A, Oliver DO, Morris PJ. Oral versus intravenous high-dose steroid treatment of renal allograft rejection. Lancet 1978; 1:117-118.
41. Orta-Sibu N, Chantler C, Bewick M, Hancock G. Comparison of high-dose intravenous methylprednisolone with low-dose oral prednisolone in acute renal allograft rejection in children. Br Med J 1982; 285: 255-260.
42. Woods JE, Anderson CF, DeWeerd JH, et al. High-dosage intravenously administered methylprednisolone in renal transplantation. A preliminary report. JAMA 1973; 223: 896-899.
43. Webel ML, Ritts RE, Taswell HF, Donadio JV, Woods JE. Celular immunity after intravenous administration of methylprednisolone. J Lab Clin Med 1974; 83: 383-392.
44. Fan PT, Yu DTY, Targoff C, Bluestone R. Effect of corticosteroids on the human immune response. Suppression of mitogen-induced lymphocyte proliferation by "pulse" methylprednisolone. Transplantation 1978; 26: 266-267.
45. Kauffman HM, Stromstad SA, Sampson D, Stawicki AT. Randomized steroid therapy of human kidney transplant rejection. Transplant Proc 1979; 11: 36-38.
46. Cosimi AB. The clinical value of antilymphocyte antibodies. Transplant Proc 1981; 15: 462-468.
47. Shield CF, Cosimi AB, Tolkoff-Rubin N, Rubin RH, Herrin J, Russell PS. Use of antithymocyte globulin for reversal of acute allograft rejection. Transplantation 1979; 28: 461-464.
48. Filo RS, Smith EJ, Leapman SB. Therapy of acute cadaveric renal allograft rejection with adjunctive antithymocyte globulin. Transplantation 1980; 30: 445-449.
49. Ortho Multicenter Transplant Study Group. A randomized clinical trial of OKT3 monclonal antibody for acute rejection of cadaveric renal transplants. N Engl J Med 1985; 313: 337-341.
50. Tesi RJ, Elkhammas EA, Henry ML, Ferguson RM. OKT3 for primary therapy of first rejection episode in kidney transplants. Transplantation 1993; 55: 1023-1029.
51. Kamath S, Dean D, Peddi VR, et al. Efficacy of OKT3 as primary therapy for histologically confirmed acute renal allograft rejection. Transplantation 1997; 64: 1428-1432.
52. Kauffman HM, Sampson D, Fox PS, Stawicki AT. High dose (bolus) intravenous methylprednisolone at the time of kidney homotransplantation. Ann Surg 1977; 186: 631-634.
53. McGeown MG, Douglas JF, Brown WA et al. Low dose steroid from the day following renal transplantation. Proc EDTA 1979; 16: 395-400.
54. Ponticelli C, De Vecchi AF, Tarantino A, et al. A search for optimizing corticosteroid administration to renal transplant patients. Kidney Int 1983; 23 (suppl 14): S85-S89.
55. Hayry P, Ahonen J, Kock B, et al. Glucocorticoids in renal transplantation. II. Impact of high- versus low-dose postoperative methylprednisolone administration on graft survival and on the frequency and type of complications. Scand J Immunol 1984; 19: 211-218.
56. D'Apice AJF, Becker GJ, Kincaid-Smith P, et al. A prospective randomized trial of low-dose versus high-dose steroids in cadaveric renal transplantation. Transplantation 1984; 37: 373-377.
57. Dumler F, Levin NW, Szego G, Vulpetti AT, Preuss LE. Long-term alternate day steroid therapy in renal transplantation. Transplantation 1982; 34: 78-82.
58. De Vecchi A, Cantaluppi A, Montagnino G, Tarantino A, Maestri O, Ponticelli C. Long-term comparison between single-morning daily and alternate-day steroid treatment in cadaver kidney recipients. Transplant Proc 1980; 12: 327-330.
59. Diethelm AG, Sterling WA, Hartley MW, Morgan JM. Alternate-day prednisone therapy in recipients of renal allografts. Arch Surg 1976; 111: 867-870.

60. Bell MJ, Martin LW, Gonzales LL, McEnery PT, West CD. Alternate-day single-dose prednisone therapy: a method of reducing steroid toxicity. J Pediatric Surg 1972; 7: 223-229.
61. Curtis JJ, Galla JH, Kotchen TA, Lucas B, McRoberts JW, Luke RG. Prevalence of hypertension in a renal transplant population on alternate-day steroid therapy. Clin Nephrol 1976; 5: 123-127.
62. Curtis JJ, Galla JH, Woodford SY, Lucas BA, Luke RG. Effect of alternate-day prednisone on plasma lipids in renal transplant recipients. Kidney Int 1982; 22: 42-47.
63. Cattran DC, Steiner G, Wilson DR, Fenton SSA. Hyperlipidemia after renal transplantation: natural history and pathophysiology. Ann Intern Med 1979; 91: 554-559.
64. Drukker A, Turner C, Start K, et al. Hyperlipidemia after renal transplantation in children on alternate day corticosteroid therapy. Clin Nephrol 1986; 26: 140-145.
65. McEnery PT, Gonzalez LL, Martin LW, West CD. Growth and development of children with renal transplants. Use of alternate-day steroid therapy. J Pediatr 1973; 83: 806-814.
66. Feldhoff C, Goldman AI, Najarian JS, Mauer SM. A comparison of alternate day and daily steroid therapy in children following renal transplantation. Int J Pediatr Nephrol 1984; 5: 11-14.
67. Hricik DE, Lautman J, Bartucci MR, Moir EJ Mayes JT, Schulak JA. Variable effects of steroid withdrawal on blood pressure reduction in cyclosporine-treated renal transplant recipients. Transplantation 1992; 53: 1232-1235.
68. Popovtzer MM, Pinnggera W, Katx FH, et al. Variations in arterial blood pressure after kidney transplantation. Relation to renal function, plasma renin activity, and the dose of prednisone. Circulation 1973; 47: 1297-1305.
69. Bennett WM, Porter GA. Cyclosporine-associated hypertension. Am J Med 1988; 85: 131-133.
70. Hricik DE, Mayes JT, Schulak JA. Independent effects of cyclosporine and prednisone on post-transplant hypercholesterolemia. Am J Kidney Dis 1991; 18: 353-358.
71. Kasiske BL, Tororice KL, Heim-Duthoy KL, Awni WM, Rao KV. The adverse impact of cyclosporine on serum lipids in renal transplant recipients. Am J Kidney Dis 1991; 17: 700-707.
72. Yoshimura N, Nakai I, Ohmori Y, et al. Effect of cyclosporine on the endocrine and exocrine pancreas in kidney transplant recipients. Am J Kidney Dis 1988; 12: 11-17.
73. Mejia G, Arbelaez M, Henao JE, Arango JL, Garcia A. Cyclosporine-associated diabetes mellitus in renal transplants. Clin Transplant 1989; 3: 260-264.
74. Dlugosz BA, Bretan PN, Novick AC, et al. Causes of death in kidney transplant recipients: 1970 to present. Transplant Proc 1989; 21: 2168-2170.
75. Hill MN, Grossman RA, Feldman HI, Hurwitz S, Dafoe DC. Changes in causes of death after renal transplantation, 1966 to 1987. Am J Kidney Dis 1991; 17: 512-518.
76. Naik RB, Abdeen H, English J, Chakraborty J, Slapak M, Lee HA. Prednisolone withdrawal after 2 years in renal transplant patients receiving only this form of immunosuppression. Transplant Proc 1979; 11: 39-41.
77. Steinman TI, Zimmerman CE, Monaco AP, et al. Steroids can be stopped in kidney transplant recipients. Transplant Proc 1981; 13 :323-324.
78. Thaysen JH, Lokegaard H. Permanent withdrawal of prednisone in kidney transplantation. Scand J Urol Nephrol 1977; 42 (suppl): 198-203.
79. First MR, Munda R, Kant KS, Fidler JP, Alexander JW. Steroid withdrawal following HLA-identical related donor transplantation. Transplant Proc 1981; 13: 319-321.

80. European Multicentre Trial. Cyclosporin A as sole immunosuppressive agent in recipients of kidney allografts from cadaver donors. Lancet 1982; 2: 57-60.
81. Griffin PJA, Gomes Da Costa CA, Salaman JR. A controlled trial of steroids in cyclosporine-treated renal transplant recipients. Transplantation 1987; 43: 505-508.
82. MacDonald AS, Daloze P, Dandavino R, et al. A randomized study of cyclosporine with and without prednisone in renal allograft recipients. Transplant Proc 1987; 19: 1865-1867.
83. Johnson RWG, Mallick NP, Bakran A, et al. A randomized study of cyclosporine with and without prednisone in renal allograft recipients. Transplant Proc 1989; 21: 1581-1582.
84. Albert FW, Schmidt U. Cyclosporine therapy with or without steroids in cadaveric kidney transplantation – a prospective randomized one-center study. Transplant Proc 1985; 17: 2669-2670.
85. Thiel G, Harder F, Loertscher R, et al. Cyclosporine alone or in combination with prednisone in cadaveric renal transplantation. Transplant Proc 1984; 16: 1187-X.
86. Tarantino A, Aroldi A, Stucchi L, et al. A randomized prospective trial comparing cyclosporine monotherapy with triple-drug therapy in renal transplantation. Transplantation 1991; 52: 53-57.
87. Ponticelli C, Tarantino A, Montagnino G. Controlled trials with cyclosporine in kidney transplantation. Transplant Proc 1994; 26: 2490-2492.
88. Bry W, Warvariv V, Bohannon L, et al. Cadaveric renal transplant without prophylactic prednisone therapy. Transplant Proc 1991; 23: 994-996.
89. Reisman L, Lieberman KV, Burrows L, et al. Follow-up of cyclosporine-treated pediatric renal allograft recipients after cessation of prednisone. Transplantation 1990; 49: 76-80.
90. Klare B, Strom TM, Hahn H, et al. Remarkable long-term prognosis and excellent growth in kidney-transplant children under cyclosporine monotherapy. Transplant Proc 1991; 23: 1013-1017.
91. Tejani A, Butt KMH, Rajpoot D, et al. Strategies for optimizing growth in children with kidney transplants. Transplantation 1989; 47: 229-233.
92. David-Neto E, Vilares S, Lando V, et al. Conversion from azathioprine/prednisone to azathioprine/cyclosporin promotes catch-up growth in pediatric renal allograft recipients. Clin Transplant 1990; 4: 229-234.
93. Wolpaw T, Deal CL, Fleming-Brooks S, et al. Factors influencing vertebral bone density after renal transplantation. Transplantation 1994; 58: 1186-1189.
94. Ingulli E, Tejani A, Markell M. The beneficial effects of steroid withdrawal on blood pressure and lipid profile in children post-transplantation in the cyclosporine era. Transplantation 1993; 55: 102-110.
95. Kupin W, Venkat KK, Oh OK, et al. Complete replacement of methylprednisolone by azathioprine in cyclosporine-treated primary cadaveric renal transplant recipients. Transplantation 1988; 45: 53-57
96. Pirsch JD, Armbrust MJ, Knechtle SJ, et al. Effect of steroid withdrawal on hypertension and cholesterol levels in living related recipients. Transplant Proc 1991; 23: 1363-1364.
97. Hricik DE, Lautman J, Bartucci MR, et al. Variable effects of steroid withdrawal on blood pressure reduction in cyclosporine-treated renal transplant recipients. Transplantation 1992; 53: 1232-1235.
98. Hricik DE, Mayes JT, Schulak JA. Independent effects of cyclosporine and prednisone on post-transplant hypercholesterolemia. Am J Kidney Dis 1991; 28: 353-358.
99. Hricik DE, Bartucci, Mayes JT, et al. The effects of steroid withdrawal on the lipoprotein profiles of cyclosporine-treated kidney and kidney-pancreas transplant recipients. Transplantation 1992; 54: 868-871.

100. Hariharan S, Schroeder TJ, Weiskittel P, et al. Prednisone withdrawal in HLA identical, one haplotype matched live related donor and cadaver renal transplant recipients. Kidney Int 1993; (suppl 43):S30-S35.
101. Hricik DE, Bartucci MR, Moir EJ, et al. Effects of steroid withdrawal on post-transplant diabetes mellitus in cyclosporine-treated renal transplant recipients. 1991; 51: 374-377.
102. Fabrega AJ, Cohan J, Meslar P, et al. Effects of steroid withdrawal on long-term renal allograft recipients with post transplantation diabetes mellitus. Surgery 1994; 116: 792-797.
103. Fabrega AJ, Meslar P, Cohan J, et al. Long-term (24 month) follow-up of steroid withdrawal in renal allograft recipients with post-transplant diabetes mellitus. Transplantation 1995; 60: 1612-1614.
104. Schulak JA, Mayes JT, Moritz CE, et al. A prospective randomized trial of prednisone versus no prednisone maintenance therapy in cyclosporine-treated and azathioprine-treated renal transplant recipients. Transplantation 1990; 49: 327-332.
105. Maiorca R, Cristinelli L, Brunori G, et al. Prospective controlled trial of steroid withdrawal after six months in renal allograft patients treated with cyclosporine. Transplant Proc 1988; 20 (Suppl 3): 121-125.
106. Ratcliffe PJ, Firth JD, Higgins RM, et al. Randomized controlled trial of complete steroid withdrawal in renal transplant patients receiving triple immunosuppression. Transplant Proc 1993; 25: 590.
107. Sinclair NR, Canadian Multicenter Transplant Study Group. Low dose steroid therapy in cyclosporine-treated renal transplant recipients with well-functioning grafts. Can Med Assoc J 1992; 147: 645-655.
108. Hilbrands LB, Hoitsma AJ, Koene RAP. Randomized prospective trial of cyclosporine monotherapy versus azathioprine-prednisone from three months after renal transplantation. Transplantation 1996; 61: 1038-1046.
109. Flechner SM, Kerman RH, Van Buren CT, et al. The use of cyclosporine in living-related renal transplantation: donor-specific hyporesponsiveness and steroid withdrawal. Transplantation 1984; 38: 685-690.
110. Cristinelli C, Brunori G, Sett G, et al. Withdrawal of methylprednisolone at the sixth month in renal transplant recipients treated with cyclosporine. Transplant Proc 1987; 19: 2021-2023.
111. O'Connell P, D'Apice A, Walker R, et al. Cessation of steroids in renal allograft recipients on combined cyclosporine A, azathioprine, and prednisolone. Transplant Proc 1988; 20: 11-13.
112. Walker RG, D'Apice AJF, Powell HR, et al. Triple low-dose immunosuppression with cessation of steroids in pediatric renal transplantation. Transplant Proc 1988; 20: 7-10.
113. Gulanikar AC, Belitsy P, MacDonald AS. Randomized controlled trial of steroids versus no steroids in stable cyclosporine-treated renal graft recipients. Transplant Proc 1991; 23: 990-991.
114. Hricik DE, O'Toole MA, Schulak JA, et al. Steroid-free immunosuppression in cyclosporine-treated renal transplant recipients: a meta-analysis. J Am Soc Nephrol 1993; 4: 1300-1305.
115. Stratta RJ, Armbrust MJ, Oh CS, et al. Withdrawal of steroid immunosuppression in renal transplant recipients. Transplantation 1988; 45: 323-328.
116. Hricik DE, Whalen CC, Lautman J, et al. Withdrawal of steroids after renal transplantation – clinical predictors of outcome. Transplantation 1992; 53: 41-45.
117. Hricik DE, Kupin WL, First MR. Steroid-free immunosuppression after renal transplantation. J Am Soc Nephrol 1994; 4(Suppl): S10-S16.

118. Hricik DE, Seliga RM, Fleming-Brooks S, et al. Determinants of long-term allograft function following steroid withdrawal in renal transplant recipients. Clin Transplant 1995; 9: 419-423.
119. Tarantino A, Montagnino G, Ponticelli C. Corticosteroids in kidney transplant recipients: safety issues and timing of discontinuation. Drug Saf 1995; 13: 145-156.
120. Ratcliffe PJ, Dudley CRK, Higgins RM, Firth JD, Smith B, Morris PJ. Randomised controlled trial of steroid withdrawal in renal transplant recipients receiving triple immunosuppression. Lancet 1996; 348: 643-648.
121. Hollander AMJ, Hene RJ, Hermans J, Van Es LA, Van der Woude FJ. Late prednisone withdrawal in cyclosporine-treated kidney transplant patients: a randomized study. J Am Soc Nephrol 1997; 8: 294-301.
122. Ghandour FZ, Knauss TC, Schulak JA, et al. Influence of steroid withdrawal on proteinuria in renal allograft recipients. Clin Transplant 1997; 11: 395-398.
123. Isoniemi HM, Krogerus L, von Willebrand E, et al. Histopathologic findings in well-functioning, long-term allografts. Kidney Int 1992; 41: 155-160.
124. Offerman G, Schwarz A, Krause PH. Long-term effects of steroid withdrawal in kidney transplantation. Transplant Int 1993; 6: 290-292.
125. Opelz G. Effect of the maintenance immunosuppressive drug regimen on kidney transplant outcome. Transplantation 1994; 58: 443-446.
126. Shapiro R, Jordan ML, Scantlebury VP, et al. Outcomes after steroid withdrawal in renal transplant patients receiving tacrolimus-based immunosuppression. Transplant Proc 1998; 30: 1375-1377.
127. Woodle ES, Buell J, Siegel C, Kulkarni S, Kopelan A, Grewal HP. Corticosteroid withdrawal under tacrolimus primary and rescue therapy in renal transplantation: the Chicago experience. Transplant Proc 1999; 31(Suppl):84S-85S.
128. Grinyo JM, Gil-Vernet S, Seron D, et al. Steroid withdrawal in mycophenolate mofetil-treated renal allograft recipients. Transplantation 1997; 63: 1688-1690.
129. Kupin W, Venkat KK, Goggins M. Improved outcome of steroid withdrawal in mycophenolate mofetil-treated primary cadaveric renal transplant recipients. Transplant Proc 1999; 31:1131-1132.
130. Lebranchu Y for the M55002 Study Group. Comparison of two corticosteroid regimens in combination with Cellcept and cyclosporine A for prevention of acute allograft rejection: 12-month results of a double-blind, randomized, multicenter study. Transplant Proc 1999; 21:249-251.
131. Steroid Withdrawal Study Group. Prednisone withdrawal in kidney transplant recipients on cyclosporine and mycophenolate mofetil – a prospective randomized study. Transplantation 1999; 68: 1865-1874.
132. Kahan BD. Am Soc Transplant Phys. 1998; p243

MYCOPHENOLATE MOFETIL AND AZATHIOPRINE

John D. Pirsch and Elias David-Neto

Introduction

Antimetabolites have been used as adjunctive immunosuppression for renal transplantation since the early 1960s. Azathioprine was one of the first antimetabolites to be used in chronic immunosuppression protocols having been shown to be effective in renal transplantation in dogs [1] and subsequently in humans [2]. Azathioprine remained a mainstay of chronic immunosuppression protocols until the mid-1990s when it was shown in double-blind randomized trials that mycophenolate mofetil (MMF) had better efficacy for the prevention of acute rejection following renal transplantation [3-5]. Although MMF has replaced azathioprine in chronic immunosuppression protocols, many centers still use azathioprine, particularly in low-risk patients.

Azathioprine

The purine metabolism inhibitors were initially examined for chemotherapeutic purposes and came into clinical medicine through the work of Elion et al. in 1951 [6]. The effects of the drug 6-mercaptopurine (6-MP) were then evaluated in homografts by Schwartz and Dameshek [7] and later for skin and kidney transplants. In 1961, Elion et al. described the 6-MP 1-methyl-4-nitro-5-imidazolyl analogue known as azathioprine (AZA) [8]. In 1963, Merrill et al. reported the first cadaver kidney transplant using AZA for immunosuppression [9].

Mohamed Sayegh and Giuseppe Remuzzi (editors), Current and Future Immunosuppressive Therapies Following Transplantation, 85-110.
© 2001 Kluwer Academic Publishers. Printed in the Netherlands.

Until the introduction of cyclosporin A in the 1980s, AZA was the sole immunosuppressive drug for transplantation and its use with steroids has been known as "conventional therapy."

Metabolism and Mode of Action

After ingestion and absorption, AZA is rapidly and almost totally converted to 6-mercaptopurine (6-MP). AZA is considered a pro-drug which has its immunosuppressive effect due to its conversion to 6-MP. This cleavage of AZA to 6-MP occurs via glutathione-S-transferase in erythrocytes [10].

6-MP is metabolized via three different pathways. The first is an anabolic pathway which converts 6-MP into its active nucleotides, 6-thioinosinic acid and 6-thioguanine acid, by the enzyme hypoxanthine-guanine-phophoribosyl transferase (HGPRT). The 6-thioguanine nucleotide seems to be the most active metabolite of 6-MP and responsible for its major action. It interferes in the metabolism of inosine-monophosphate (IMP) to adenosine-monophosphate (AMP), adenosine-triphosphate (ATP) and in the RNA and DNA synthesis in the salvage pathway. Patients with the Lesch-Nyhan syndrome lack the enzyme HGPRT and, therefore, are resistant to the 6-MP action.

The second catabolic pathway involves the action of the enzyme xanthine-oxidase (XO) which converts 6-MP into thiouric acid. This enzyme is stable in humans and its deficiency is rare. The xanthine-oxidase enzyme is also the site of action of allopurinol. Patients under AZA can develop serious myelotoxicity with the concomitant use of allopurinol. However, in kidney transplantation, allopurinol in small doses enhances the action of AZA in preventing rejection episodes in both adults [11] and children [12]. The probable mechanisms of this interaction between allopurinol and AZA is that by blocking XO more 6-MP is available for the conversion to thioguanine. On the other hand, drugs that are not metabolized by XO, like cyclophosphamide, also can induce bone marrow toxicity when given in association with allopurinol. The best marker for AZA bone marrow suppression is erythrocyte thioguanine nucleotides [13]. It is interesting to note, however, that the concentration of 6-thioguanine in red blood cells does not differ whether patients are treated with AZA or AZA plus allopurinol [10].

The third 6-MP catabolic pathway involves the production of the inactive metabolite 6-methyl-MP by the enzyme thiopurine methyltransferase (TPMT). Due to the genetic polymorphism of the TPMT enzyme, there are three different phenotypes for the TPMT activity: high (> 26 pmol/hr/mgHb), intermediate (15-26 pmol/hr/mgHb), and low (<15 pmol/hr/mgHb) [14]. It is estimated that 85% of the Caucasian population has a high activity of the TPMT enzyme while 11-23% is intermediate and 0.3% has a complete lack of the TPMT activity [15]. These patients are more susceptible to AZA myelotoxicity.

In the Afro-Brazilian population, the distribution of phenotypes is similar to Caucasians. However, there are individuals with a very high activity among this race (65-84 pmol/hr/mgHb). In the same study, all of the 32 Brazilians of Japanese origin had high TPMT activity (29-48 pmol/hr/mgHb) [16]. The occurrence of these three different phenotypes is now recognized as the probable cause of the ineffective action of AZA in preventing rejection episodes in some patients compared to others who do well with this drug. The pre-transplant evaluation of the TPMT activity before transplantation may distinguish a group of patients who need higher doses of AZA [15]. The confirmation of this data and the availability of clinical tests for TPMT activity may renew interest in AZA as an immunosuppressive drug as effective as its competitor, MMF, in the current search for an efficient and economic immunosuppressive regimen for organ transplantation.

Clinical Studies

In clinical practice, AZA has been used in doses of 2-5 mg/kg/day during the pre-CyA era along with many steroid protocols. During the CyA era, CyA was added to the classical conventional protocol and its dose was reduced to 1-2 mg/kg/day. The rationale for this dose reduction was based on the theoretical reason that toxicity could be avoided by giving lesser amounts of three synergic drugs (AZA, CyA, and prednisone). In most transplant centers, AZA is usually started at 2 mg/kg/day and the dose is tailored according to the total peripheral leukocyte counts and the plasma levels of the liver enzymes.

In contrast to MMF, AZA interferes with the RNA and DNA synthesis not only of lymphocytes but also other leukocytes, erythrocytes, and platelet precursor cells. Therefore, high AZA doses can lead to anemia and low platelet and leukocyte counts. The macrocytic anemia can be misinterpreted as folate and vitamin B12 deficiency. Leukopenia varies according to dose used but occurs in around 30% of patients [17]. Dose reduction or temporary withdrawal of AZA usually reverts the myelo-toxic effect in a few days. Tailoring of drug dosage according to myelo-toxicity has been used to individualize AZA dose. Most centers use a leukocyte count less than 4000 cells/ml as indicator for dose reduction.

Beyond its myelotoxic effect, AZA is considered a hepatotoxic drug. Even after many years of use, the mechanism(s) of AZA-induced liver injury is not clear. It seems to be related to hepatocyte injury [18], interlobular bile duct injury [19] and rarely endothelial cell damage [20]. Despite association of liver toxicity with AZA, the current doses of AZA used clinically do not appear to have significant hepatotoxicity. It is likely that at least some of the hepatotoxicity attributed to AZA in the past was due to undiagnosed hepatitis C disease. Viral liver disease may result in decreased catabolism of AZA and its toxic metabolites which can be related to the liver injury. Therefore, use of regular doses of AZA is seldom toxic to the liver but is very harmful when associated with viral disease [21].

For many years it was not clear whether one could avoid the AZA hepatotoxic effect, in hepatitis C and/or B transplanted patients by reducing the AZA dose until the liver enzymes decrease either to a normal level or to the lowest achievable level. In a prospective randomized study of renal transplant patients with hepatitis C and/or B, David-Neto et al. verified that AZA, in long-term follow-up, even in lower doses (that are able to reduce or normalize the liver enzymes), is harmful to the liver. The group of patients with low AZA dose developed cirrhosis more frequently and died from liver dysfunction and infection more often than patients who had AZA withdrawn [22].

AZA plus steroids therapy had been used since 1965 until CyA became available for organ transplantation. However, this combination (AZA/steroids) is associated with poorer graft survival in cadaveric renal transplantation. In the Collaborative Transplant Study, including thousands of patients transplanted between 1988 and 1997 in more than 200 centers worldwide, Opelz showed a 5-year graft survival of only 50% for the AZA plus steroids regimen compared with 72% for the CyA-based regimens [23].

In view of the new potent immunosuppressive drugs available, the role of AZA in the triple-therapy regimen has been questioned. It is unclear whether the addition of AZA to calcineurin-inhibitors plus steroid regimens adds any advantage to double-drug therapy with CyA and prednisone. To address these question, Amenabar et al., in a randomized trial in cadaveric renal transplantation, reported that the addition of AZA to CyA/steroids decreased the incidence of steroid-resistant rejection episodes and did not increase the incidence of infectious episodes. However, 10% of the patients discontinued AZA due to side-effects [17]. In a tacrolimus-based regimen for renal transplantation, Shapiro et al. showed that the addition of AZA did not add advantages for the 2-year patient and graft survival, although diminished the incidence of acute rejection episodes [24].

In the long-term, after the early risk of rejection during the first year, registry studies suggest that a regimen of AZA with CyA, without steroids, appeared to be associated with the best patient and graft survival rates [25]. This data has been questioned since patients who successfully wean off steroids may have less immunologic risk or did not have previous rejection episodes. The obvious benefit of CyA/AZA immunotherapy is to achieve efficient immunosuppression without the steroid side-effects, particularly in children needing improvement in linear growth [26-31]. Currently, it is estimated that only 9% of the recipients of cadaveric kidneys with triple-therapy have steroids weaned and are maintained on the CyA-AZA regimen [23].

However, steroid avoidance and immunotherapy with AZA/CyA in the early period after renal transplantation was associated with a high incidence of acute rejection episodes in children [32] and was abandoned by most centers. In adults, however, the South Australian Renal

Transplant service adopted this regimen for "low-risk" recipients (PRA<50% in all sera). Of the 121 patients who were initiated on double-therapy, 53 (44%) did not receive steroids after transplantation (either live or cadaveric), 44 (36%) required steroids for rejection and were later successfully weaned, and 24 (20%) were maintained on long-term steroids. They reported a 1- and 5-year graft survival of 91% and 78%, respectively [33].

Currently, MMF has been shown to be more effective than AZA in preventing rejection episodes. Therefore, AZA has lost its role as an immunosuppressive drug for the early phase after transplantation. Even if one considers high acquisition costs of MMF, this is offset by high costs of treating rejection in the first 6 mos. after transplantation [34].

However, AZA may have a role in replacing MMF after the early period of transplantation, particularly in the low-risk group of recipients. In a recent multicenter trial, 477 renal transplant patients receiving MMF/CyA/steroids were randomized to receive either AZA (group I) or MMF (group II) for 9 months. The 1-year results were compared between these two groups and with a third group that received CyA/AZA/steroids for the entire year (group III). Group III showed the highest treatment failure. Twenty-three patients in group I were unable to be switched from MMF to AZA. In the remaining 135 patients who were switched, the number of rejection episodes was higher than in patients who were maintained on MMF (group II) for the entire first year (10 vs 1). However, 7 out of the 10 rejection episodes were mild and responded well to steroids only. Graft losses and death rate were similar for the two MMF groups [35].

The Brazilian MMF Collaborative Study compared the addition of either MMF (n=123) or AZA (n=121) to the CyA/prednisone regimen in low-risk, first-transplant recipients of cadaveric (n=124) or live-donor kidneys (n=120). This study found no differences in the rate of biopsy-proven rejection episodes in the first year (AZA 18% vs MMF 22%), and in 1-year graft and patient survival rates for the subgroup of living-donors, although the number of rejection episodes were higher in the cadaveric group receiving AZA (37% vs 19%, p=0.02) [36].

Analyzing this data, it is possible to speculate that the low-risk renal transplant patients receiving CyA/MMF/steroids who have never experienced a rejection episode during the first 3-6 months can have MMF switched for AZA, with a very low risk of severe rejection.

The regimen of AZA and steroids, without CyA, continues to be successfully used in HLA-identical live-donor kidney-transplant recipients. Bartucci et al. successfully converted 11 of 12 recipients of an HLA-identical live-donor kidney to AZA. These patients had excellent renal function and low mixed-lymphocyte culture against the donor cells after 1 year of transplantation [37].

Mycophenolate Mofetil

Mycophenolate mofetil (MMF) is a morpholinoethyl ester of mycophenolic acid. MMF is a prodrug [38,39]. It is rapidly hydrolyzed in the stomach and small intestine into the active drug which is mycophenolic acid (MPA). MPA is a selective and noncompetitive inhibitor of inosine monophosphate dehydrogenase (IMPDH) which is an essential enzyme in the de novo pathway of purine biosynthesis for mammalian cells. By inhibiting IMPDH, there is depletion of guanine monophosphate and ultimately guanine triphosphate. This results in the inhibition of DNA synthesis in cells that are exposed to MMF. One of the critical features of the drug is that lymphocytes are particularly susceptible to IMPDH inhibition compared to other mammalian cells. This has been shown to be due to the lack of an effective salvage pathway for the production of guanosine nucleotides [38-41].

Mycophenolic acid (MPA) was first isolated from a penicillin culture in 1898 by Gosio [42] and again was isolated in 1913 by Alsberg and Black [43] who named the isolate "mycophenolic acid." The drug was initially investigated as a potential antibiotic; however, it was soon discovered that the drug had both antitumor and immunosuppressive properties. Early trials were performed in the 1970s as a treatment for psoriasis [44,45]. The drug appeared to have good clinical efficacy, but was limited by side effects such as diarrhea and myelosuppression. In the early 1990s, Allison and Eugui rekindled interest in the possible role for mycophenolic acid as an immunosuppressant for transplant patients [46,47]. A prodrug of mycophenolic acid (mycophenolate mofetil) was available at Syntex Corporation. *In vitro* studies demonstrated that MMF depleted intracellular pools of GTP and had a profound effect on the proliferation of human peripheral lymphocytes. The early *in vitro* work led to animal studies, which were later confirmed in man in controlled clinical trials. These studies resulted in the approval of MMF in 1994 for the prevention of acute rejection in kidney transplantation.

Mechanism of Action

There are two major pathways of purine biosynthesis in lymphocytes and other mammalian cells: the de novo pathway and salvage pathway (**Figure 1**) [41]. In the de novo pathway, 5-phosphoribosyl-1-pyrophosphate (PRPP) synthetase catalyzes a reaction between ribose-5-phosphate and ATP to form 5-phosphoribosyl-1-pyrophosphate (PRPP) (**Figure 1**). PRPP is a precursor of inosine monophosphate which in the presence of inosine monophosphate dehydrogenase (IMPDH) forms guanosine monophosphate [48]. Guanosine monophosphate is a precursor of guanosine diphosphate (GDP), guanosine triphosphate (GTP), and deoxyguanine diphosphate (dGTP), and is an essential nucleotide for RNA synthesis. MPA is an inhibitor of IMPDH and prevents the

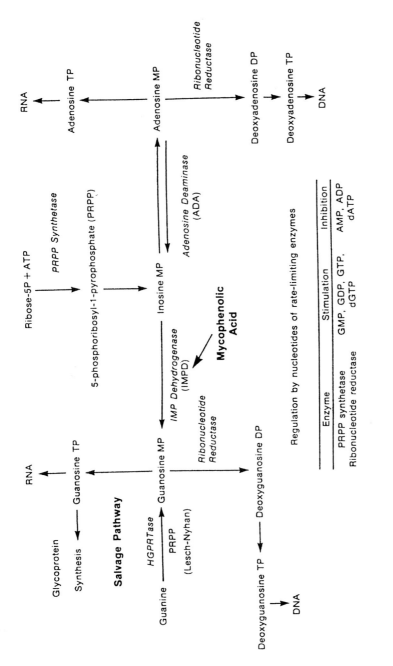

Figure 1. De novo pathways of purine biosynthesis. MPA inhibits IMP dehydrogenase, thereby depleting GMP, GTP and dGTP. Lymphocytes lack an effective salvage pathway for the production of guanine nucleotides which leads to more efficient inhibition by MPA than other mammalian cells. (From Allison AC, Eugui EM, Sollinger HW. Mycophenolate mofetil (RS-61443): mechanisms of action and effects in transplantation. Transpl Rev 1993;7:129-139. Permission requested.)

conversion of inosine monophosphate to guanosine monophosphate. Most mammalian cells have a salvage pathway whereby guanosine monophosphate can also be derived from guanine directly. This is catalyzed by hypoxanthine-guanine phosphoribosyl transferase (HGPRTase). Lymphocytes appear to be particularly dependent on the de novo pathway for the synthesis of guanine nucleotides compared to other cell types [49]. Because of the high specificity of MPA for IMPDH in lymphocytes, MPA is a very specific lymphocyte inhibitor.

IMPDH exists in two isoforms (types I and II). The type II isoform is 4 to 5 times more sensitive to MPA than is type I, but both isoforms are inhibited by MPA [50]. The type II isoform is increased during proliferation of lymphocytes. This may also explain the relative specificity of MPA inhibition in lymphocytes compared to other cell types.

In Vitro Studies

MPA has been shown *in vitro* to deplete both GTP and dGTP levels [38,39,49,51]. This effect is reversed upon addition of guanosine or deoxyguanosine in the presence of MPA. In addition, MPA has been shown to inhibit humoral responses *in vitro*. Nanomolar amounts of MPA completely inhibited polyclonally-activated human B lymphocytes and secondary responses of human spleen cells to REF tetanus toxoid [52,53]. MPA depletion of GTP also inhibits the transfer of fucose and mannose to glycoproteins which are important precursors of some adhesion molecules [54,55]. *In vitro* experiments have demonstrated that MPA, by depleting GTP, inhibits the glycosylation of adhesion molecules and binding of activated lymphocytes to endothelial cells.

Animal Models

MMF has been evaluated extensively in a number of transplant animal models. Recently, it has been studied to determine if there is a therapeutic effect in animal models of glomerulonephritis.

Morris et al. performed the first animal studies with MMF [56]. They examined the effect of MMF on the survival of allograft rat hearts which were heterotopically transplanted to the abdomen of recipients. MMF clearly prolonged survival in this model. MMF could also be shown to reverse advanced rejection in the same model when given in higher doses [57]. This early work in mice was extended at the Univer-ity of Wisconsin in renal allograft models in dogs [58-61]. When MMF was used alone or in combination with cyclosporine and methyl-predniso-lone, allograft survival in dogs was prolonged significantly over control animals [58]. To examine whether MMF had a beneficial effect on treatment of ongoing rejection, kidney allografts were performed in dogs that were then allowed to reject [59]. High-dose MMF was then given which reversed rejection in 14 of 16 dogs. Additional work in dogs

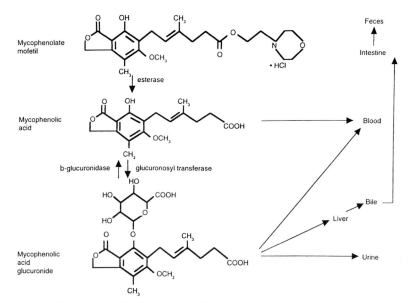

Figure 2. Structure of the morpholinoethyl ester of mycophenolic acid, mycophenolate mofetil (CellCept), and its conversion by esterase activity to mycophenolic acid. The principal metabolite is the mycophenolic acid glucuronide (MPAG), which can undergo enterohepatic recycling. (From Allison AC, Eugui EM. Purine metabolism and immunosuppressive effects of mycophenolate mofetil (MMF). Clin Transplant 1996;10:77-84. Permission requested.)

demonstrated that MMF prolonged heterotopic intestinal transplant [60] and liver allograft survival [61] significantly over control animals.

In addition to allotransplantation models, MMF has also been shown to be effective in several xenograft models. O'Hair et al. studied cardiac I xenografts from cynomolgus monkeys to baboons [62]. Baboons receiving MMF, prednisone, and cyclosporine had no evidence of chronic vascular rejection compared to animals treated with azathio-prine. Other models examining hamster-to-rat heart [63,64] and liver xeno-transplantation [64] and pig-to-rabbit cardiac xenografts [65] have demonstrated prolonged survival in animals treated with MMF compared to other standard antirejection therapies. MMF also prevented rejection of both allo- [66] and islet pancreatic xenografts in experimental models [66-70].

Recent studies have examined the role of MMF in animal models of glomerulonephritis. MMF inhibited mesangial proliferation in a rat model of experimental mesangial proliferative glomerulonephritis [71]. In a rat model of Heymann nephritis, MMF prevented the induction of the disease by suppressing Th2 cytokines [72]. MMF was shown to reduce severity of murine lupus glomerulonephritis in a mouse model [73,74] and halt the progression of non-immune renal injury in rats [75].

Human Studies - Pharmacokinetics

MMF is a morpholinoethyl ester of mycophenolic acid. MMF is rapidly absorbed and desterified after oral dosing. The plasma MPA concentration peaks in approximately 1 hour with a second peak at 6 to 12 hours [76]. The latter peak is probably due to enterohepatic cycling of the major metabolite which is mycophenolic acid glucuronide (MPAG). MMF is extensively and tightly bound to human serum albumin with only 1.25% of free MPA in plasma. It is believed that the free form is the pharmacologically active fraction for the inhibition of inosine monophosphate dehydrogenase (IMPDH). The mean plasma elimination half-life for radioactive-labeled MMF in healthy volunteers was approximately 17 hours. The major site of excretion is in urine and is almost exclusively MPAG. Over 96% of MPAG is excreted in the urine with 5.5% recovered in the feces [76]. Despite the rapid conversion of MPA to its metabolite MPAG, only MPA appears to have immunologic activity.

Multiple pharmacokinetic evaluations have been performed in healthy individuals and renal transplant recipients. The pharmacokinetics of MPA are significantly different in patients who have undergone recent transplantation compared to late renal transplant patients (**Table 1**). Early renal transplant patients have substantially lower C_{max} and AUC_{12} values with prolonged T_{max}. The T_{max} of MPAG is also prolonged in the early transplant recipient. The longer T_{max} for early transplant recipients suggests poor absorption. In contrast, late renal transplant patients have a substantially higher C_{max}, a shorter T_{max}, and a higher AUC_{12}. Overall, the available data indicates that in the early post-transplant period the mean plasma MPA AUC is approximately 30-50% lower than for the same dose in the late transplant period.

The effect of post-transplant renal impairment and metabolism of MPA has been examined in transplant recipients with delayed graft function (DGF) [76]. In patients with DGF, the mean plasma interval AUC_{12} values of MPA are similar to those in patients without DGF;

Table 1. Pharmacokinetic parameters for mycophenolic acid (mean ± SD) following administration of single-dose mycophenolate mofetil*

Study Group	Dose (g bid)	T_{max} (h)	C_{max} (μg/mL)	AUC (μg•h/mL)
Healthy volunteers	1.5	0.90 ± 0.4	32.8 ± 8.2	51.5 ±15.1
Renal transplants				
<40 days	1	1.31 ± 0.76	8.16 ± 4.5	27.0 ± 10.9
<40 days	1.5	1.21 ± 0.81	13.5 ± 8.18	38.4 ± 15.4
>3 months	1.5	0.9 ± 0.24	24.1 ± 12.1	65.0 ± 35.4

*Sources: Bullingham et al. [76]
Hoffmann-LaRoche Inc. CellCept (mycophenolate mofetil capsules) package insert

however, the MPAG AUC_{12} may be 6- to 8-fold higher in patients with DGF than in recipients without DGF. Despite the higher concentrations of MPAG, there does not appear to be correlation between the higher MPAG levels and adverse events. It should also be noted that hemodialysis has no apparent effect on MPA or MPAG concentrations.

There has been limited studies of metabolism of MPA in recipients with hepatic impairment [76]. The metabolism of MPA in patients with cirrhosis is variable and related to the severity of hepatic dysfunction. Patients with mild impairment had similar pharmacokinetics to healthy volunteers. Patients with moderate impairment had a higher C_{max} and AUC compared to patients with mild impairment of hepatic function. However, patients with severe hepatic impairment had similar pharmacokinetics compared to patients with mild hepatic impairment or healthy individuals. This may be explained by an increased renal clearance which was noted in the patients with severely impaired liver function which counterbalanced the effect of hepatic impairment.

The pharmacokinetics of MPA appear to be mildly affected by coadministration with aluminum/magnesium hydroxide, intravenous ganciclovir, oral contraceptives, and the administration of cholestyramine. There appears to be a modest effect on the pharmacokinetics of MPA with food; however, the relative changes are minor.

Both tacrolimus and cyclosporine appears to affect MMF metabolism. Zucker et al. found that renal transplant recipients receiving tacrolimus and MMF had significantly higher levels of MPA (C_{min} and AUC) compared to those receiving cyclosporine and MMF (50.2 ± 16.5 vs 32.1 ± 16.7 mcg h/ml AUC, $p < 0.02$) [77]. The major metabolite of MPA (MPAG) was significantly lower in tacrolimus recipients, suggesting a specific inhibition of the metabolism of MPA to MPAG. Recently, an effect of cyclosporine on the metabolism of MPA was reported [78]. MPA trough levels were measured in stable renal transplant recipients after withdrawal of cyclosporine. MPA levels increased significantly after cyclosporine was withdrawn compared to patients on triple therapy (MMF, prednisone, cyclosporine) or patients who had prednisone withdrawn. This study suggests that cyclosporine lowers MPA trough levels. This observation might explain the lower MPA trough and AUC values in cyclosporine-MMF recipients compared to tacrolimus-MMF recipients.

Kidney Transplantation

The first human study of MMF was in primary cadaveric renal transplants receiving prednisone and cyclosporine for maintenance immunosuppression [79]. Forty-nine recipients were entered into the study in eight dosing groups (100-3500 mg/d). In this study, there was a reduction in rejection episodes and need for OKT3 in patients who received greater than 2 grams per day of MMF. This study indicated that doses of 2 grams per day and above may be efficacious in the prevention of acute rejection. Another early trial examined the benefit of MMF for refractory kidney transplant rejection [80]. Seventy-five patients were entered in this trial with rejection refractory to OKT3 therapy. Of patients entered, 69% had stabilization of renal function following initiation of MMF therapy. Rescue rejection was more successful when patients were entered with a creatinine of 4 mg/dL or lower (79% vs 52%). In both of the initial studies of MMF, it became apparent that GI toxicity and leukopenia were the major clinical side effects.

These initial preliminary studies led to a number of clinical trials examining the effects of MMF on the prevention and treatment of acute rejection. The clinical program included three worldwide studies which examined the efficacy of MMF for the prevention of acute rejection and two additional studies examining the role of MMF in the treatment of rejection, both as initial treatment and as rescue therapy.

The rejection-prevention studies were quite similar in design and were conducted in parallel fashion worldwide [3-5]. All studies were randomized, double-blind, and controlled, and examined the role of MMF for the prevention of acute rejection starting from day of transplant. The MMF-treatment arms were similar in all three studies with one group receiving 2 grams a day of MMF and the other group 3 grams a day of MMF. The studies differed in the use of a third concomitant agent. The U.S. and Tricontinental trials used azathioprine 1 to 2 mg/kg/day as a control [3,5]. The European [4] trial was controlled with placebo. The U.S. trial differed from the European and Tricontinental trial with the inclusion of induction therapy with ATGAM for all recipients. The primary efficacy endpoint was the prevention of acute rejection at 6 months with longer term follow-up out to 3 years [81-83].

The results of the 6-month and 3-year rejection efficacy in patient and graft survival are shown in **Table 2**. For all of the studies, MMF, either at 2 or 3 grams, was significantly superior for the prevention of acute rejection over azathioprine (in the U.S. and Tricontinental trials) or placebo. There was a significantly lower incidence of treatment failure in the MMF-treated recipients compared to control. The toxicity profiles were similar with a higher incidence of gastrointestinal events and leukopenia for patients treated with MMF. There was also a slightly higher incidence of cytomegalovirus (CMV) disease in recipients receiving MMF, but no dramatic increase in other opportunistic infections. Although these studies were primarily designed to examine the role of the prevention of acute rejection, longer term follow-up was examined at the 1- and 3-year post-study initiation time points [81-83]. Despite an improvement in the overall prevention of acute rejection, the 1- and 3-year graft and patient survivals did not differ between the two groups. It should be noted, however, that these studies were not statistically powered to determine efficacy for long-term patient and graft survival.

Table 2. The results of the controlled, randomized, double-blind trials of mycophenolate mofetil in cadaveric renal transplantation.

Study	Concomitant therapy	Study drugs	Number enrolled	Biopsy-proven rejection (6 mos)	Biopsy-proven rejection or treatment failure (6 mos)	Graft loss (excluding death)		Death	
						6 mos	3 yrs	6 mos	3 yrs
U.S. Renal Transplant Mycophenolate Mofetil Study Group [3,81]	ATGAM, prednisone, cyclosporine	MMF 2 gm	167	19.8	31.1[a]	1.8	13.4	3.6	10.6
		MMF 3 gm	166	17.5	31.3	6.7	17.0	5.5	12.2
		AZA 1-2 mg/kg	166	38	47.6	8.6	17.1	3.0	11.9
European Mycophenolate Mofetil Cooperative Study Group [4,82]	prednisone, cyclosporine	MMF 2 gm	165	17	30.3[b]	4.2	8.7	2.4	7.3
		MMF 3 gm	160	13.8	38.8	6.3	12.8	3.1	8.2
		placebo	166	46.4	56	9.0	16.0	3.6	11.1
Tricontinental Myco-phenolate Mofetil Renal Transplantation Study Group [5,83]	prednisone, cyclosporine	MMF 2 gm	173	19.7	38.2[c]	4.0	14.6	0.5	4.7
		MMF 3 gm	164	15.9	34.8	1.8	8.5	1.8	9.1
		AZA 1-2 mg/kg	166	35.5	50.0	3.0	15.4	1.2	8.6

[a] AZA vs MMF 2 gm (p=0.0015); AZA vs MMF 3 gm (p=0.0021)
[b] p<0.001 for both MMF groups compared to placebo
[c] AZA vs MMF 2 gm (p=0.0287); AZA vs MMF 3 gm (p=0.0045)

Two additional studies were performed to evaluate the efficacy of MMF for both the treatment of first acute renal allograft rejection and for the treatment of refractory acute cellular renal transplant rejection. In the refractory acute rejection trial [84], a total of 150 patients with refractory rejection were enrolled and randomized to receive either oral MMF (1.5 gm twice daily, n=77) or IV methylprednisolone (5 mg/kg for 5 days, n=73). All of the patients enrolled in this trial had refractory acute rejection after prior treatment with OKT3, ALG, or ATG for at least 7 days. The primary efficacy variable was graft and patient survival at 6 months. Graft loss and death were reduced by 42% in the MMF-treatment group. Nineteen patients (26%) in the IV steroid group experienced graft loss or died compared with 11 patients (14.3%) in the MMF group (p=0.08). MMF also decreased the number of subsequent full courses of immunosuppressive treatment. 35.6% of patients in the IV steroid group and 24.7% of patients in the MMF group received subsequent treatment. As expected, there was a high rate of opportunistic infection in this study with nearly 35% of patients in each treatment group developing an opportunistic infection, mostly with CMV. This study demonstrated that the addition of MMF in this setting can reverse refractory acute rejection.

The other major study examined the efficacy of MMF in the treatment of first renal allograft rejection [85]. This was a comparative trial comparing the addition of MMF (1.5 gm twice daily) in patients with first acute rejection with a rapid taper of corticosteroids. The control group consisted of patients with rejection who were treated with intravenous corticosteroids at 5 mg/kg/day and continued on azathioprine. At 6 months, 16.8% of the MMF-treated and 41% of the azathioprine-treated patients required at least one course of antilymphocyte therapy (p<0.001). The number of subsequent courses of acute anti-rejection therapy was less in the MMF-treated group (24.8%) versus the azathioprine-treated control group (58.3%) (p<0.001). Use of antilymphocyte therapy was significantly lower (MMF, 29.2%, vs azathioprine, 51.9%, p=0.0006). As in all the MMF-treated patients, there were more adverse events, particularly GI toxicity, leukopenia and CMV infection.

Taken together all of these studies demonstrated significant efficacy for the use of MMF in both the prevention of acute rejection and treatment of first acute rejection or refractory acute rejection. The major limitation of these trials is efficacy in the long-term transplant patient; however, these clinical trials were not designed to assess the efficacy of long-term treatment with MMF on patient and graft survival.

Other Immunosuppressive Drug Combinations

MMF has been used in a variety of protocols using different immunosuppressive drug regimens. The use of MMF and tacrolimus in renal transplantation has been prospectively studied in Europe [86] and the

United States [87]. The European study randomized 223 patients in three groups: tacrolimus/corticosteroids (n=82); tacrolimus/ cortico-steroids/MMF 1 g (n=79); or tacrolimus/corticosteroids/MMF 2 g (n=71). Rejection rates were 32.8%, 13.8%, and 5.6% (p<0.05), respectively. Forty percent of the 2 g MMF group had a reduction in dose. The incidence of post-transplant diabetes mellitus (PTDM) was less than 4%. Similar findings were noted in the U.S. trial which randomized 176 tacrolimus/prednisone-treated patients to azathioprine (n=59), MMF 1 g (n=59), and MMF 2 g (n=58). Biopsy-proven rejection incidences at 1 year were 32.2%, 32.2%, and 8.6%, respectively. The 2 g MMF group had a 25% mean reduction in dose by 12 months, primarily due to GI toxicity. The incidence of PTDM in this study was 11.9%. These studies suggest that the 2 g dose MMF in combination with tacrolimus is poorly tolerated by most patients. This is likely due to the higher MPA exposure when MMF is combined with tacrolimus compared to cyclosporine.

Another large clinical experience was reported by Shapiro et al. who randomized 208 renal transplant recipients to receive tacrolimus/ pred-nisone (n=106) or tacrolimus/prednisone/MMF (n=102) [88]. The incidence of rejection was 44% and 27% (p=0.014), respectively. Thirty-six percent of patients were taken off steroids. The incidence of PTDM was 7.0% in the double-therapy group vs 2.9% in triple-therapy group.

Steroid-withdrawal with MMF has been reported recently in a double-blind controlled trial [89]. Stable renal transplant recipients receiving MMF, prednisone and cyclosporine were randomized at 3 months to undergo blinded-steroid withdrawal. Patients randomized had no previous rejection episodes. One-hundred-thirty-four patients were withdrawn from steroids; 132 were maintained on steroids. At 1 year post-transplant, rejection or treatment failure occurred in 9.8% of maintenance group and 30.8% of withdrawal group (p=0.0007). Rejection alone occurred in 4.9% versus 22.4% (p=0.0007), maintenance versus withdrawal, respectively. Black recipients had a higher rate of rejection or treatment failure compared to non-blacks (39.6% vs 16%, p<0.001). Graft loss and renal function was equivalent for the two groups. The steroid-withdrawal group had significantly lower cholesterol levels and fewer antihypertensive medications after withdrawal. This study suggested that steroid withdrawal was safe for non-black, low-risk recipients receiving MMF and cyclosporine.

Chronic Rejection

Because of MMF's ability to inhibit both B- and T cell proliferation and activation, there has been considerable interest on the potential role of MMF in chronic rejection. Several animal studies have been performed which have shown inhibition of early chronic rejection in both rat kidney allografts [90] and rat aortic allografts [91,92]. However, there has been no systematic study which has shown a benefit of MMF in the prevention of acute rejection. A recent study examined addition of MMF in patients with the diagnosis of chronic allograft nephropathy [93]. All the patients were receiving cyclosporine and had slow progressive deterioration of renal function. In this trial, the cyclosporine dose was reduced by 50%, azathioprine was discontinued, MMF was added. The mean loss of renal function was less after conversion of patients to MMF and reduction of cyclosporine. Renal function improved in 21 of 28 patients with only one patient having continued deterioration of renal function. Although this study does not prove that MMF is effective at treating acute rejection, it does suggest that it can be used as a cyclosporine-sparing agent in patients with chronic transplant nephropathy.

Therapeutic Drug Monitoring

MPA is easily assayed using high-performance liquid chromatography (HPLC) [94]. Data from early trials suggested that there was a pharmacokinetic/pharmacodynamic correlation between the AUC_{12} of mycophenolic acid and the incidence of rejection [95]. Patients who experienced rejection in those trials had lower AUC_{12} levels of MPA than patients who did not have rejection. These results suggested that therapeutic drug monitoring (TDM) of plasma concentrations of MPA might be advantageous. A randomized double-blind multicenter plasma concentration controlled study of the efficacy of oral MMF for the prevention of acute rejection was published recently [96]. One-hundred-fifty-four adult recipients of primary or secondary cadaveric grafts were randomly allocated in a double-blind fashion to receive MMF treatment aimed at three predefined target MPA AUC values (16.1, 32.2, and 60.6 mcg/hr/ml). Concomitant immunosuppression consisted of cyclosporine and MMF. Of the 150 patients who were eligible for analysis, the incidence of acute rejection was 27.5% in the low group, 14.9% in the intermediate group, and 11.5% in the high MPA AUC group. There was a highly statistically significant relation between median ln(MPA AUC) and the occurrence of biopsy-proven rejection ($p<0.001$). The mean dose of MMF was highly significant ($p=0.001$) for the development of adverse events. It is worth noting that the mean doses of MMF in the low, intermediate, and high group were approximately 1 gm, 2-2.5 gm, and 3-4 gm, respectively. This observation suggests that therapeutic drug monitoring may be helpful in decreasing the risk of rejection and improving efficacy of MMF.

Other Solid Organ Transplants

Heart transplantation. There have been a number of uncontrolled clinical experiences with the use of MMF in heart transplant recipients [97-99]. The initial studies were quite promising, particularly when

MMF was used in the treatment of acute rejection. A double-blind, placebo controlled trial was undertaken which randomized 650 patients undergoing their first heart transplant to receive MMF (3,000 per day) or azathioprine (1.5 to 3 mg/kg/day) [100]. Concomitant therapy consisted of cyclosporine and corticosteroids. The primary efficacy end-point was the incidence of acute rejection and survival at 6 and 12 months. The use of MMF in this trial demonstrated a significant reduction in mortality at 1 year (18 (6.2%) versus 33 deaths (11.4%), $p=0.031$) and a significant reduction in treatment for rejection (65.7% versus 73.7%, $p=0.026$). Fewer MMF patients had greater than grade IIIA rejection or required antilymphocyte therapy. MMF was well tolerated with the exception of GI and hematologic toxicity and there was no increase in malignancy in patients treated with MMF, but there was a higher incidence of opportunistic infection including herpes simplex and herpes zoster.

Liver transplantation. The early experience with MMF for liver transplant recipients was in the treatment of refractory human liver rejection [101-103]. In one study of liver recipients with resistant rejection, 21 of 23 patients responded when MMF was added to the regimen [101]. The experience with MMF was expanded by Stegall et al. who randomized 71 patients to either tacrolimus (n=35) and MMF or cyclosporine (n=36) and MMF with rapid steroid withdrawal at 14 days [104]. Both groups had similar rejection rates (46% for cyclosporine-MMF and 42.3% for tacrolimus-MMF). Patient and graft survival were similar with no immunologic graft losses in either group. Very similar results were obtained in another prospective study comparing MMF and tacrolimus versus cyclosporine and MMF [105]. In this study, only 19% of patients experienced acute rejection.

A large clinical experience was reported by Jain et al. which compared the efficacy and toxicity of tacrolimus and steroids (double-drug therapy) versus tacrolimus, steroids and MMF (triple-drug therapy) in primary adult liver transplant recipients [106]. This study demonstrated similar patient and graft survival and rejection rates in both groups with a trend toward a lower incidence of rejection and decreased neph-rotoxicity in recipients of triple therapy. Similar results were noted in a retrospective pilot study by Eckhoff et al. who examined the outcome of patients receiving MMF, tacrolimus, and steroids with MMF taper and discontinuation at 3 months [107]. Major findings in this study were a lower rate of rejection and slightly less long-term nephrotoxicity.

A large randomized double-blind controlled trial comparing MMF (n=278) and azathioprine (n=287) in liver transplant recipients was reported recently [108]. Concomitant immunosuppression consisted of cyclosporine and corticosteroids. At 6 months, acute rejection occurred in 47.7% of azathioprine recipients and 38.1% of MMF recipients (p=0.02). Graft loss and death at 1 year were similar. Adverse events were similar and resulted in withdrawal rates of nearly 50% in both groups.

Recently the conversion of liver transplant recipients with renal insufficiency from cyclosporine to MMF has been examined [109,110]. Most patients are able to tolerate cyclosporine reduction or withdrawal when MMF is added with improvement in renal function.

<u>Pancreas transplantation.</u> Stegall et al. in a small controlled study compared tacrolimus, prednisone and MMF to cyclosporine, prednisone and MMF in simultaneous pancreas-kidney (SPK) recipients [111]. The overall incidence of rejection was only 11% in both groups which was a significant reduction in the incidence of acute rejection compared to historical controls. Gruessner et al. examined the use of MMF in 61 SPK, 44 pancreas-after-kidney (PAK), and 15 pancreas transplant alone (PTA) recipients. All groups had excellent patient and graft survival [112]. The major benefit of MMF was seen in the SPK recipients with a 15% incidence of rejection compared to a historical rate of 43% with azathioprine. There was no difference in rejection rates for PAK or PTA.

In a large retrospective of 358 consecutive SPK transplants at the University of Wisconsin, Odorico et al. compared the rejection and graft survival rates with patients treated with MMF (n=109) or azathioprine (n=249) [113]. The MMF-treated patients demonstrated a significantly reduced incidence of rejection (31% vs 75%, p=0.0001). There was a decrease in steroid refractory rejection, 15% compared to 52% for historical controls (p=0.01), and there was overall better kidney and pancreas survival. Finally, Kaufman et al. confirmed the beneficial rate of the use of MMF in SPK recipients in an uncontrolled clinical trial [114]. Of 50 consecutive patients treated with MMF and tacrolimus, the overall rejection rate was 16%. Although these studies were nonran-domized and uncontrolled, the dramatic decrease in rejection incidence paralleled the findings from the kidney-alone controlled trials.

<u>Lung transplantation.</u> There have been a few small nonrandomized trials in lung transplantation which demonstrated a decreased incidence of acute rejection per 100 patient days [115-117]. A larger experience with reported by Reichenspurner et al. [118]. Seventy-eight patients undergoing lung transplantation were evaluated in this analysis comparing 34 patients treated with cyclosporine and azathioprine versus 30 patients receiving tacrolimus and azathioprine and 12 patients receiving tacrolimus with MMF. All of the patients received prednisone. There was a marked decrease in the incidence of acute rejection in the tacrolimus groups, either with MMF or azathioprine. There was also more freedom from acute rejection in patients treated with MMF. The overall survival rates were improved for patients re-ceiving tacrolimus therapy with or without azathioprine or MMF. To date, there has not been a controlled randomized trial on lung trans-plantation comparing MMF to either placebo or azathioprine.

Intestinal transplantation. There is only one published report of the use of MMF in intestinal transplantation [119]. Tzakis et al. examined the use of MMF in 27 primary intestinal transplants and four patients in whom MMF was added for rescue therapy. In the primary group, there were 47 episodes of rejection in 25 patients, and in the rescue group, seven episodes of rejection in three patients. There was no comparator group, so it is difficult to ascertain whether this is an improvement in the rejection incidence in this very difficult transplant population. As expected, there were a number of significant complications, including diarrhea and leukopenia which were possibly due to the use of MMF.

Other clinical uses. Mycophenolic acid was initially evaluated as a therapy for psoriasis [44,45]. Some of the initial clinical studies showed that the drug was effective in ameliorating disease in about 65% of patients who were treated with the drug. The clinical experience for the dermatologic application of MMF has been expanded and single case reports in refractory pyoderma gangrenosum [120], bullous pemphigoid and pemphigus vulgaris [121,122], and idiopathic nodular panniculitis have been reported [123]. Other possible indications for MMF include treatment of refractory myasthenia gravis [124], Takayasu arteritis [125], refractory uveitis [126], and lupus nephritis [127,128].

One major indication for the use of MMF may be in inflammatory bowel disease. A recent randomized study comparing azathioprine plus prednisolone or MMF plus prednisolone demonstrated that disease activity with highly active Crohn's disease was suppressed to a greater degree with MMF and cortisone compared to azathioprine and cortisone [129]. Despite the GI toxicity associated with MMF use, no cases of diarrhea occurred on MMF treatment. Whether or not MMF will be effective for other types of inflammatory bowel disease, including ulcerative colitis, is unknown.

Conclusion

The introduction of MMF into the clinical practice of transplantation was a major accomplishment in the 1990s. As a specific inhibitor of purine synthesis, MMF has a distinct advantage over azathioprine. The clinical MMF program was rationally designed and progressed from the known scientific actions of the drug to clinical trials in man in less than 5 years. MMF has gained widespread use in all aspects of solid organ transplantation and its use is expanding into other immunologic disease states. However, much remains to be learned from the experimental and clinical use of the drug. Goals for the future should include a better understanding of the pharmacology and therapeutic monitoring of MMF, the benefits in long-term transplant recipients, the role for MMF in other immunologic disease states, and use with newer immunosuppressants such as rapamycin.

References

1. Calne RY, Alexandre GPJ, Murray JE. A study of drugs in prolonging survival of homologous renal transplants in dogs. Ann NY Acad Sci 1962;99:743-61.
2. Murray JE, Merrill JP, Harrson JH, et al. Prolonged survival of human-kidney homografts by immunosuppressive drug therapy. N Engl J Med 1963;268:1315-23.
3. Sollinger HW for the US Renal Transplant Mycophenolate Mofetil Study Group. Mycophenolate mofetil for the prevention of acute rejection in primary cadaveric renal allograft recipients. Transplantation 1995;60:225-32.
4. European Mycophenolate Mofetil Cooperative Study Group. Placebo-controlled study of mycophenolate mofetil combined with cyclosporin and corticosteroids for prevention of acute rejection. Lancet 1995;345:1321-5.
5. The Tricontinental Mycophenolate Mofetil Renal Transplantation Study Group. A blinded, randomized clinical trial of mycophenolate mofetil for prevention of acute rejection in cadaveric renal transplantation. Transplantation 1996;61:1029-37.
6. Elion GB, Hitchings GH, Vanderwerff J. Antagonists of nucleic acid derivatives. J Biol Chem 1951;192:505.
7. Schwartz R, Dameshek H. The effects of 6-mercaptopurine on homografts reactions. J Clin Invest 1960;39:952.
8. Elion GB, Callahan S, Bibier S, Hitchings GH, Rundles RW. A summary of investigations with 6-(1'-methyl-4'nitro-5'imidazolyl)thiopurine. Cancer Chemother 1961;14:93.
9. Merrill JP, Murray JE, Takacs FJ, Hager ED, Wilson RE, Dammin GJ. Successful transplantation of kidney from a human cadaver. J Am Med Assoc 1963;185:347.
10. el-Gamel A, Evans C, Keevil B, et al. Effect of allopurinol on the metabolism of azathioprine in heart transplant patients. Transplant Proc 1998;30:1127-9.
11. Chocair PR, Duley JA, Cameron JS, et al. Does low-dose allopurinol, with azathioprine, cyclosporin and prednisolone, improve renal transplant immunosuppression? Adv Exp Med Biol 1994;370:205-8.
12. Dervieux T, Medard Y, Baudouin V, et al. Thiopurine methyltransferase activity and its relationship to the occurrence of rejection episodes in paediatric renal transplant recipients treated with azathioprine. Br J Clin Pharmacol 1999;48:793-800.
13. Lennard L, Singleton HJ. High-performance liquid chromatographic assay of the methyl and nucleotide metabolites of 6-mercaptopurine: quantitation of red blood cell 6-thioguanine nucleotide, 6-thioinosinic acid and 6-methylmercaptopurine metabolites in a single sample. J Chromatogr 1992;583:83-90.
14. Chocair PR, Duley JA, Simmonds HA, Cameron JS. The importance of thiopurine methyltransferase activity for the use of azathioprine in transplant recipients. Transplantation 1992;53:1051-6.
15. Escousse A, Guedon F, Mounie J, Rifle G, Mousson C, D'Athis P. 6-Mercaptopurine pharmacokinetics after use of azathioprine in renal transplant recipients with intermediate or high thiopurine methyl transferase activity phenotype. J Pharm Pharmacol 1998;50:1261-6.
16. Chocair PR, Duley JA, Sabbaga E, Arap S, Simmonds HA, Cameron JS. Fast and slow methylators: do racial differences influence risk of allograft rejection? Q J Med 1993;86:359-63.
17. Amenabar JJ, Gomez-Ullate P, Garcia-Lopez FJ, Aurrecoechea B, Garcia-Erauzkin G, Lampreabe I. A randomized trial comparing cyclosporine and steroids with cyclosporine, azathioprine, and steroids in cadaveric renal transplantation. Transplantation 1998;65:653-61.
18. Arber N, Zajicek G, Nordenberg J, Sidi Y. Azathioprine treatment increases hepatocyte turnover. Gastroenterology 1991;101:1083-6.

19. Pol S, Cavalcanti R, Carnot F, et al. Azathioprine hepatitis in kidney transplant recipients. A predisposing role of chronic viral hepatitis. Transplantation 1996;61:1774-6.
20. Haboubi NY, Ali HH, Whitwell HL, Ackrill P. Role of endothelial cell injury in the spectrum of azathioprine-induced liver disease after renal transplant: light microscopy and ultrastructural observations. Am J Gastroenterol 1988;83:256-61.
21. Farge D, Parfrey PS, Forbes RD, Dandavino R, Guttmann RD. Reduction of azathioprine in renal transplant patients with chronic hepatitis. Transplantation 1986;41:55-9.
22. David-Neto E, da Fonseca JA, de Paula FJ, Nahas WC, Sabbaga E, Ianhez LE. Is azathioprine harmful to chronic viral hepatitis in renal transplantation? A long-term study on azathioprine withdrawal. Transplant Proc 1999;31:1149-50.
23. Opelz G. Evaluation of immunosuppressive induction regimens in renal transplantation. Collaborative Transplant Study. Transplant Proc 1998;30:4029-30.
24. Shapiro R, Jordan ML, Scantlebury VP, et al. A prospective randomized trial of FK506-based immunosuppression after renal transplantation. Transplantation 1995;59:485-90.
25. Opelz G. Influence of treatment with cyclosporine, azathioprine and steroids on chronic allograft failure. The Collaborative Transplant Study. Kidney Int Suppl 1995;52:S89-92.
26. David-Neto E, Vilares S, Lando V, et al. Conversion from azathioprine/prednisone to azathioprine/cyclosporin promotes catch-up growth in pediatric renal allograft recipients. Clin Transplantation 1990;4:229.
27. David-Neto E, Nahas W, Sampaio EC, Ianhez LE, Sabbaga E, Arap S. CSA/AZA, in the absence of prednisone, improves linear growth in renal transplanted children. Transplant Int 1992;5(Suppl 1):S3.
28. David-Neto E, Ianhez LE, Nahas WC, Krasilcic S, Sabbaga E, Arap S. Do steroids matter in one-haplotype pediatric renal allograft recipients on cyclosporine/azathioprine? Transplant Proc 1994;26:95-6.
29. Birkeland SA, Larsen KE, Rohr N. Pediatric renal transplantation without steroids. Pediatr Nephrol 1998;12:87-92.
30. Fine RN. Growth hormone treatment of children with chronic renal insufficiency, end-stage renal disease and following renal transplantation--update 1997. J Pediatr Endocrinol Metab 1997;10:361-70.
31. Kimmel SG, Zangari A, Acal L, Bilik R, Zaki A, Superina RA. Growth in children after liver transplantation. American Society of Transplant Surgeons 23rd Annual Scientific Meeting, May 14-16, 1997, Chicago, IL (abstract).
32. David-Neto E, Furusawa EA, Schwartzman BS, et al. Are steroids essential in pediatric living-related renal transplantation? A long-term single-center prospective study of CYA/AZA vs CYA/AZA/PRED. (Abstract). Pediatr Transplant 1998;2(Suppl 1):29.
33. Faull RJ, Bannister KM, Russ GR, Mathew TH, Clarkson AR. Excellent long-term survival of low-risk, first renal allografts using cyclosporine/azathioprine double therapy. Transplant Proc 1999;31:1155-6.
34. Khosla UM, Martin JE, Baker GM, Schroeder TJ, First MR. One-year, single-center cost analysis of mycophenolate mofetil versus azathioprine following cadaveric renal transplantation. Transplant Proc 1999;31:274-5.
35. Sadek S, Vogt B, Beauregard-Zollinger L, Prestele H, Group PINS. Short-term combination of mycophenolate mofetil with cyclosporine as a safe therapeutic option for renal transplant recipients. Transplant 2000 - First Joint Meeting of the American Society of Transplant Surgeons and American Society of Transplantation, May 13-17, 2000, Chicago, IL (abstract submitted).
36. David-Neto E, Gonçalves LF, Noronha IL, et al. One-year results of the Brazilian Trial on the addition of mycophenolate mofetil (CellCept) vs azathioprine to cyclosporin-A and steroids for the prevention of acute renal allograft rejection.

XVIII International Congress of the Transplantation Society, August 27-September 1, 2000, Rome, Italy (abstract submitted).

37. Bartucci MR, Flemming-Brooks S, Koshla B, Knauss TC, Hricik DE, Schulak JA. Azathioprine monotherapy in HLA-identical live donor kidney transplant recipients. J Transpl Coord 1999;9:35-9.
38. Allison AC, Kowalski WJ, Muller CD, Eugui EM. Mechanisms of action of mycophenolic acid. Ann NY Acad Sci 1993;696:63-87.
39. Allison AC, Eugui EM. The design and development of an immunosuppressive drug, mycophenolate mofetil. Springer Semin Immunopathol 1993;14:353-80.
40. Sollinger HW, Eugui EM, Allison AC. RS-61443: mechanism of action, experimental and early clinical results. Clin Transplant 1991;5(Spec issue):523-6.
41. Allison AC, Eugui EM, Sollinger HW. Mycophenolate mofetil (RS-61443): mechanisms of action and effects in transplantation. Transplant Rev 1993;7:129-39.
42. Gosio B. Ricerche bacteriologiche e chimiche sulle alterazioni del mais. Riv Igiene e Sanita Pubblica 1896;7:825-68.
43. Alsberg CL, Black OF. Contribution to the study of maize deterioration: biochemical and toxocological investigations of *Penicillium puberulum* and *Penicillium stoloniferum*. US Dept Agr Plant Industry Bull 1913;270:7-48.
44. Farber EM, Pearlman D, Abel EA. An appraisal of current systemic chemotherapy for psoriasis. Arch Dermatol 1976;112:1679-88.
45. McDonald CJ. Chemotherapy of psoriasis. Int J Dermatol 1975;14:563-74.
46. Allison AC, Eugui EM. Immunosuppressive and long-acting anti-inflammatory activity of mycophenolic acid and derivative, RS-61443. Br J Rheumatol 1991;30(Suppl 2):57-61.
47. Allison AC, Almquist SJ, Muller CD, Eugui EM. *In vitro* immunosuppressive effects of mycophenolic acid and an ester pro-drug, RS-61443. Transplant Proc 1991;23(2 Suppl 2):10-4.
48. Ransom JT. Mechanism of action of mycophenolate mofetil. Ther Drug Monit 1995;17:681-4.
49. Eugui EM, Allison AC. Immunosuppressive activity of mycophenolate mofetil. Ann NY Acad Sci 1993;685:309-29.
50. Hager PW, Collart FR, Huberman E, Mitchell BS. Recombinant human inosine monophosphate dehydrogenase type I and type II proteins. Purification and characterization of inhibitor binding. Biochem Pharmacol 1995;49:1323-9.
51. Allison AC, Eugui EM. Immunosuppressive and other effects of mycophenolic acid and an ester prodrug, mycophenolate mofetil. Immunol Rev 1993;136:5-28.
52. Eugui EM, Almquist SJ, Muller CD, Allison AC. Lymphocyte-selective cytostatic and immunosuppressive effects of mycophenolic acid *in vitro*: role of deoxyguanosine nucleotide depletion. Scan J Immunol 1991;33:161-73.
53. Eugui EM, Mirkovich A, Allison AC. Lymphocyte-selective antiproliferative and immunosuppressive effects of mycophenolic acid in mice. Scand J Immunol 1991;33:175-83.
54. Allison AC, Kowalski WJ, Muller CJ, Waters RV, Eugui EM. Mycophenolic acid and brequinar, inhibitors of purine and pyrimidine synthesis, block the glycosylation of adhesion molecules. Transplant Proc 1993;25(3 Suppl 2):67-70.
55. Blaheta RA, Leckel K, Wittig B, Zenker D, Oppermann E, Harder S, et al. Inhibition of endothelial receptor expression and of T cell ligand activity by mycophenolate mofetil. Transpl Immunol 1998;6:251-9.
56. Morris RE, Hoyt EG, Eugui EM, Allison AC. Prolongation of rat heart allograft survival by RS-61443. Surg Forum 1989;40:337-8.
57. Morris RE, Hoyt EG, Murphy MP, Eugui EM, Allison AC. Mycophenolic acid morpholinoethylester (RS-61443) is a new immunosuppressant that prevents and halts heart allograft rejection by selective inhibition of T- and B-cell purine synthesis. Transplant Proc 1990;22:1659-62.

58. Platz KP, Sollinger HW, Hullett DA, Eckhoff DE, Eugui EM, Allison AC. RS-61443 – a new, potent immunosuppressive agent. Transplantation 1991;51:27-31.
59. Platz KP, Bechstein WO, Eckhoff DE, Suzuki Y, Sollinger HW. RS-61443 reverses acute allograft rejection in dogs. Surgery 1991;110:736-41.
60. D'Alessandro AM, Rankin M, McVey J, Hafez GR, Sollinger HW, Kalayoglu M, et al. Prolongation of canine intestinal allograft survival with RS-61443, cyclosporine, and prednisone. Transplant Proc 1993;25:1207-9.
61. Bechstein WO, Schilling M, Steele DM, Hullett DA, Sollinger HW. RS-61443/cyclosporine combination therapy prolongs canine liver allograft survival. Transplant Proc 1993;25(1 Pt 1):702-3.
62. O'Hair DP, McManus RP, Komorowski R. Inhibition of chronic vascular rejection in primate cardiac xenografts using mycophenolate mofetil. Ann Thorac Surg 1994;58:1311-5.
63. Fujino Y, Kawamura T, Hullett DA, Sollinger HW. Evaluation of cyclosporine, mycophenolate mofetil, and brequinar sodium combination therapy on hamster-to-rat cardiac xenotransplantation. Transplantation 1994;57:41-6.
64. Murase N, Starzl TE, Demetris AJ, Valdivia L, Tanabe M, Cramer D, et al. Hamster-to-rat heart and liver xenotransplantation with FK506 plus antiproliferative drugs. Transplantation 1993;55:701-8.
65. Yatscoff RW, Wang S, Keenan R, Chackowsky P, Koshal A. Efficacy of rapamycin, RS-61443, and cyclophosphamide in the prolongation of survival of discordant pig-to-rabbit cardiac xenografts. Transplant Proc 1994;26:1271-3.
66. Hao L, Lafferty KJ, Allison AC, Eugui EM. RS-61443 allows islet allografting and specific tolerance induction in adult mice. Transplant Proc 1990;22:876-9.
67. Wennberg L, Wallgren AC, Karlsson-Parra A, Kozlowski T, Sundberg B, Tibell A, et al. Efficacy of various immunosuppressive drugs in preventing pig-to-rat islet xenograft rejection. Transplant Proc 1995;27:266-7.
68. Beger C, Menger MD. RS-61443 prevents microvascular rejection of pancreatic islet xenografts. Transplantation 1997;63:577-82.
69. Wennberg L, Groth CG, Tibell A, Zhu S, Liu J, Rafael E, et al. Triple drug treatment with cyclosporine, leflunomide and mycophenolate mofetil prevents rejection of pig islets transplanted into rats and primates. Transplant Proc 1997;29:2498.
70. Song Z, Wennberg L, Bennet W, Sundberg B, Groth CG, Korsgren O. FK506 prevents islet xenograft rejection: a study in the pig-to-rat model. Transplant Proc 1999;31:981.
71. Ziswiler R, Steinmann-Niggli K, Kappeler A, Daniel C, Marti HP. Mycophenolic acid: a new approach to the therapy of experimental mesangial proliferative glomerulonephritis. J Am Soc Nephrol 1998;9:2055-66.
72. Penny MJ, Boyd RA, Hall BM. Mycophenolate mofetil prevents the induction of active Heymann nephritis: association with Th2 cytokine inhibition. J Am Soc Nephrol 1998;9:2272-82.
73. Jonsson CA, Svensson L, Carlsten H. Beneficial effect of the inosine monophosphate dehydrogenase inhibitor mycophenolate mofetil on survival and severity of glomerulonephritis in systemic lupus erythematosus (SLE)-prone MRL/pr/lpr mice. Clin Exp Immunol 1999;116:534-41.
74. van Bruggen MCJ, Walgreen B, Rijke TPM, Berden JHM. Attenuation of murine lupus nephritis by mycophenolate mofetil. J Am Soc Nephrol 1998;9:1407-15.
75. Remuzzi G, Zoja C, Gagliardini E, Corna D, Abbate M, Benigni A. Combining an antiproteinuric approach with mycophenolate mofetil fully suppresses progressive nephropathy of experimental animals. J Am Soc Nephrol 1999;10:1542-9.
76. Bullingham RES, Nicholls AJ, Kamm BR. Clinical pharmacokinetics of mycophenolate mofetil. Clin Pharmacokinet 1998;34:429-55.
77. Zucker K, Rosen A, Tsaroucha A, de Faria L, Roth D, Ciancio G, et al. Unexpected augmentation of mycophenolic acid pharmacokinetics in renal transplant patients

receiving tacrolimus and mycophenolate mofetil in combination therapy, and analogous *in vitro* findings. Transpl Immunol 1997;5:225-32.

78. Gregoor PJ, de Sevaux RG, Hene RJ, Hesse CJ, Hilbrands LB, Vos P, et al. Effect of cyclosporine on mycophenolic acid trough levels in kidney transplant recipients. Transplantation 1999;68:1603-6.

79. Sollinger HW, Deierhoi MH, Belzer FO, Diethelm AG, Kauffman RS. RS-61443 – a phase I clinical trial and pilot rescue study. Transplantation 1992;53:428-32.

80. Sollinger HW, Belzer FO, Deierhoi MH, Diethelm AG, Gonwa TA, Kauffman RS, et al. RS-61443 (mycophenolate mofetil). A multicenter study for refractory kidney transplant rejection. Ann Surg 1992;216:513-9.

81. US Renal Transplant Mycophenolate Mofetil Study Group. Mycophenolate mofetil in cadaveric renal transplantation. Am J Kidney Dis 1999;34:296-303.

82. European Mycophenolate Mofetil Cooperative Study Group. Mycophenolate mofetil in renal transplantation: 3-year results from the placebo-controlled trial. Transplantation 1999;68:391-6.

83. Mathew TH for the Tricontinental Mycophenolate Mofetil Renal Transplantation Study Group. A blinded, long-term, randomized multicenter study of mycophenolate mofetil in cadaveric renal transplantation: results at three years. Transplantation 1998;65:1450-4.

84. The Mycophenolate Mofetil Renal Refractory Rejection Study Group. Mycophenolate mofetil for the treatment of refractory, acute, cellular renal transplant rejection. Transplantation 1996;61:722-9.

85. The Mycophenolate Mofetil Acute Renal Rejection Study Group. Mycophenolate mofetil for the treatment of a first acute renal allograft rejection. Transplantation 1998;65:235-41.

86. Forsythe J for the European Multicentre Tacrolimus/MMF Study Group. Tacrolimus and mycophenolate mofetil in cadaveric renal transplant recipients. Transplant Proc 1999;31(Suppl 7A):69S-71S.

87. Miller J, Mendez R, Pirsch JD, Jensik SC for the FK506/MMF Dose-Ranging Kidney Transplant Study Group. Safety and efficacy of tacrolimus in combination with mycophenolate mofetil (MMF) in cadaveric renal transplant recipients. Transplantation 2000;69:875-80.

88. Shapiro R, Jordan ML, Scantlebury VP, Vivas C, Marsh JW, McCauley J, et al. A prospective, randomized trial of tacrolimus/prednisone versus tacrolimus/ prednisone/mycophenolate mofetil in renal transplant recipients. Transplantation 1999;67:411-5.

89. Steroid Withdrawal Study Group. Prednisone withdrawal in kidney transplant recipients on cyclosporine and mycophenolate mofetil – a prospective randomized study. Transplantation 1999;68:1865-74.

90. Azuma H, Binder J, Heemann U, Schmid C, Tullius SG, Tilney NL. Effects of RS61443 on functional and morphological changes in chronically rejecting rat kidney allografts. Transplantation 1995;59:460-6.

91. Raisanen-Sokolowski A, Vuoristo P, Myllarniemi M, Yilmaz S, Kallio E, Hayry P. Mycophenolate mofetil (MMF, RS-61443) inhibits inflammation and smooth muscle cell proliferation in rat aortic allografts. Transpl Immunol 1995;3:342-51.

92. Steele DM, Bechstein WO, Kowalski J, et al. RS-61443 inhibits intimal hyperplasia in aortic allografts. Surg Forum 1992;43:383-5.

93. Weir MR, Anderson L, Fink JC, Gabregiorgish K, Schweitzer EJ, Hoehn-Saric E, et al. A novel approach to the treatment of chronic allograft nephropathy. Transplantation 1997;64:1706-10.

94. Shaw LM, Korecka M, Aradhye S, Grossman R, Barker C, Naji A, et al. Scientific principles for mycophenolic acid therapeutic drug monitoring. Transplant Proc 1998;30:2234-6.

95. Nicholls AJ. Opportunities for therapeutic monitoring of mycophenolate mofetil dose in renal transplantation suggested by the pharmacokinetic/pharmaco-

dynamic relationship for mycophenolic acid and suppression of rejection. Clin Biochem 1998;31:329-33.

96. van Gelder T, Hilbrands LB, Vanrenterghem Y, Weimar W, de Fijter JW, Squifflet JP, et al. A randomized double-blind, multicenter plasma concentration controlled study of the safety and efficacy of oral mycophenolate mofetil for the prevention of acute rejection after kidney transplantation. Transplantation 1999;68:261-6.

97. Renlund DG, Gopinathan SJ, Kfoury AG, Taylor DO. Mycophenolate mofetil (MMF) in heart transplantation: rejection prevention and treatment. Clin Transplant 1996;10:136-9.

98. Kirklin JK, Bourge RC, Naftel DC, Morrow WR, Deierhoi MH, Kauffman RS, et al. Treatment of recurrent heart rejection with mycophenolate mofetil (RS-61443): initial clinical experience. J Heart Lung Transplant 1994;13:444-50.

99. Ensley RD, Bristow MR, Olsen SL, Taylor DO, Hammond EH, O'Connell JB, et al. The use of mycophenolate mofetil (RS-61443) in human heart transplant recipients. Transplantation 1993;56:75-82.

100. Kobashigawa J, Miller L, Renlund D, Mentzer R, Alderman E, Bourge R, et al. A randomized active-controlled trial of mycophenolate mofetil in heart transplant recipients. Transplantation 1998;66:507-15.

101. Klintmalm GB, Ascher NL, Busuttil RW, Deierhoi M, Gonwa TA, Kauffman R, et al. RS-61443 for treatment-resistant human liver rejection. Transplant Proc 1993;25:697.

102. Platz KP, Mueller AR, Neuhaus R, Keck HH, Lobeck H, Neuhaus P. FK506 and mycofenolate mofetil rescue for acute steroid-resistant and chronic rejection after liver transplantation. Transplant Proc 1997;29:2872-4.

103. Hebert MF, Ascher NL, Lake JR, Emond J, Nikolai B, Linna TJ, et al. Four-year follow-up of mycophenolate mofetil for graft rescue in liver allograft recipients. Transplantation 1999; 67:707-12.

104. Stegall MD, Wachs ME, Everson G, Steinberg T, Bilir B, Shrestha R, et al. Prednisone withdrawal 14 days after liver transplantation with mycophenolate: a prospective trial of cyclosporine and tacrolimus. Transplantation 1997;64:1755-60.

105. Fisher RA, Ham JM, Marcos A, Shiffman ML, Luketic VA, Kimball PM, et al. A prospective randomized trial of mycophenolate mofetil with Neoral or tacrolimus after orthotopic liver transplantation. Transplantation 1998;66:1616-21.

106. Jain AB, Hamad I, Rakela J, Dodson F, Kramer D, Demetris J, et al. A prospective randomized trial of tacrolimus and prednisone versus tacrolimus, prednisone, and mycophenolate mofetil in primary adult liver transplant recipients. Transplantation 1998;66:1395-8.

107. Eckhoff DE, McGuire BM, Frenette LR, Contreras JL, Hudson SL, Bynon JS. Tacrolimus (FK506) and mycophenolate mofetil combination therapy versus tacrolimus in adult liver transplantation. Transplantation 1998;65:180-7.

108. Mamelok RD, Kalayoglu M, Klintmalm G, Langnas AN, Levy GA, McDiarmid SV, et al. A randomized, double-blind comparative study of mycophenolate mofetil (MMF) and azathioprine (AZA), in combination with cyclosporine and corticosteroids in liver transplant recipients. American Association for the Study of Liver Diseases 50th Annual Meeting, November 5-9, 1999, Dallas, TX (abstract).

109. Papatheodoridis GV, O'Beirne J, Mistry P, Davidson B, Rolles K, Burroughs AK. Mycophenolate mofetil monotherapy in stable liver transplant patients with cyclosporine-induced renal impairment: a preliminary report. Transplantation 1999;68:155-7.

110. Herrero JI, Quiroga J, Sangro B, Girala M, Gomez-Manero N, Pardo F, et al. Conversion of liver transplant recipients on cyclosporine with renal impairment to mycophenolate mofetil. Liver Transpl Surg 1999;5:414-20.

111. Stegall MD, Simon M, Wachs ME, Chan L, Nolan C, Kam I. Mycophenolate mofetil decreases rejection in simultaneous pancreas-kidney transplantation

when combined with tacrolimus or cyclosporine. Transplantation 1997;64:1695-1700.

112. Gruessner RWG, Sutherland DER, Drangstveit MB, Wrenshall L, Humar A, Gruessner AC. Mycophenolate mofetil in pancreas transplantation. Transplantation 1998;66:318-23.

113. Odorico JS, Pirsch JD, Knechtle SJ, D'Alessandro AM, Sollinger HW. A study comparing mycophenolate mofetil to azathioprine in simultaneous pancreas-kidney transplantation. Transplantation 1998;66:1751-9.

114. Kaufman DB, Leventhal JR, Stuart J, Abecassis MM, Fryer JP, Stuart FP. Mycophenolate mofetil and tacrolimus as primary maintenance immunosuppression in simultaneous pancreas-kidney transplantation. Transplantation 1999; 67:586-93.

115. Ross DJ, Waters PF, Levine M, Kramer M, Ruzevich S, Kass RM. Mycophenolate mofetil versus azathioprine immunosuppressive regimens after lung transplantation: preliminary experience. J Heart Lung Transplant 1998;17:768-74.

116. O'Hair DP, Cantu E, McGregor C, Jorgensen B, Gerow-Smith R, Galantowicz ME, et al. Preliminary experience with mycophenolate mofetil used after lung transplantation. J Heart Lung Transplant 1998;17:864-8.

117. Zuckermann A, Klepetko W, Birsan T, Taghavi S, Artemiou O, Wisser W, et al. Comparison between mycophenolate mofetil- and azathioprine-based immunosuppressions in clinical lung transplantation. J Heart Lung Transplant 1999; 18:432-40.

118. Reichenspurner H, Kur F, Treede H, Meiser BM, Deutsch O, Welz A, et al. Optimization of the immunosuppressive protocol after lung transplantation. Transplantation 1999;68:67-71.

119. Tzakis AG, Weppler D, Khan MF, Koutouby R, Romero R, Viciana AL, et al. Mycophenolate mofetil as primary and rescue therapy in intestinal transplantation. Transplant Proc 1998;30:2677-2679.

120. Nousari HC, Lynch W, Anhalt GJ, Petri M. The effectiveness of mycophenolate mofetil in refractory pyoderma gangrenosum. Arch Dermatol 1998;134:1509-11.

121. Grundmann-Kollmann M, Korting HC, Behrens S, Kaskel P, Leiter U, Krahn G, et al. Mycophenolate mofetil: a new therapeutic option in the treatment of blistering autoimmune diseases. J Am Acad Dermatol 1999;40:957-60.

122. Grundmann-Kollmann M, Kaskel P, Leiter U, Krahn G, Behrens S, Peter RU, et al. Treatment of pemphigus vulgaris and bullous pemphigoid with mycophenolate mofetil monotherapy. Arch Dermatol 1999;135:724-5.

123. Enk AH, Knop J. Treatment of relapsing idiopathic nodular panniculitis (Pfeifer-Weber-Christian disease) with mycophenolate mofetil. J Am Acad Dermatol 1998;39:508-9.

124. Hauser RA, Malek AR, Rosen R. Successful treatment of a patient with severe refractory myasthenia gravis using mycophenolate mofetil. Neurology 1998; 51:912-3.

125. Daina E, Schieppati A, Remuzzi G. Mycophenolate mofetil for the treatment of Takayasu arteritis: report of three cases. Ann Intern Med 1999;130:422-6.

126. Kilmartin DJ, Forrester JV, Dick AD. Rescue therapy with mycophenolate mofetil in refractory uveitis. Lancet 1998;352:35-6.

127. Glicklich D, Acharya A. Mycophenolate mofetil therapy for lupus nephritis refractory to intravenous cyclophosphamide. Am J Kidney Dis 1998;32:318-22.

128. Dooley MA, Cosio FG, Nachman PH, Falkenhain ME, Hogan SL, Falk RJ, et al. Mycophenolate mofetil therapy in lupus nephritis: clinical observations. J Am Soc Nephrol 1999;10:833-9.

129. Neurath MF, Wanitschke R, Peters M, Krummenauer F, zum Buschenfelde KHM, Schlaak JF. Randomised trial of mycophenolate mofetil versus azathioprine for treatment of chronic active Crohn's disease. Gut 1999;44:625-8.

CYCLOSPORINE FORMULATIONS

Venkataraman Ramanathan and J. Harold Helderman

Introduction

Borel et al in 1972 discovered the immunosuppressive properties of cyclosporine (CyA) and since then this fungal metabolite extracted from Tolypocladium inflatum, has revolutionized the field of clinical transplantation. Approved in 1983 by Food and Drug Administration (FDA) for widespread clinical use, this drug has improved the graft survival and has been the cornerstone in most immunosuppression protocols. The more selective inhibition of T lymphocyte immunity by CyA was unique when it was discovered compared to its predecessor drugs like steroids and azathioprine. Since its use in clinical practice, marked improvements in outcome have been accomplished in one year and in chronic renal allograft survival and routinely successful heart, liver, pancreas, and lung transplants are possible. Cyclosporine is a cyclic polypeptide consisting of 11 aminoacids and molecular weight of approximately 1200 ($C_{62} H_{111} N_{11} O_{12}$) The cyclic structure is necessary for its immunosuppressive effect.

Pharmacokinetics

Cyclosporine is slowly and incompletely absorbed from the upper small intestine after oral administration resulting in approximately 33% bioavailability. Hence conversion between the oral and IV forms of the drug requires a 3:1 dose ratio. Oral absorption is bile-dependent. Cholestasis and biliary diversion procedures after liver transplantation result in impaired drug absorption. Also conditions like gastroparesis,

Mohamed Sayegh and Giuseppe Remuzzi (editors), Current and Future
Immunosuppressive Therapies Following Transplantation, 111-121.
© 2001 Kluwer Academic Publishers. Printed in the Netherlands.

intestinal resection, diarrhea and malabsorption decrease the bioavailability. The microemulsion form is better absorbed and bile independent resulting in better levels and may be particularly useful in patients with GI or liver disorders.

One-third of cyclosporine is bound to lipoproteins and the binding is important for the transfer of the drug through the plasma membranes. Low cholesterol levels may exaggerate the toxicity of the drug. Conversely, high cholesterol reduces the effect. The remaining two-thirds is bound to RBC.   Hence it is important to recognize if the concentration is measured in serum, plasma or whole blood. Due to RBC binding, whole blood drug levels will be threefold higher than plasma levels. Metabolism is via the cytochrome P450 IIIA4 enzyme system in the GI tract and liver. First metabolism is in the intestinal wall cytochrome system and the variability in the absorption may be accounted by the heterogeneity in the cytochrome activity. Extensive metabolism (99%) occurs in the gut and liver and at least 25 metabolites are recognized. Certain metabolites appear to contribute at least in part to the immunosuppressive activity although CyA as unchanged drug is chiefly responsible for its action. Major route of elimination is via the biliary tract and enterohepatic recirculation can occur in some patients resulting in biphasic peak. Since only 1% of CyA is excreted unchanged in urine, dose adjustment is not needed for renal impairment.   Similarly the dose need not be adjusted for dialysis patients since the drug is not significantly dialyzed. African-American patients may require larger doses of CyA due to higher clearance.

Evidence is available that area under the curve (AUC) is the key factor in determining the efficacy and safety of CyA. The peak blood level occurs between 1 ½ and 3 hrs followed by metabolism to a trough at 12 hours. The trough level is called C_{min} and the peak is called C_{max}. The integrated area under the curve (AUC) has been used as a means or a measure of drug exposure for both toxicity and efficacy. Even for the same C_{min}, the AUC can be different in individual patients. There is intra-patient and inter-patient variability in absorption and metabolism resulting in different pharmacokinetic profiles. Neoral has less variable pharmacokinetic profile compared to Sandimmune.   Monitoring AUC routinely can be cumbersome and hence in clinical practice C_{min} is used as a surrogate marker for drug efficacy and toxicity.   With Sandimmune, only 4 times out of 10, the C_{min} relates to the drug exposure as evaluated by the AUC while with Neoral the C_{min} is more correlative of AUC.   The coefficient of variation (r value) is 0.4 for Sandimmune whereas the r value is 0.85 for Neoral. Healthy volunteers showed a ratio of 0.6 between the AUC values of Sandimmune compared with same dose of Neoral [1]. USA multicenter, randomized, blinded study showed a moderately greater absorption with Neoral [2]. In other studies, Neoral resulted in significantly lower degree of intra-patient variability in AUC levels.   Considering that there is an association between intrapatient variability and incidence of chronic allograft nephropathy, this may prove to be significant in the long term. A review of global database of switch studies [3] was done addressing the question if there were any pharmacokinetic advantages to switch stable patients from one formulation to another. Patients who absorbed Sandimmune well did not get a significant pharmacological advantage for the switch to Neoral, while "poor absorbers" of Sandimmune did the best with the microemulsion form. "Poor absorbers" are patients who required more than 8 mg/kg/day of Sandimmune to achieve target blood levels. No differences in rejections or patient losses were noted in either of the groups. The question arises if the incidence of side effects would be more with Neoral with increased drug exposure. In the double-blind study, when the physician or the patient did not know the formulation, there were no differences in the creatinine values to either of the drugs.

Mechanism of Action

The interaction between the antigen presenting cells and CD3-T cell receptor (TCR) complex permits the passage of signals into the T cell. This interaction initiates a cascade of events that results in stimulation of the calcineurin pathway required for the transcription of IL-2 gene (Signal 1). Signal 2 or that derived from co-stimulatory pathway, involves the interaction of a series of ligand-receptor pairs such as CD28 on T cells with ligands on the APC such as B7-1 and B7-2. Both signals are required for optimal IL-2 gene transcription. Stimulation of signal 1 alone induces anergy in T cells, a state of unresponsiveness even with appropriate signals. The other important function of co-stimulatory pathway is prevention of apoptosis or passive cell death. CD28 stimulation directly induces the expression of *bcl*-x_L, a cell survival gene in antigen-activated T cells [4]. An indirect effect can be mediated through IL-2 that up regulates the expression of Bcl-2 in T cells. IL-2 has dual signals in T cells. The first signal induces proliferation and the second signal primes the cells to undergo apoptosis after Fas ligation. This is possibly mediated by increased expression of Fas-ligand. Another significant co-stimulatory pathway is mediated through the CD40 on APC that binds to CD40-ligand on activated T cells. Signal 3 starts with IL-2 receptor stimulation that results in proliferation of T cell.

The signal of TCR stimulation induces key enzymes in the T cell. Phosphotyrosine kinase mediates the appearance of phosphorylated tyrosine residues on a number of proteins. This leads to formation of inositol 1,4,5 triphosphate (IP3) and diacylglycerol (DAG) from phosphatidylinositol via a cascade of events [4]. IP3 stimulates the release of ionized calcium from intracellular stores. Cytoplasmic calcium forms a complex with the calcium-dependent regulatory protein called calmodulin (**Figure 1**). The calcium-calmodulin activates calcineurin.

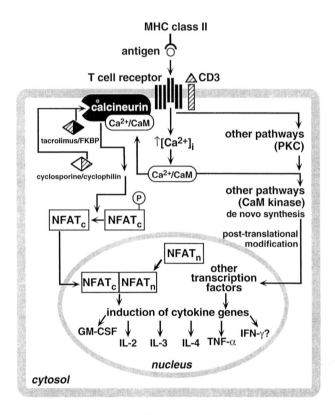

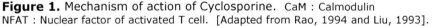

Figure 1. Mechanism of action of Cyclosporine. CaM : Calmodulin
NFAT : Nuclear factor of activated T cell. [Adapted from Rao, 1994 and Liu, 1993].

Calcineurin is activated when intracellular calcium ion levels rise following T cell receptor binding and dephosphorylates the cytosolic component of the transcription factor, nuclear factor of activated T cells
(NF-AT$_c$). Activated NF-AT$_c$ migrates to the nucleus and binds to NF-AT$_n$
forming the active transcription factor, NF-AT. In the nucleus, NF-AT
binds cooperatively with *c-fos* and *c-jun*, products of cellular proto-
oncogenes, to the distal NF-AT binding sites in the promoter sequence
of the IL-2 gene and enhances transcription of this gene. Hence activation of NF-AT occurs in at least two stages: a CyA-sensitive stage
involving modification and /or translocation of the pre-existing NF-AT
complex, and a CyA–insensitive stage involving the addition of newly
synthesized *fos* or *fos/jun* proteins to the pre-existing complex [5].

 CyA binds to the immunophilin, cyclophilin, which is a peptidyl-prolyl
cis-trans isomerase. The isomerase activity is not relevant to the
immunosuppression. The discovery, purification, and ultimately cloning
of gene encoding cyclophilin shed light on the mechanism of T cell

inhibition by CyA. The immunophilin-cyclosporine complex binds and inhibits the calcium-activated serine/threonine phophatase calcineurin. CyA by inhibiting the calcineurin enzyme, impairs the expression of T cell activation genes, including those for IL-2 and its receptor and the proto-oncogenes H-*ras* and c-*myc*. Transforming growth factor-beta (TGF-β) is implicated in inhibiting IL-2 and the generation of cytotoxic T lymphocytes and CyA increases the expression of TGF-β.

Formulation

Sandimmune soft gelatin capsules are available as 25mg, 50 mg, and 100mg capsules. Sandimmune oral solution is supplied in 50 ml bottles containing 100 mg of CyA per ml. A dosage syringe is provided for dispensing the drug. It contains the drug in an olive oil vehicle and 12.5% alcohol. Sandimmune injection is supplied as a 5 ml sterile ampoule containing 50 mg of CyA per ml and is manufactured by Sandoz Pharmaceuticals Corporation, East Hanover, NJ. It is a sterile solution of the drug in castor oil and 32.9% alcohol.

Neoral is an oral formulation of CyA that immediately forms a homogenous transparent microemulsion in an aqueous environment with a droplet size smaller than 100 nm in diameter. Neoral is supplied as 25 mg and 100mg soft gelatin capsules and is manufactured by Sandoz Pharmaceuticals corporation, NJ. In this formulation, the molecular structure of CyA is unaltered, and aqueous dilution results in formation of an emulsion without reprecipitation of the drug. Neoral oral solution is supplied in 50mL bottles containing 100 mg/ml. It is dispersed in a mixture of propylene glycol (hydrophilic solvent) and corn oil monoglycerides, diglycerides, and triglycerides (lipophilic solvent); when dispersed, castor oil serves as a surfactant, and tocopherol as an antioxidant. There is a concern of acceleration of oxidation of LDL with calcineurin inhibitors, CyA and tacrolimus. The presence of antioxidant, tocopherol may confer protection against LDL oxidation and its deleterious effects.

Another formulation, SangCya oral solution was marketed by Sangstat and was considered to be bioequivalent to Neoral oral solution and at the same time less expensive than Neoral. The product was recently withdrawn from the market because of clinical evidence that the generic drug's bioavailability was reduced relative to Neoral oral solution when the drug was administered with apple juice.

Abbott's Gengraf capsules, a generic CyA form, was approved by FDA for the prevention of organ rejection in kidney, liver and heart transplants. Gengraf was granted an AB rating by the FDA that designates that the product is therapeutically equivalent to, or interchangeable with the reference drug, Neoral. The effect of food and the steady-state pharmacokinetics of Gengraf were comparable to Neoral. Eon's generic CyA was also approved with a similar AB rating by FDA.

Drug Monitoring

Determination of the pharmacokinetics of CyA is dependent on the biologic fluid analyzed and the assay used. As explained earlier, the whole blood levels of CyA is approximately threefold higher than plasma or serum level since 2/3 of CyA is bound to RBC. Plasma and serum concentrations are comparable. Different methods are available for measuring CyA concentration. High-pressure liquid chromatography (HPLC) of CyA is technically difficult, expensive and slow. It is specific for measuring the parent molecule and each specific metabolite for which a standard is available. When radioimmunoassay (RIA) methods that employ monoclonal or polyclonal antibodies are used for monitoring CyA concentrations, cross-reactivity of the anti-sera with circulating metabolites of CyA has resulted in higher CyA concentrations than when HPLC is used. Both specific (for unchanged drug) and non-specific RIA methods are available. Other methods currently employed

Table 1. Drugs Altering CyA Concentration

Increase CyA Concentration		Decrease CyA Concentration	
Calcium channel blockers		*Antimicrobials*	
	Diltiazem		Rifampin & Rifabutin
	Nicardipine		INH
	Verapamil		Nafcillin
Antifungals		*Anticonvulsants*	
	Ketoconazole		
	Carbamazepine		
	Itraconazole		
	Phenobarbitol		
	Fluconazole		Phenytoin
Antibiotics		*Other drugs*	
	Erythromycin		Octreotide
	Clarithromycin		Ticlopidine
Glucocorticosteroids			
	High dose steroids		
Retroviral drugs			
	Indinavir		
	Nelfinavir		
	Ritonavir		
Grapefruit juice			

include nonspecific or specific fluorescence polarization immunoassay (FPIA) and a specific enzyme multiplied immunoassay technique (EMIT). FPIA method is widely used because it is technically simple and rapid. While the polyclonal assay measures both parent compound and metabolites, the monoclonal assay employs antiserum that measures the parent compound and only a few cross-reacting metabolites. Even with specific assays targeted only against the parent compound, some cross-reactivity occurs with CyA metabolites leading to different reference ranges for CyA concentrations. Hence it is important for the transplant center to create its own reference ranges. The pharmacokinetics of the drug is significantly impaired in the presence of liver disease. The serum level of CyA becomes uninterpretable since even sophisticated monoclonal immunoassays can measure minute quantities of the metabolites of CyA. The ratio of the parent compound to metabolites can vary significantly in this scenario. Under such circumstances, measurement of e parent compound with HPLC method is useful to guide dose adjustment.

Drug Interactions

Concentrations of CyA may be influenced by drugs that affect the microsomal enzymes, particularly cytochrome P-450 IIIA4. Substances that inhibit this enzyme system will result in higher CyA concentra-tions while the drugs that induce the system will result in lower CyA concentrations (**Table 1**). Even though the percentage change in the serum level of CyA is known for some drugs, monitoring the CyA concentration is important when drugs that interfere with the microsomal enzyme system are added.

Enhanced renal dysfunction occurs when CyA is combined with known nephrotoxic drugs like non-steroidals, aminoglycosides and amphotericin. Vasoconstriction induced by CyA potentiates the toxicity of these drugs. CyA interacts with lovastatin, a HMGCoA reductase inhibitor and causes myopathic syndrome with elevated creatinine phosphokinase. This interaction is noted with high doses of lovastatin. Reduced urate clearance by CyA leads to hyperuricemia. Cyclosporine interaction with colchicine can result in severe colchicine toxicity manifested by myoneuropathy, hepatic dysfunction and GI disturbances. The nephrotoxicity of CyA is potentiated by colchicine. Gingival hyperplasia is noted when combined with nifedipine.

Side Effects

The principal adverse reaction of CyA is renal dysfunction. General toxicity syndromes associated with CyA are detailed in **Table 2**.

Table 2: General Toxicity

Cosmetic
Hirsutism, acne
Gingival Hyperplasia
GI
Nausea, vomiting, abdominal pain and diarrhea
Endocrine
Diabetes mellitus
Hepatic
$\uparrow$ bilirubin, cholestatic picture
Neurologic
Seizures, tremors, paresthesia and headache
Hypercholesteremia
$\uparrow$ LDL-C levels
Bone loss

Renal Effects

In addition to hypertension and electrolyte imbalance, CyA causes three major types of nephrotoxic syndromes:
- Acute vasoconstriction
- Chronic fibrosis
- Direct endothelial injury

Acute Vasoconstriction

CyA is a potent vasoconstrictor of both afferent and efferent arteriole and Kf or ultrafiltration coefficient is decreased. This combination causes a "pre-renal" picture and a dose-dependent increase in serum creatinine. An imbalance between the renal vasoconstrictors and vasodilators creates this scenario. Vasodilators like prostaglandin and nitric oxide are decreased while the vasoconstrictors like endothelin and thromboxane are increased with CyA. CyA stimulates sympathetic activity in kidneys thereby increasing vasoconstriction. Intact innervation to the kidney with non-renal transplants may account for the increased nephrotoxicity noticed in these patients with CyA compared to renal transplants. Vasoconstriction is seen in all vasculature leading to systemic hypertension. Salt retaining potential further worsens blood pressure. Changes in intracellular calcium homeostasis causing hypertension accounts for the efficacy of calcium-channel blockers in blood pressure control in CyA treated patients.

Chronic Injury

Calcineurin inhibitors have had a paradoxical impact on the long-term transplant outcomes even though they have reduced the acute rejection episodes. Chronic ischemia secondary to vasoconstriction and arterial damage leads to ischemic scarring and collapse of the glomeruli. Renal biopsy shows obliterative arteriopathy, tubular atrophy and vacuolization, and "stripped" interstitial fibrosis. Tranforming growth factor-β (TGF-β) and osteopontin have been implicated for interstitial fibrosis. TGF-β, a potent pro-fibrotic agent, and osteopontin (a macrophage chemoattractant) are elevated in CyA treated patients. Angiotensin II stimulates TGF-β and this raises a question if introduction of low dose angiotensin converting enzyme inhibitors or angiotensin II receptor blockers can ameliorate chronic nephrotoxicity of CyA. If introduced early post-transplant, a rise in serum creatinine due to these drugs can further confuse the clinical picture. A long-term clin-ical trial is needed to confirm this hypothesis. Until recently, it was difficult to differentiate chronic cyclosporine toxicity from chronic allo-graft nephropathy. The interstitial matrix accumulation and collagen deposition is different in these two conditions. Collagen types I and III accumulation in the interstitium is uniquely found in chronic CyA toxicity while collagen 4A3 and laminin β2, particularly in the proximal tubular basement membrane, accumulates in chronic rejection [6]. Hence by screening for type of collagen, the pathologist can now diagnose precisely the presence of either chronic rejection or CyA toxicity.

Direct Endothelial Toxicity

Lesions similar to thrombotic thrombocytopenia purpurahemolytic uremic syndrome (TTP-HUS) are seen due to direct endothelial toxicity and occasionally can be restricted to the kidneys. Damage can be severe leading to graft loss in some patients. For unknown reasons, conversion from one calcineurin inhibitor to another can lead to remission, even though both CyA and FK506 have been implicated as etiologic agents.

CyA leads to electrolyte imbalance manifested by hyperkalemia, hypomagnesemia, renal tubular acidosis and hypophosphatemia. The causes of hyperkalemia include reduction of GFR, aldosterone deficiency and resistance, reduced salt delivery to distal tubules and a direct effect causing "chloride shunt". An increased absorption of chloride along with sodium is postulated resulting in loss of electrogenic gradient for secretion of potassium. Hypomagnesemia and hypophos-phatemia are secondary to renal wasting. Decreased renal urate excretion leads to hyperuricemia.

Future

Since 1988, there has been a substantial increase in short-term and long-term survival of kidney grafts from both living and cadaveric donors [7] and this may be attributable to calcineurin inhibitors. Newer agents may be able to achieve same clinical results and trials with reduced dose of calcineurin inhibitors or total avoidance are currently underway. Until then, calcineurin inhibitors like CyA will remain as the backbone of immunosuppression.

References

1. Kovarik JM, Mueller EA, Van Bree JB et al: Transplantation 58: 658, 1994.
2. Kahan BD, Dunn J, Fitts C et al: Transplantation 59: 505, 1995.
3. Helderman J.H.: Lessons from the Neoral Global Database. Transplant Proc 30(5): 1721-2, 1998.
4. Gudmundsdottir H and Turka LA: New therapies for transplant rejection. J Am Soc Nephrol 10: 1356-65, 1999.
5. Jain J, McCaffrey PG, Valge-Archer VE & Rao A: Nuclear factor of activated T cells contains Fos and Jun. Nature 356: 801-4, 1992.
6. Abrass CK, Berfield AK, Stehman-Breen C, Alpers CE and Davis CL: Unique changes in Interstitial extracellular matrix composition are associated with rejection and cyclosporine toxicity in human renal allograft biopsies. Am J Kidney Dis 33: 11-20, 1999.
7. Hariharan S. Improved graft survival after renal transplantation in the United States, 1988 to 1996. N Engl J Med 342:605-12. 2000.

TACROLIMUS

Ron Shapiro

Introduction

Tacrolimus (Prograf, Fujisawa, Deerfield, IL, USA) is a macrocyclic lactone with a molecular weight of 822 daltons. (**Figure 1**) [1]. It was the first immunosuppressive agent to be discovered as a result of a deliberate search, rather than as the accidental byproduct of the investigation of antineoplastic or antibiotic agents. It was isolated in 1984 from fermentation broth of the soil organism streptomyces Tsukubaensis [2]. In 1986, Ochiai described its immunosuppressive capabilities in experimental transplantation at the Transplantation Society Congress in Helsinki, Finland [3]. In 1987, a great deal of pre-clinical data was presented in Gothenburg, Sweden, [4] and in 1989, the first clinical reports were presented in Barcelona, Spain. [5] Since then, it has been used as an immunosuppressive agent in the trans-plantation of all solid organs. This chapter will start by discussing the mechanism of action of tacrolimus, and then go on to summarize its use as both primary immunosuppressive agent and as rescue agent in adult and pediatric sold organ transplantation (emphasizing the most recent multi-center and selected single center trial data), its dosage, its use in combination with other immunosuppressive agents, and, finally, its side-effect profile.

Mechanism of Action

The mechanism of action of tacrolimus is similar to that of cyclosporine, in that it is a predominantly T cell-specific calcineurin inhibitor [6,7].

Mohamed Sayegh and Giuseppe Remuzzi (editors), Current and Future
Immunosuppressive Therapies Following Transplantation, 123-142.
© 2001 Kluwer Academic Publishers. Printed in the Netherlands.

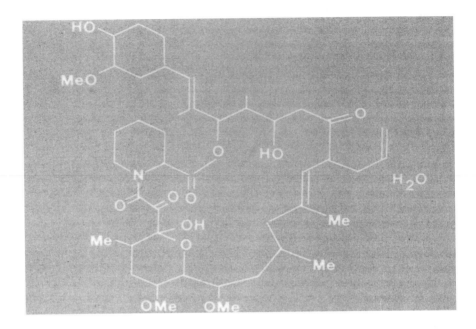

Figure 1. Structure of Tacrolimus

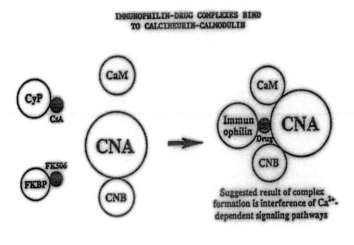

Figure 2. Mechanism of Action (a): Tacrolimus binds to FKBP; the complex of Tacrolimus/FKBP binds to calcineurin.

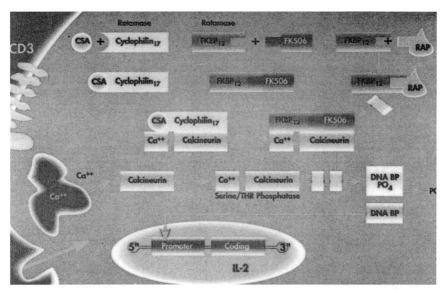

Figure 3. Mechanism of Action (b): Tacrolimus-induced inhibition of calcineurin phosphatase inhibits dephosphorylation of NF-AT, rendering it incapable of migrating to the nucleus to initiate 1L-2 transcription.

Like cyclosporine, tacrolimus is a prodrug; to be effective it must bind intracytoplasmically with its specific binding protein, FKBP (**Figure 2**) [8,9]. The tacrolimus/FKBP complex then binds to calcineurin (at a site different from that of the cyclosporine / cyclophilin complex) [10]. This binding, which a calcium-dependent event, blocks the phosphatase activity of calcineurin and thus inhibits the dephosphorylation of Nuclear Factor of Activated T Cells (NFAT) (**Figure 3**). [7-9] This blocks the migration of NFAT into the nucleus to initiate IL-2 transcription (calcineurin apparently also participates in this migration) [7,10]. There are probably other mechanisms of action of tacrolimus, but the calcineurin inhibition is perhaps the most important and best understood.

Clinical Immunosuppression – Primary

Liver

Tacrolimus has been used as a primary immunosuppressive agent in both single-center and multi-center trials of orthotopic liver transplantation (**Table 1**). The first trials, in Pittsburgh, [11-14] were followed by two pivotal multi-center trials, in the United States and Europe, comparing tacrolimus with the original formulation of cyclosporine [15,16]. These trials, in fact, led to FDA approval of tacrolimus in 1994.

Table 1. Liver Transplantation – Primary

American Multi-Center Trial (5-year data)	Tacrolimus	Cyclosporine	P
Patient Survival - Overall	79.0%	73.1%	NS
Patient Survival - Hepatitis C	78.1%	69.5%	0.041
Graft Survival - Overall	71.8%	66.4%	NS
Rejection	68%	76%	0.0002
Steroid-Resistant Rejection	19%	36%	0.001
Cholesterol (mg/dl)	182	210	0.0005

Five-year actuarial outcomes of the American multi-center trial demonstrated 79.0% patient survival and 71.8% graft survival in patients randomized to tacrolimus, and 73.1% patient survival and 66.4% graft survival in the patients randomized to cyclosporine; these differences were not statistically significant [17]. In the subset of patients with hepatitis C, 5-year patient survival rates were better in tacrolimus-treated patients, 78.1%, than in cyclosporine-treated patients, 69.5% (p = 0.041). The incidences of biopsy-proven rejection and steroid-resistant rejection were lower in tacrolimus-treated patients, 68% and 19%, than in the cyclosporine-treated patients, 76% (p < 0.0002) and 36% (p < 0.001). Renal function and the incidences of post-transplant lymphoproliferative disorder (PTLD) and post-transplant diabetes mellitus (PTDM) were comparable. Cholesterol levels were lower in the tacrolimus-treated patients, 182 mg/dl, then in the cyclosporine-treated patients, 210 mg/dl (p = 0.0005).

Single-center data from the University of Pittsburgh on 1000 patients receiving tacrolimus-based therapy showed outcomes generally similar to those from the American multi-center trial [18]. However, some two-thirds of successfully transplanted patients were able to be weaned off steroids, and outcomes in pediatric patients were particularly good, with 7-year actuarial patient survival rates of 80%-90%.

Table 2. Kidney Transplantation – Primary

American Multi-Center Trial (3-year data)	Tacrolimus	Cyclosporine	P
Patient Survival	91.7%	92.3%	NS
Graft Survival	81.9%	77.8%	NS
Rejection	27.8%	44.4%	0.001
Steroid-Resistant Rejection	10.7%	25.1%	0.001

Kidney

After initial single-center reports from Pittsburgh suggesting its utility in renal transplantation [19-23], tacrolimus was studied in a phase II [24,25] and then a phase III American multi-center trial, and was compared with the original formulation of cyclosporine (**Table 2**) [26-28]. All patients received induction antibody therapy, azathioprine, and steroids. A parallel European trial, without antibody induction, was also performed [29-30]. Three-year actuarial data from the American multi-center trial showed comparable patient and graft survival, 91.7% and 81.9%, respectively, in the tacrolimus-treated patients, and 92.3% and 77.8%, respectively, in the cyclosporine-treated patients [28]. The incidences of rejection and steroid-resistant rejection were lower in the tacrolimus-treated patients, 27.8% and 10.7%, than in the cyclosporine-treated patients, 44.4% and 25.1% (p < .001) [26]. Crossover from cyclosporine to tacrolimus because of refractory acute rejection was also more common, and was seen in 16.2% of cases. Cholesterol levels were lower in the tacrolimus-treated patients, as was the incidence of hypertension [26,28,31] Renal function was similar between the two groups, as was the incidence of malignancy. The incidence of PTDM was significantly higher at 1 and 3 years in the tacrolimus-treated patients, 19.9% and 11.3%, than in the cyclosporine-treated patients, 4% (p<0.001 - **Table 3**) [28]. Subsequent trials have shown a lower incidence of PTDM, 7.0%, in a multi-center trial of patients receiving tacrolimus and mycophenolate mofetil (MMF), [32] and an initial and final incidence of 7.0% and 2.9% in a single-center trial of patients receiving tacrolimus and steroids with or without MMF (**Table 3**) [33].

Table 3. Kidney Transplantation -- Post-Transplant Diabetes Mellitus (PTDM)

	Tacrolimus		Cyclosporine		P
	Initial	Final	Initial	Final	
American Multi-Center Trial	19.9%	11.8%	4%*	4%	0.001
Multi-center Trial**(Tacrolimus/MMF vs. Neoral/MMF)	7.0%		7.0%***		
Pittsburgh Trial (Tacrolimus with or without MMF)	7.0%	2.9%			

*Standard formulation of cyclosporine
**A 3rd arm, tacrolimus/azathioprine had an incidence of 14%.
***Microemulsion formulation of cyclosporine

Table 4. Kidney Transplantation - Pediatric – Primary

Pittsburgh Data	N = 82	
Patient Survival	1-year	99%
	4-year	94%
Graft Survival	1-year	98%
	4-year	84%
Steroid Withdrawal		66%
Anti-hypertensive Medication Withdrawal		86%
Post-Transplant Lymphoproliferative Disorder	12/89 – 12/92*	17%
	1/93 – 12/96	4%

*2 additional cases of late lymphoma in this subgroup

There are to date no multi-center pediatric trials of tacrolimus in renal transplantation, and only a small number of single-center experiences, the largest of which is from Pittsburgh (**Table 4**) [34,35]. One and 4-year actuarial patient and graft survival rates of 99% and 94%, and 98% and 84%, respectively, have been reported [35]. Steroids were discontinued in some two-thirds of successfully transplanted patients, with significant catch-up growth, and antihypertensive medications were withdrawn in over 80% of patients. Early EBV-related PTLD has been a particularly worrisome problem in this group, although the incidence has declined from 17% to 4%, as more experience has been acquired with the agent. In addition, there were 2 additional cases of late PTLD, both of which required chemotherapy to eradicate the lymphoma. The outcomes in the children that did develop PTLD have been quite good, with 5-year patient and graft survival rates of 100% and 89%, respectively [36].

Pancreas

Tacrolimus has also been used as a primary immunosuppressive agent in pancreatic transplantation, most commonly in simultaneous pancreas/kidney transplantation (SPK) but also in pancreas after kidney transplantation (PAK), and pancreas transplantation alone (PTA) (**Table 5**) [37-42]. While single-center, multi-center, and regis-try reports have all been published, no large multi-center, randomized trials have been performed to compare tacrolimus with cyclosporine. Matched pair analysis using historical controls has suggested better outcomes under tacrolimus-based therapy [37], but registry data has suggested better outcomes with tacrolimus only in PAK patients [38].

Table 5. Pancreas – Primary

1 Year Graft Survival	Tacrolimus		Cyclosporine	
	Review	Registry	Review*	Registry
Simultaneous Kidney/Pancreas	88%**	81%	73%	82%
Pancreas After Kidney	85%	84%***	65%	65%
Pancreas Transplant Alone	68%	64%	70%	66%

*Matched pair historical control
**p = 0.0002
***p = 0.04

Heart

The first single-center reports of tacrolimus in heart transplantation also came from Pittsburgh [43], with subsequent reports suggesting less rejection in tacrolimus-treated patients than in cyclosporine-treated patients (**Table 6**) [44]. A multi-center trial showed no difference in patient or graft survival, but did show a lower incidence of hypertension and lower cholesterol levels in the tacrolimus-treated patients [45].

Table 6. Heart – Primary

Rejection	Tacrolimus	Cyclosporine	Cyclosporine//RATG
Pittsburgh (N=243)	53%[+]	78%	47%
Multi-center (N=85) Rejection	60%	65%	
Cholesterol (mg/dl)	186 ± 40*	212 ± 46	
Hypertension (N)	13**	24	
Hyperglycemia	14%	12%	

*p<0.02
**p=0.05
[+]p<0.01 (vs cyclosporine)

Lung

There are no multi-center reports of primary lung transplantation under tacrolimus-based therapy. A single-center trial, again from Pittsburgh, comparing tacrolimus with the original formulation of cyclosporine, showed no difference in patient survival, but did show a trend toward

less acute rejection (**Table 7**) and a lower incidence of obliterative bronchiolitis in the tacrolimus-treated patients than in the cyclosporine-treated patients, and more crossovers from cyclosporine to tacrolimus [46].

Table 7. Lung – Primary

Pittsburgh (N=133)	Tacrolimus	Cyclosporine
Rejection/100 patient days	0.85	10.9
Obliterative Bronchitis	22%*	38%
Crossover (N)	T→C**	C→T
	2	13

*p=0.015
**p=0.02

Clinical Immunosuppression – Rescue

Liver

Early reports from Pittsburgh suggested that successful rescue with tacrolimus was possible in liver transplant patients with either acute or chronic rejection (**Table 8**) [47,48]. Subsequent reports in pediatric patients confirmed the long-term utility of rescue for acute rejection, with 5-year patient and graft survival rates of 90%, but showed worse results after rescue for chronic rejection, with 5-year patient and graft survival rates of 70% and 55%, respectively [49].

Table 8. Liver – Rescue

	Survival		Time
	Patient	Graft	
Pittsburgh			
Early Report			
Acute Rejection	83%	78%	9 months
Chronic Rejection	100%	67%	9 months
Late Report (Pediatric)			
Acute Rejection	90%	90%	5 years
Chronic Rejection	70%	55%	5 years
Multi-center (Adult)			
Chronic	84.4%	69.9%	1 year
	81.2%	48.5%	2 years

A multi-center trial of rescue for chronic rejection after liver transplantation showed 1- and 2-year actuarial patient survival rates of 84.4% and 81.2%, and 1- and 2-year actuarial graft survival rates of 69.9% and 48.5% [50].

Table 9. Kidney – Rescue

1 Year Survival	Patient (mg/dl)	Graft Creatinine	Serum	CMV Rejection	Recurrent
Pittsburgh	92%	74%	2.3	4%	4%
Multi-center	93%	75%	2.2	4%	16%

Pittsburgh	Pediatric Survival	
	Patient	Graft
1 year	100%	75%
2 years	100%	68%

Kidney

Rescue for acute rejection in both adults and children was described initially by the Pittsburgh group [51-54], and confirmed by other single-center studies [55-58] and by a multi-center trial (**Table 9**) [59]. None of these trials was randomized, although there have been remarkably similar outcomes in the Pittsburgh studies and in the multi-center trial reports, with 1-year patient survival rates of 92%-100% and graft survival rates of 74%-75%.   Chronic rejection is probably a contraindication to rescue with tacrolimus.

A multi-center trial of conversion from cyclosporine to tacrolimus for hypercholesterolemia was performed, with no change in renal function and a significant fall in cholesterol levels [60]. In addition, there are reports of conversion for cyclosporine-associated hirsutism and gum hyperplasia, with good outcomes [61].

Pancreas

A multi-center report described a non-randomized experience with rescue therapy in SPK, PAK, and PTA recipients, with success rates of 89%, 69%, and 58%, respectively (**Table 10**) [37].

Table 10. Pancreas – Rescue

	1 Year Graft Survival
Simultaneous Pancreas/Kidney (SPK)	89%
Pancreas After Kidney (PAK)	69%
Pancreas Transplant Alone (PTA)	58%

Heart

There are small multi-center and single-center experiences with tacrolimus rescue in heart transplant recipients, with uniform success [43, 63].

Lung

There are small multi-center and single-center experiences with tacrolimus as a rescue agent after lung transplantation [46,62]. In general, a marked decrease in rejection has been seen after conversion to tacrolimus.

Dosage

Most centers using tacrolimus-based immunosuppression have used the oral formulation exclusively. As an example, the multi-center kid-ney trials have started with oral tacrolimus 0.2-0.3 mg/kg/day in divided doses [24-30] (**Table 11**). Various trials have started tacrolimus either immediately after transplantation or waited until good kidney function has been achieved; in the latter situation, antibody induction has been employed. Initial target levels have been 10-20 ng/ml for the first 3 months, and 5-15 ng/ml thereafter [26-30]. The only two programs to advocate intravenous tacrolimus have been the Pittsburgh and the Miami groups. The former have routinely employed a continuous infusion for 1-2 days of 0.025-0.05 mg/kg/day in adults (0.05-0.10 mg/kg/day in children for 3-5 days), aiming for levels of 20 –25 ng/ml for the first two weeks, 15-20 ng/ml by one month, 10-15 ng/ml by 3 months, and 5-12 ng/ml (5-9 ng/ml in children) chronically [33,35]. The Miami group has used a short course of intravenous tacrolimus, 1 mg/24 hours, in a series of SPK recipients, with good results [41]. In both instances, antibody induction has not been used.

Table 11. Dosage

	Initial Dose (mg/kg/d)	Target Levels (ng/ml)
Multi-center Trials	0.2 – 0.3 po 5 – 15 (chronic)	10 – 20 (1st 3 months)
Pittsburgh	0.025 – 0.05 IV (0.05 – 0.1 pediatric) continuous Infusion then 0.3 po	20 – 25 (1st week) 15 – 20 (1 month) 10 – 15 (3 months) 5 – 12 (chronic) (5-9 pediatric)

Tacrolimus in Combination with Other Immunosuppressive Agents

Tacrolimus/Steroids

With rare exceptions, tacrolimus has always been used with steroids. One trial of tacrolimus monotherapy has been reported, with quite favorable results, from a program that has had a tradition of using cyclosporine monotherapy as well (**Table 12**) [63]. Virtually every other transplant program has used tacrolimus in combination with steroids. The Pittsburgh program has routinely attempted to wean steroids completely and has reported success in approximately two-thirds of successfully transplanted patients [35,64]. In adult kidney recipients, the 3-year patient and graft survival rates in patients weaned off steroids were 98% and 94%, respectively; in patients who were unable to come off steroids (and who had a number of risk factors, including more delayed graft function, more acute rejection, and older donor age), the 3-year actuarial patient and graft survival rates were 80% and 50% [64]. In pediatric patients, over 90% of patients were weaned off steroids, although only 70% were able to remain off steroids chronically [36]. In children weaned off steroids, the 5-year actuarial patient and graft survival rates, were 96% and 82% (without any difference in outcomes in the patients who had to resume steroids), while in children who were never able to be taken off steroids, the 5-year actuarial patient and graft survival rates were 83% and 33%, respectively [36].

A small series from the University of Chicago has attempted routine steroid withdrawal by one week after transplantation, with excellent initial results [65].

Tacrolimus/Azathioprine

Tacrolimus has been used routinely with azathioprine in the American multi-center kidney trial, without any apparent problems (**Table 13**) [26,27. A single-center randomized trial of tacrolimus and steroids, with or without azathioprine, actually showed worse outcomes in the patients randomized to azathioprine, with 3-year graft survival rates of 76%, versus 84% in the patients randomized to tacrolimus/steroids [66,67].

Tacrolimus/Mycophenolate Mofetil (MMF)

In renal transplantation, the combination of tacrolimus and MMF has been evaluated in a prospective, randomized, multi-center trial [32,68], a prospective, randomized, single-center trial [33], and a non-randomized, single-center trial (**Table 13**) [69]. All three have

Table 12. Steroid Withdrawal/Avoidance

Manchester (England)	Avoidance			
	Recruited	Entered	Remained in Trial	Rejection
	N=45	30	26	29%

	Withdrawal		
Pittsburgh*	Withdrawn	Never Withdrawn	
Adults (N=379)	76%	24%	
Median time to withdrawal (months)	10		
Patient Survival			
1-year	99%	91%	
3-year	98%	80%	
Graft Survival			
1-year	98%	77%	
3-year	94%	50%	

Pittsburgh**	Withdrawn	Withdrawn/ Restarted+	Never Withdrawn
Pediatric (N=80)	70%	22.5%	7.5%
Median time to withdrawal (months)	5.7		
Patient Survival			
1-year	100%	100%	100%
5-year	96%	100%	83%
Graft Survival			
1-year	100%	100%	100%
5-year	82%	83%	33%

Chicago (N=52)	Steroid withdrawal at one week	
Patient Survival	100%	(F/U=18 months)
Graft Survival	96%	
Rejection	25%	
Steroid-Resistant Rejection	12%	
Off Steroids	76%	

*18/397 (4.5%) and
**2/82 (2.4%) patients lost their allografts < 3 weeks after transplantation and were excluded from the analysis
+39% of patients withdrawn and restarted were eventually withdrawn again

Table 13. Tacrolimus / Other Agents

Azathioprine		
Pittsburgh (N=397)	*Tacrolimus/Prednisone*	*Tacrolimus/AZA/Pred*
Patient Survival		
1-year	97%	94%
3-year	94%	90%
Graft Survival		
1-year	90%	88%
3-year	84%[+]	76%

Mycophenolate Mofetil (MMF)		
Miami (N=170)	*Tacrolimus/Prednisone*	*Tacrolimus/MMF/Pred*
Patient Survival 1-year	96%	98%
Graft Survival 1-year	94%	97%
Rejection	21.4%	8.2%**
Pittsburgh (N=208)		
Patient Survival* 1-year	95%	98%
Graft Survival* 1-year	92%	93%
Rejection	44%	27%***
Steroid-Resistant Rejection	7.5%	2.9%

Multicenter (N=176)	Tac/AZA	*Tac/MMF/1gm*	*Tac/MMF/2gm*
Rejection	36%	35%	9%****
Steroid Resistant-Rejection	9%	13%	3%

	Patient	*Graft*
1-Year Survival (overall)	95%	94%

Multicenter (N=223)	*Tac/MMF/Pred*	*Tac/AZA/Pred*	*Neoral/MMF/Pred*
Patient Survival 1-Year	94%	89%	96%
Graft Survival 1-Year	89%	87%	88%
Acute Rejection	15%	17%	20%
Steroid Resistant Rejection	4%	12%	11%

[+]p=0.031   *Patients <60 years, without delayed graft function
**p=0.003   ***p=0.014   ****p=.0075

confirmed the efficacy of the combination, with rejection rates as low as 8%-10% in patients receiving antibody induction [32,68,69]. The combination of tacrolimus and MMF has also been described in pancreas transplantation, with similar claims of efficacy [39-42]. A prospective, randomized trial in liver transplantation has shown a small, but not significant reduction in the incidence of rejection [70].

Tacrolimus/Sirolimus

There are very preliminary clinical data from the Halifax group (based on promising pre-clinical data) utilizing the combination of low dose tacrolimus, sirolimus, and steroids in liver and kidney/pancreas recipients [71-73]. These data suggest that this combination is exceptionally effective in preventing rejection. Anecdotal reports of the combination of tacrolimus and sirolimus for the rescue of rejecting renal allografts have been described but not yet reported.

Side Effects

Tacrolimus is comparably nephrotoxic when compared with cyclosporine, and histopathologic findings have been similar [74-78]. Neurotoxicity is manifested principally by tremor, insomnia, and paresthesia of the extremities; these tend to be dose-dependent and reversible with dosage reduction [79]. Diabetogenicity (**Table 3**) has been described above; [26,28,32,33] as more experience has been acquired with tacrolimus, the incidence of PTDM has not been different from that reported under cyclosporine-based immunosuppression. Viral complications and malignancies have been similar in both incidence and classification, with the exception of the increased incidence of EBV-related PTLD (**Table 4**) in pediatric renal allografts recipients early in the experience with tacrolimus (described above) [34,35]. As in the case of PTDM, the incidence of PTLD has declined with time.

Summary

Tacrolimus has been used as a primary and rescue immunosuppressive agent in the transplantation of all solid organs. In general, the various studies have suggested that it is comparable to or better than cyclosporine-based therapy, in terms of patient and graft survival. Tacrolimus clearly seems to be associated with lower rejection rates, lower steroid requirements, less hypertension, and lower cholesterol levels than cyclosporine. Tacrolimus is comparable to cyclosporine in terms of nephrotoxicity and neurotoxicity. Early concerns about the increased diabetogenicity of tacrolimus have not been confirmed in more recent reports, and problems with EBV-related PTLD have become less of an issue over time, as more experience has been acquired with the drug. It is important to point out that relatively few studies have been performed comparing tacrolimus with the microemulsion form-ulation of cyclosporine. The combination of tacrolimus and MMF seems to be effective in reducing the rate of acute rejection. The combination of tacrolimus and sirolimus remains to be explored in depth, but early reports are promising.

In conclusion, tacrolimus is an effective immunosuppressive agent in solid organ transplantation, and offers a number of important advantages over conventional immunosuppressive agents.

References

1. Thomson AW.   Mechanisms of action of immunosuppressive agents. Renal Transplantation (Eds. R Shapiro, RL Simmons, TE Starzl), Appleton & Lange, pgs. 163-175, 1997.
2. Goto T, Kino T, Hatanaka H, et al.   Discovery of FK-506, a novel immunosuppressant isolated from streptomyces tsukubaensis.   Trans Proc, 14(5):4-8, 1987.
3. Ochiai T, Nakajima K, Nagata M, et al. Trans Proc, 19:1284, 1987.
4. Iwasaki Y.   FK-506 – a potential breakthrough in immunosuppression. Transplantation Proceedings (TE Starzl, L Makowka, S Todo), Grune & Stratton; Harcourt Brace Jovanovich, Inc, Vol XIX, #5, Suppl. 6, 1987.
5. Starzl TE, Todo S, Fung JJ, Groth C.   FK 506 – a potential breakthrough in immunosuppression—clinical implications. Trans Proc, XXII(1), (Eds. TE Starzl, S Todo, JJ Fung, C Groth), Appleton & Lange, 1990.
6. Thomson AW, Starzl TE.   Immunosuppressive Drugs: developments in anti-rejection therapy. Boston, Little, Brown, 1994.
7. Sigal NH, Dumont FJ.   Cyclosporin A, FK-506, and rapamycin: pharmacologic probes of lymphocyte signal transduction.   Annu Rev Immunol, 10:519-560, 1992.
8. Schreiber SL, Liu J, Albers MW, et al.   Immunophilin-ligand complexes as probes of intracellular signaling pathways. Trans Proc, 23(6):2839-2844, 1991.
9. Ullman KS, Flanagan WM, Cothesy B, Kuo P, Northrop JP, Crabtree GR.   Site of action of cyclosporine and FK 506 in the pathways of communication between the T-lymphocyte antigen receptor and the early activation genes. Trans Proc, 23(6):2845, 1991.
10. Halloran P, personal communication.
11. Starzl TE, Todo S, Fung J, Demetris AJ, Venkataramman R, Jain A. FK 506 for liver, kidney, and pancreas transplantation. Lancet, 2(8670):1000-1004, 1989.
12. Todo S, Fung JJ, Starzl TE.   Liver, kidney, and thoracic organ transplantation under FK506. Ann Surg, 212:295, 1990.
13. Fung JJ, Abu-Elmagd K, Jain A, et al.   A randomized trial of FK506 vs. cyclosporine. Trans Proc, 23:2977, 1991.
14. Todo S, Fung JJ, Starzl TE, et al.   Single-center experience with primary orthotopic liver transplantation under FK506 immunosuppression. Ann Surg, 222:270-280, 1995.
15. The U.S. Multi-center FK506 Liver Study Group. A comparison of tacrolimus (FK 506) and cyclosporine for immunosuppression in liver transplantation. N Eng J Med, 331(17):1110-1115, 1994.
16. European FK506 Multicentre Liver Study Group.   Randomised trial comparing tacrolimus (FK506) and cyclosporin in prevention of liver allograft rejection. Lancet, 344(8920):423-428, 1994.
17. Wiesner RH. A long-term comparison of tacrolimus (FK506) versus cyclosporine in liver transplantation.   A report of the United States FK506 Study Group. Transplantation, 66(4):493-499, 1998.
18. Jain A, Reyes J, Kashyap R, et al. Liver transplantation under tacrolimus in infants, children, adults, and seniors: long-term results, survival, and adverse events in 1000 consecutive patients. Trans Proc, 30(4):1403-1404, 1998
19. Starzl TE, Fung JJ, Jordan M, et al. Kidney transplantation under FK506. Trans Proc, 23:920, 1993.
20. Shapiro R, Todo S, Starzl TE.   Kidney transplantation under FK506 immunosuppression. Trans Proc, 23:920, 1991.
21. Shapiro R, Jordan ML, Scantlebury V, et al.   FK506 in clinical kidney transplantation. Trans Proc, 23:3065, 1991.

22. Shapiro R, Jordan M, Scantlebury V, et al. A prospective, randomized trial of FK506 in renal transplantation: a comparison between double and triple drug therapy. Clin Transplant, 8:508, 1994.

23. Shapiro R, Jordan ML, Scantlebury VP, et al. A prospective, randomized trial of FK506-based immunosuppression after renal transplantation. Transplantation, 59:485-490, 1995.

24. Laskow DA, Vincenti F, Neylan J, Mendez R, Matas A. Phase II FK506 multi-center concentration control study: one-year follow-up. Trans Proc, 22:809, 1995.

25. Vincenti F, Laskow DA, Neylan JF, Mendez R, Matas AJ. One-year follow-up of an open-label trial of FK506 for primary kidney transplantation. A report of the U.S. Multi-center FK506 Kidney Transplant Group. Transplantation, 61(11):1576-1581, 1996.

26. Pirsch JD, Miller J, Deierhoi MH, et al. A comparison of tacrolimus (FK506) and cyclosporine for immunosuppression after cadaveric renal transplantation. Transplantation, 63:977-983, 1997.

27. Miller J, Pirsch JD, Deierhoi R. FK506 in kidney transplantation: results of the U.S.A. randomized comparative phase III study. Trans Proc, 29:304-305, 1997.

28. Jensik SC. Tacrolimus (FK 506) in kidney transplantation: three-year survival results of the US multi-center, randomized, comparative trial. FK 506 Kidney Transplant Study Group. Trans Proc, 30(4):1216-1218, 1998.

29. Schleibner S, Krauss M, Wagner K, et al. FK506 versus cyclosporin in the prevention of renal allograft rejection: European pilot study—six-week results. Transplant Int, 8:86-90, 1995.

30. Mayer AD, Dmitrewski J, Squifflet JP, et al. Multi-center randomized trial comparing tacrolimus (FK506) and cyclosporine in the prevention of renal allograft rejection: a report of the European Tacrolimus Multi-center Renal Study Group. Transplantation, 64(3):436-443, 1997.

31. Laskow DA. Hypertension in renal transplant recipients: 2-year results from the FK506 multi-center, randomized comparative trial. The International Congress of Immunosuppression, December 11-13, 1997.

32. Miller J. Tacrolimus and mycophenolate mofetil in renal transplant recipients: one year results of a multi-center, randomized dose ranging trial. FK506/MMF Dose-Ranging Kidney Transplant Study Group. Transplantation Proceedings. 31(1-2):276-7, 1999 Feb-Mar.

33. Shapiro R, Jordan ML, Scantlebury VP, et al. A Prospective, Randomized Trial of Tacrolimus/Prednisone versus Tacrolimus/Prednisone/Mycophenolate Mofetil in Renal Transplant Recipients. Transplantation, 67(3):411-415, 1999.

34. Shapiro R, Scantlebury VP, Jordan ML, et al. Tacrolimus in pediatric renal transplantation. Transplantation, 62(12):1752-1758, 1996.

35. Shapiro R, Scantlebury VP, Jordan ML, et al. Pediatric renal transplantation under tacrolimus-based immunosuppression. Transplantation, 67(2):299-303, 1999.

36. Chakrabarti P, Wong HY, Scantlebury VP, et al. Outcome after steroid withdrawal in pediatric renal transplant patients receiving tacrolimus-based immunosuppression. Presented at the 18th Annual Scientific Meeting of the American Society of Transplantation, May, 1999.

37. Gruessner RW. Tacrolimus in pancreas transplantation: a multi-center analysis. Tacrolimus Pancreas Transplant Study Group. Clin Trans, 11(4):299-312, 1997.

38. Gruessner A, Sutherland DER. Pancreas transplantation in the United States (US) and non-US as reported to the United Network for Organ Sharing (UNOS) and the International Pancreas Transplant Registry (IPTR). Clinical Transplants 1996 (J Michael Cecka, Paul I Terasaki, eds; UCLA Tissue Typing Laboratory, Los Angeles, CA) pgs 47-67, 1996.

39. Stratta RJ.   Simultaneous use of tacrolimus and mycophenolate mofetil in combined pancreas-kidney transplant recipients: a multi-center report.   The FK/MMF Multi-Center Study Group. Trans Proc, 29(1-2):654-655, 1997.
40. Bruce DS, Woodle ES, Newel KA, et al.   Effects of tacrolimus, mycophenolate mofetil, and cyclosporine microemulsion on rejection incidence in synchronous pancreas-kidney transplantation. Trans Proc, 30(2):507-508, 1998.
41. Burke GW, Ciancio G, Alejandro R, et al.   Use of tacrolimus and mycophenolate mofetil for pancreas-kidney transplantation with or without OKT3 induction. Trans Proc, 30(4):1544-1545, 1998.
42. Kaufman DB, Leventhal JR, Stuart J, Abecassis MM, Fryer JP.   Stuart JP. Mycophenolate   mofetil   and   tacrolimus   as   primary   maintenance immunosuppression in simultaneous pancreas-kidney transplantation: initial experience in 50 consecutive cases. Transplantation, 67(4):586-593, 1998.
43. Armitage JM, Kormos RL, Fung J, Starzl TE.   The clinical trial of FK 506 as primary and rescue immunosuppression in adult cardiac transplantation. Trans Proc, 23(6):3054-3057, 1991.
44. Pham SM, Kormos RL, Hattler BG, et al.   A prospective trial of tacrolimus (FK 506) in clinical heart transplantation: intermediate-term results. J Thoracic & Cardiovascular Surgery, 111(4):764-772, 1996.
45. Taylor DO, Barr ML, Radovancevic B, et al.   A randomized, multi-center comparison of tacrolimus and cyclosporine immunosuppressive regimens in cardiac transplantation: decreased hyperlipidemia and hypertension with tacrolimus.   Presented at the International Society of Heart and Lung Transplantation, 1997.
46. Keenan RJ, Konishi H, Kawai A, et al.   Clinical trial of tacrolimus versus cyclosporine in lung transplantation.   Ann Thoracic Surgery, 60(3):580-584, 1995.
47. Fung JJ, Todo S, Jain A, McCauley J, Alessiani M, Scotti C, Starzl TE.   Conversion from cyclosporine to FK 506 in liver allograft recipients with cyclosporine-related complications. Trans Proc, 22(1):6-12, 1990.
48. Demetris AJ, Fung JJ, Todo S, et al.   FK 506 used as rescue therapy for human liver allograft recipients. Trans Proc, 23(6):3005-3006, 1991.
49. Reyes J, Jain A, Mazariegos G, Kashyap N, Fung J, Starzl TE.   Conversion of pediatric liver allograft recipients from cyclosporin to tacrolimus based immunosuppression: mean seven years follow-up. Hepatology, 28(No.4, Pt 2) :pg 351A(Abstract 754), 1998.
50. Sher LS, Cosenza CA, Michel J, et al.   Efficacy of tacrolimus as rescue therapy for chronic rejection in orthotopic liver transplantation: a report of the U.S. Multi-center Liver Study Group. Transplantation, 64(2):258-263, 1997.
51. Jordan ML, Shapiro R, Vivas CA, et al.   FK506 salvage of renal allografts with ongoing rejection failing cyclosporine immunosuppression.   Trans Proc, 25(1):638-640, 1993.
52. Jordan M, Shapiro R, Vivas C, et al.   FK506 rescue for resistant rejection of renal allograft under primary cyclosporine immunosuppression.   Transplantation, 57(6):860-865, 1994.
53. Shapiro R, Jordan ML, Scantlebury VP, et al.   FK506 in pediatric kidney transplantation—primary and rescue experience.   Pediatr Nephr, 9:S43-S48, 1995.
54. Jordan ML, Naraghi R, Shapiro R, et al.   Tacrolimus rescue therapy for renal allograft rejection-five year experience. Transplantation, 63(2):223-228, 1997.
55. Mathew A, Talbot D, Minford EJ, et al.   Reversal of steroid-resistant rejection in renal allograft recipients using Fk506. Transplantation, 60:1182-1184, 1995.
56. Felldin M, Backman L, Brattstrom C, et al.   Rescue therapy with tacrolimus (FK506) in renal transplant recipients: A multi-center analysis. Trans Proc, 27:3425, 1995.

57. Ciancio G, Roth D, Burke G, et al. Renal transplantation in a new immunosuppressive era. Trans Proc, 27:812-813, 1995.
58. Corey HE, Tellis V, Schechner R, Greenstein SM. Improved renal allograft survival in children treated with FK506 (tacrolimus) rescue therapy. Pediatr Neph, 10:720-722, 1996.
59. Woodle ES, Thistlethwaite JR, Gordon JH, et al. A multi-center trial of FK506 (tacrolimus) therapy in refractory acute renal allograft rejection. A report of the Tacrolimus Kidney Transplantation Rescue Study Group. Transplantation, 62(5):594-599, 1996.
60. McCune TR, Thacker LK II, Peters TG, et al. Effects of tacrolimus on hyperlipidemia after successful renal transplantation: a Southeastern Organ Procurement Foundation multi-center clinical study. Transplantation, 65(1):87-92, 1998.
61. Busque S, Demers P, St-Louis G, et al. Conversion from neoral (cyclosporine) to tacrolimus of kidney transplant recipients for gingival hyperplasia or hypertrichosis. Trans Proc, 30:1247-1248, 1998.
62. Mentzer RM Jr., Jahania MS, Lasley RD. Tacrolimus as a rescue immunosuppressant after heart and lung transplantation. The U.S. Multi-center FK506 Study Group. Transplantation, 65(1):109-113, 1998.
63. Campbell BA, Johnson RWG, Short CD, Roberts ISD. Tacrolimus monotherapy in primary renal allograft transplantation. The International Congress on Immunosuppression, December 11-13, 1997.
64. Shapiro R, Jordan ML, Scantlebury VP, et al. Outcome after steroid withdrawal in renal transplant patients receiving tacrolimus-based immunosuppression. Trans Proc, 10, 1375-1377, 1998.
65. Grewal HP, Thistlethwaite JR Jr, Loss GE, et al. Corticosteroid cessation 1 week following renal transplantation using tacrolimus/mycophenolate mofetil based immunosuppression. Trans Proc, 30(4):1378-1379, 1998.
66. Shapiro R, Jordan ML, Scantlebury VP, et al. Tacrolimus in renal transplantation. Trans Proc, 28(4):2117-2118, 1996.
67. Shapiro R, Jordan ML, Scantlebury VP, et al. The superiority of tacrolimus in renal transplant recipients: the Pittsburgh experience. Clinical Transplants 1995. (Eds. PI Terasaki, JM Cecka) UCLA Tissue Typing Laboratory, Los Angeles, pgs 199-205, 1996.
68. Johnson C, Ahsan N, Gonwa T, et al. Randomized comparative trial of prograf (tacrolimus) in combination with azathioprine or mycophenolate mofetil versus Neoral® (cyclosporine) with mycophenolate mofetil after kidney transplantation. The 17th Annual Scientific Meeting of the American Society of Transplant Physicians, May, 1998.
69. Roth D, Colona J, Burke GW, Ciancio G, Esquenazi V, Miller J. Primary immunosuppression with tacrolimus and mycophenolate mofetil for renal allograft recipients. Transplantation, 65(2):248-252, 1998.
70. Jain AB, Hamad I, Rakela J, et al. A prospective randomized trial of tacrolimus and prednisone versus tacrolimus, prednisone and mycophenolate mofetil in primary adult liver transplant recipients. Transplantation, 66(10):1395-1398, 1998.
71. MacDonald AS. Clinical implications of immunosuppressive cytokine inhibitors. The 17th World Congress of the Transplantation Society, 1998.
72. McAlister VC, Peltekian K, Gao Z, Mahalari K, Dominuques J, MacDonald AS. Liver and kidney-pancreas transplantation using tacrolimus, sirolimus and steroid immunosuppression. Abstract, Presented at the 25th Annual meeting of the American Society of Transplant Surgeons, May, 1999.
73. Mahalau K, McAlister V, Peltikian K, Dominguez J, Gao ZH, MacDonald AS. A clinical pharmacokinetic study of tacrolimus and sirolimus combination

immunosuppression. Presented at the 18th Annual scientific Meeting of the American Society of Transplant Physicians, May, 1999.

74. McCauley J, Takaya S, Fung J, et al. The question of FK506 nephrotoxicity after liver transplantation. Trans Proc, 23:1444, 1991.

75. Starzl TE, Abu-Elmagd K, Tzakis A, Fung JJ, Porter KA, Todo S. Selected topics on Fk506, with special references to rescue of extrahepatic whole organ grafts, transplantation of "forbidden organs," side effects, mechanisms, and practical pharmacokinetics. Trans Proc, 23:914, 1991.

76. Starzl TE. FK506 versus cyclosporine. Trans Proc, 25:511, 1993.

77. Demetris AJ, Banner B, Fung JJ, Shapiro R, Jordan M, Starzl TE. Histopathology of human renal allograft function under FK506: a comparison with cyclosporine. Trans Proc, 23:944, 1991.

78. Randhawa PS, Shapiro R, Jordan ML, Starzl TE, Demetris AJ. The histopathological changes associated with allograft rejection and drug toxicity in renal transplant recipients maintained on FK506: clinical significance and comparison with cyclosporine. Am J Surg Pathol, 17:60, 1993.

79. Shapiro R, Fung JJ, Jain AB, Parks P, Todo S, Starzl TE. The side effects of FK506 in humans. Trans Proc,22(1):35,1990.

SIROLIMUS

Barry D. Kahan

Introduction

Sirolimus (SRL, Rapamune®, Wyeth-Ayerst, Radnor, PA) is a hydrophobic 31-membered macrocyclic lactone (**Figure 1**) derived from *Streptomyces hygroscopicus,* an actinomycete isolated from soil samples taken from the Vai Atari region of Rapa Nui (Easter Island). Macrocyclic lactones are lipophilic molecules bearing a large 12-, 14-, or 16-membered lactone ring substituted with hydroxyl, methyl, and ethyl groups, as well as carbonyl functions with one, two, or three carbohydrate fragments.

SRL: Molecular and Cellular Mechanisms

Though structurally similar to tacrolimus, SRL is not functionally related and exhibits a mechanism of action unique from those of calcineurin antagonists or anti-metabolites. Following unhindered entry into the cytoplasm, SRL complexes with FK-binding proteins (FKBP) to form the active inhibitor of cytosolic processes, SRL-FKBP. SRL blocks Ca^{2+}-dependent and Ca^{2+}-independent events, including transduction of proliferative and differentiation signals delivered by the lymphokines that act on T and B cells—interleukin (IL)-2, IL-3, IL-4, IL-5, IL-6, and IL-15. In addition, SRL blocks cytokine-dependent, *Staphylococcus aureus*- and soluble CD4 ligand-stimulated proliferative signals to B cells, and in addition, impedes immunoglobulin (Ig) class switching. In

Mohamed Sayegh and Giuseppe Remuzzi (editors), Current and Future Immunosuppressive Therapies Following Transplantation, 143-163.
© *2001 Kluwer Academic Publishers. Printed in the Netherlands.*

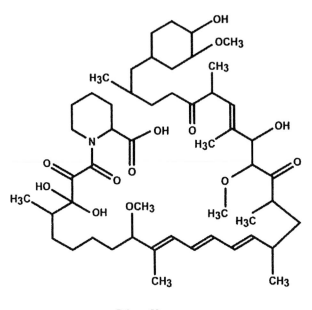

Sirolimus
(RAPA,SRL)

Figure 1. The chemical structure of SRL.

T cells, SRL inhibits the co-stimulatory pathways necessary for cytokine synthesis during the transition from the G_0 to the G_1 phase of activation, as well as the protein synthetic, and DNA transcriptional processes mediating cell-cycle progression during the G_1 phase following cytokine stimulation [1]. During the co-stimulatory cascade necessary for the G_0-G_1 progression, SRL-FKBP complexes inhibit the generation of c-Rel, a critical intermediate in the signal 1 amplification necessary for cytokine transcription [2]. During the G_1 build-up, SRL inhibits a multifunctional phosphatidyl-inositol kinase—mammalian target of rapamycin (mTOR)—that exerts a variety of actions to regulate the phosphorylation of several receptor-type, sarcoma-like (src), and cell-cycle-dependent kinases (cdk). For example, the inhibition of mTOR disrupts the dissociation of the elongation initiation factor (EIF_4), which is necessary for protein synthesis [3] and for the hyperphosphorylation of retinoblastoma protein, a critical factor in cell-cycle progression. In addition, the FKBP12-SRL-mTOR complex inhibits the $p70^{s6}$ (but not the $P85^{s6}$) kinase which leads to the hyperphosphorylation of the 40S ribosomal protein $p70^{s6}$ [4, 5]. Further, SRL inhibition of mTOR prevents activation of the downstream serine-threonine cell cycle protein kinases, such as p34^{cdc2}, facilitating the persistence of the cyclin-dependent kinase inhibitor p27^{kip1} and interrupting the formation of the active p34^{cdc2}-cyclin D hetero-complexes that form a critical "maturational promotion factor."

To a lesser extent, SRL inhibits signal transduction by a variety of other cytokines, not only *in vitro* but also apparently *in vivo* in man, including fibroblast growth factor, which may explain problems with wound healing in SRL-treated patients; colony stimulating factor, leukopenia; IL-11, thrombocytopenia; and erythropoietin, anemia. Owing to its inhibition of insulin growth factor signals, SRL disrupts cytokine-stimulated proliferation of cardiac fibroblasts [6], human endothelial cells [7], as well as non-stimulated proliferation of vascular smooth muscle cells [8], bronchial smooth muscle cells [9], or rat smooth muscle cells [10]. The effects of SRL on smooth muscle cell and vascular endothelial proliferation occur at drug concentrations 10- to 100-fold greater than those required to inhibit T and B cell maturation, and at concentrations about equal to the sensitivity of cytotoxic CD8+T, natural, lymphokine-activated, and antibody-dependent killer cells. These actions may explain the beneficial effects of SRL to interrupt obliterative vascular lesions induced by balloon catheter injury, and possibly of chronic rejection [11].

Effects on Transplant Survival in Experimental Animals

The preliminary experiments showing that SRL prolongs the survival of heterotopic vascularized rat heart allografts [12] were confirmed using grafts of rat kidney, orthotopic and heterotopic small bowel, and pancreaticoduodenal composites [13]. In addition, anecdotal experience suggested a synergistic interaction of SRL with cyclosporine (CsA, Neoral®, Sandimmune®, Sandoz, Basel, SZ) in both mongrel canine [14] and subhuman primate models.

Detailed experiments using rat heart or kidney transplantations *in vivo* and *in vitro* human lymphocyte proliferation assays revealed that SRL acts in a supra-additive (synergistic) fashion with CsA. In contrast, CsA did not display synergism with the antiproliferative agents azathioprine (Aza; Imuran, Burroughs-Wellcome, Research Triangle Park, NC), mycophenolic acid, or mizorbine [15]. Recently, both pharmacokinetic and pharmacodynamic components have been identified in the interaction of SRL and CsA. The CsA-SRL interaction included a pharmacokinetic component to mutually increase drug concentrations [16], owing to competition between SRL and CsA for metabolism by the cytochrome P450 (CYP) 3A4 system. The pharmacodynamic interaction was attributed to the actions of SRL to disrupt the co-stimulatory cascade necessary for maximal transcription of cytokine genes during the G_0-G_1 transition. In addition, SRL interrupted the transduction of the humoral signals necessary for the G_1 build-up for proliferative responses. The latter two actions are complementary to the inhibition of calcineurin phosphatase activity by complexes of CsA with its immunophilin cyclophilin.

Pharmacokinetic Properties

SRL, like other macrocyclic lactones, displays four distinct pharmacokinetic limitations. First, the low and variable bioavailability has been attributed to sensitivity to gastric acid, first-pass hepatic metabolism, and incomplete intestinal absorption. Second, the binding of drug to intracellular and plasma proteins displays significant interindividual variability, ranging from 10% to 93% at therapeutic concentrations. Third, owing to the binding of macrocyclic lactone metabolite nitrosoalkanes to CYP450 iron (II), there are widespread drug-drug pharmacokinetic interactions with co-administered pharmaceuticals at the level of CYP450 3A isozymes. The resultant formation of stable but inactive iron-metabolite complexes prolongs the half-lives of other drugs metabolized by this system. Fourth, owing to marked differences in the activities of the multidrug action efflux pump P-glycoprotein (P-gp) and CYP 3A4, both of which are located in intestinal enterocytes [17], absorption and clearance of orally-administered drug displays a large inter-subject variability. For example, an 11-fold inter-individual variation exists in the intestinal content of CYP 3A4 proteins [18, 19]. By spacing the delivery of CsA and SRL four hours apart, the prominent interactions associated with the concomitant delivery of the drugs to patients by the oral route may be reduced [20].

SRL exhibits an average terminal half-life of between 57 and 62 hours and an oral bioavailability of approximately 15%. After administration of a single oral dose of 1-34 mg/m^2, whole blood peak concentrations usually occurred within one hour (range 0.8-3 hours). SRL displays extensive tissue distribution, in specific, a volume of distribution of 5.6-16.7 L/kg in stable renal transplant recipients [21]. SRL plasma concentrations are far lower (only 3.1% of SRL is free in plasma) than SRL whole-blood concentrations, because 94.5% of SRL is bound to red blood cells and 1% is bound to lymphocytes and granulocytes. The extensive partitioning of SRL in tissues results in a greater delay to steady-state concentrations and contributes to a relatively long terminal half-life that permits once-daily dosing [22]. To expedite tissue loading, the first SRL dose is generally administered at three times the baseline amount. It also seems advisable to continue with twice the baseline amount for at least three days. For instance, the regimen to achieve maximal rejection prophylaxis is 15 mg on day 1 post-transplant, 10 mg on days' 2, 3, and 4, and then 5 mg daily thereafter. In contrast to CsA, wherein trough (C_0) measurements are not representative of overall drug exposure [23], there was a good correlation (r=0.94) between the SRL C_0 and the area under the concentration-time curve (AUC) concentrations when using a multiple-dose regimen, suggesting that SRL C_0 values represent good indicators of total drug exposure [22, 24]. At present, C_0 monitoring appears to be the most practical method available; nonetheless, this strategy is both expensive and cumbersome owing to the nature of drug measurements by high-performance liquid chromatography (HPLC) using ultraviolet detection. However, this obstacle may be addressed by an automated assay presently under development (IM®x, Abbott Diagnostics, North Chicago, IL).

During Phase I/II trials, we utilized the HPLC method and observed that acute rejection prophylaxis was practically guaranteed when the SRL C_0 were maintained between 10 and 15 ng/mL [25] and CsA exposure was set at average concentrations (C_{av}; the quotient of the AUC and the dosing interval) between 350–450 ng/mL. These CsA C_{av} concentrations were 40% lower than those used in CsA-steroid regimens without SRL [26]. Through the combination of SRL and CsA, drugs that inhibit distinct immune mechanisms, pharmacodynamic resistance may be prevented and individual drug doses may be reduced, thereby minimizing adverse side effects. Concentration-controlled protocols that maintain a SRL C_0 of <15 ng/mL have been associated with only modest drug toxicity.

During primary clinical trials, an oil-based liquid formulation of SRL that requires refrigeration for stabilization of the drug suspension was utilized; however, a solid SRL tablet has been introduced thereafter [27]. A pharmacokinetic comparison of the two formulations was conducted using 12 renal transplant recipients who had been taking the liquid formulation for more than one year. Concurrent 12-hour pharmacokinetic profiles of SRL and CsA were conducted on the last dose of liquid and again at 2-, 4-, and 8-weeks after conversion to the tablet formulation. Notably, the only significant difference between the two formulations of SRL was a higher maximum concentration (C_{max}) after administration of the liquid compared with the tablet. No significant differences were found among the pharmacokinetic parameters of CsA AUC_{0-12}, time to maximum SRL concentration (t_{max}), dose-corrected SRL C_0, and relative oral bioavailability for the liquid versus the solid formulation.

The results of initial clinical trials suggest that a 2mg dose of SRL, in conjunction with administration of CsA, is appropriate for most patients; African-Americans require a 5mg dose. Phase III trials confirmed that 2.0 or 5.0 mg SRL doses provide excellent prophylaxis of acute rejection episodes, although, some patients required dose reductions in response to toxic adverse events (*vide infra*). Conversely, it may be necessary to increase the long-term SRL dose to exploit its potential for chronic rejection prophylaxis [28]. Future clinical trials will seek to exploit the synergistic therapeutic interactions of and minimize the toxicities of CsA and SRL by exploring individual dose reduction.

Clinical Results

Phase I, II, and III Studies of Sirolimus Therapy and Acute Rejection Prophylaxis

Based on the findings of the Phase I study of quiescent renal transplant recipients [29], we conducted an open-label, single-center, dose-escalation Phase I/II trial to examine the safety and efficacy of *de novo* use of SRL to full therapeutic doses of CsA in mismatched living donor renal transplants [25]. The first cohort of 20 patients was divided into five groups of four patients that were treated with multiple ascending doses of SRL (0.5, 1.0, 2.0, 3.0, and 5.0 mg/m^2/day) in combination with CsA and prednisone (Pred) according to our customary steroid-tapering schedule. Because we were concerned about the metabolic effects of long-term steroid treatment and since only 1/20 patients experienced an acute rejection episode (an African American recipient of a spousal transplant in the 0.5 mg/m^2/day dose group), we began to withdraw steroids (at a minimum of five months post-transplant) from the immunosuppressive regimen of this cohort. No rebound acute rejection episodes occurred. We examined the possibility of early withdrawal of patients from steroids by treating two additional cohorts of 10 patients each with 7 mg/m^2/day SRL in addition to CsA, and either 1-week or 1-month post-transplant courses of Pred. Each cohort contained one patient who experienced a rejection episode. Thus, a total of three rejection episodes occurred (two of them in patients off steroids), among the 40 patients in this trial, yielding an overall 7.5% incidence of acute rejection episodes. This result was significantly better than the 32% acute rejection rate in an historical CsA-Pred cohort [25].

A multi-center Phase II trial demonstrated that the addition of SRL to the CsA-Pred regimen allowed a significant reduction in doses of the Sandimmune® formulation of CsA among non-African-American patients; despite the reduced CsA exposure, the incidence of acute rejection episodes was only 12% [30]. In light of these findings, we conducted a single-center *de novo* trial using markedly reduced doses of CsA, namely, a C_{av} target of 250 ng/mL rather than the usual target of 550 ng/mL [26], revealing excellent prophylaxis of acute rejection episodes among cadaveric kidney recipients of all races (unpublished data).

Another Phase II multi-center trial focused on the efficacy of SRL therapy without calcineurin inhibitors. The study compared two immunosuppressive regimens, namely, SRL-Aza-Pred (41 patients) versus CsA-Aza-Pred (42 patients). At 12 months, the incidence of biopsy-confirmed acute rejection episodes was 41% versus 38%, respectively [31]. The CsA group experienced three graft losses (one rejection and two thromboses), and the SRL group experienced one graft loss (rejection plus sepsis). No deaths took place in either group. In the SRL group, the more frequently observed laboratory abnormalities included reduced platelet and leucocyte counts, and increased cholesterol and triglyceride levels. Interestingly, they found at least transiently improved renal function in the SRL cohort as compared to the CsA cohort. These results suggest that SRL may be as effective as CsA in preventing acute rejection episodes in renal transplant patients receiving Aza and steroids. In the selection of a maintenance regimen, the clinician must determine whether the potential benefit of SRL monotherapy on renal function merits the increased risk of an acute rejection episode.

One pivotal Phase III multi-center, randomized, blinded, double dummy, clinical trial in 719 renal transplant recipients was conducted at 38 centers across the United States. The trial compared the safety and efficacy of 2 (n=284) versus 5 (n=274) mg/day doses of SRL compared with the anti-proliferative agent Aza (n=161) in combination with a protocol-stipulated regimen of CsA Neoral® and Pred [25]. Administration of both doses of SRL resulted in a significant reduction in the overall rate of efficacy failure, including occurrence of an acute rejection episode, graft loss, or death within six months, compared to Aza, namely, 17.3% (p=0.003), 17.9% (0.009), and 29.2%, respectively. Not only was there a reduced incidence of efficacy failure, but also, the acute rejection episodes were fewer in incidence and milder in severity as estimated by the Banff grade and by the number of patients who required antibody therapy. At one year, graft and patient survivals were similar among all three treatment groups.

The second pivotal Phase III global multi-center, randomized, blinded trial utilized a single dummy. This study included 576 recipients treated worldwide with 2 (n=227) or 5 (n=219) mg/day SRL or with a placebo (n=130), in addition to a baseline immunosuppressive regimen of the microemulsion formulation of CsA (Neoral®; Novartis, Basel, Switzerland) and steroids [32]. The incidence of biopsy-proven rejection among the groups was reduced by SRL therapy: namely, 19% (p=0.076) and 11% (p=0.001) compared to 37% with placebo. During the initial six months, there were no differences in graft (88-93%) or patient survival (95-98%) rates among the three treatment groups. A significant reduction in the overall severity of acute rejection episodes was found among patients receiving 5 but not 2 mg/day SRL compared to placebo. Further, the need to treat steroid-resistant episodes of acute rejection with antibody therapy was significantly decreased in the 2 mg/day SRL group (2.2%) compared to placebo (7.7%, p=0.025).

These two pivotal studies of SRL demonstrate its ability to enhance the prophylactic effect of a CsA-Pred regimen in primary renal allograft recipients.

Other Possible Indications for SRL

Induction immunosuppression. Owing to its lack of nephrotoxic properties [33], SRL proffers a baseline for administration in an induction immunosuppressive regimen. In view of the high incidence of acute rejection episodes (41%) that occurred using a SRL-Aza-steroid regimen [31], we combined anti-IL-2R monoclonal antibodies (mAb) with SRL [34], to yield a regimen free of nephrotoxic calcineurin inhibitors for use when there were adverse donor (or recipient) factors that placed the patient at high risk for delayed graft function. For example, factors included cold ischemia time greater than 36 hours, donor age less than 10 years, peri-operative complications (for example, myocardial infarction), or adverse procurement conditions (premature cardiac arrest, hypotension). The two IL-2 regimens use either treatment on alternate weeks with five doses of daclizumab (Zenapax®, Roche, Nutley, NJ), administered at doses of 1 mg/kg [35], or treatment with two 20 mg doses of basiliximab (Simulect®, Novartis, East Hanover, NJ) administered on days 0 and 4 [36]. SRL therapy was initiated at 15 mg on day 1, 10 mg on days 2, 3, 4, and then dose-selected to achieve a C_0 value >10 ng/ml. Once the serum creatinine value fell below 2.5 mg/dl, low doses of CsA (50-100 mg bid) were administered. Not one of the initial six patients experienced an episode of acute rejection [33], in marked contradistinction to the 50% rejection rate observed when induction therapy combined MMF and daclizumab with steroids.

Steroid withdrawal. Steroid withdrawal was performed in two cohorts of patients that received *de novo* treatment with SRL/CsA: namely, 40 recipients of HLA-mismatched living donors (the Phase IIA trial) and 35 recipients of cadaver donor renal transplants (the Phase IIB trial). The minimum follow-up periods were 18 and 12 months, respectively. In the Phase IIA trial, eight of the 40 patients were ineligible for steroid withdrawal [25], owing to patient request, previous chronic steroid therapy, or compromised renal function. Among the 32 eligible patients, 25 were successfully withdrawn from steroids (78%). The two episodes (8%) of acute rejection occurred when steroids were withdrawn at one week or at one month. After a six-month period of SRL/CsA/Pred therapy, both of the patients who had experienced acute rejection episodes were successfully withdrawn the second time, such that all 25 patients were off steroids at 12 months. Between months 12 and 18, one patient experienced a flare-up of pre-existent lupus erythematosus and was returned to steroid treatment, such that 24 patients were off steroids at 18 months. At twelve months, patients in the Phase IIA trial who had been withdrawn from steroids showed significantly reduced white blood cell counts (probably owing to an absence of steroid stimulation of leukocytes), and, more notably, significant reductions in serum cholesterol and triglyceride values. The mean triglyceride value was 251 mg/dl for the SRL/CsA compared to 365 mg/dl for the SRL-CsA-Pred group (p=0.02), and the mean values for the cholesterol were 244 versus 278 mg/dl (p=0.05), respectively. In the Phase IIB trial, eight of the 35 cadaver recipients were ineligible for steroid withdrawal owing to drop-outs or to the occurrence of an acute rejection episode. Among the 27 patients entered into the steroid withdrawal protocol (77%) [37], four patients experienced episodes of acute rejection after steroid withdrawal (15%), and four additional patients required the reinstatement of steroid treatment owing to medical reasons. The remaining 19 patients (54%) were rejection- and steroid-free at one year, although the cohort was not sufficiently large enough to detect a significant improvement in triglyceride or cholesterol levels. In summary, 77% of renal transplant recipients tolerated steroid withdrawal from a SRL/CsA regimen, with 12-month success rates of 96% among living and 54% among cadaver donor kidney recipients. Large multi-center trials of the effects of steroid withdrawal are planned during the Phase IV development of SRL.

Refractory renal allograft rejection. As evidenced by the persistence of vascular rejection (Banff Grade IIB or III) on renal transplant biopsy, despite treatment with antilymphocyte antibodies, refractory rejection almost inevitably progresses to transplant loss. After an impressive result of the first case of SRL treatment of refractory rejection in a patient experiencing such severe, ongoing renal dysfunction after combined OKT3/AMGEN/corticosteroid therapy that she required ongoing dialysis [38], we entered an additional 17 adult patients who had failed treatment with *at least one* 14-day course of OKT3, combined with a *second* 7-day course of OKT3 (n=13) and/or a 14-day course of ATGAM (n=8). In addition, five patients were treated for rescue with mycophenolate mofetil (MMF, Syntex, CA). SRL therapy was initiated at 7 mg/m^2 for five days and continued thereafter at 5 mg/m^2. CsA doses were not modified; steroids were tapered off or withdrawn as tolerated [39]. The actuarial two-year patient survival rate was 85%; one patient died suddenly of an unknown cause but with a functioning graft (creatinine 1.5 mg/dl), and one patient, owing to pre-existent congestive cardiomyopathy. Two additional grafts were lost: one owing to persistent rejection, and one abandoned owing to overwhelming, presumably infectious, diarrhea. At the end of the previous therapy with antilymphocyte antibodies (and at the time of the confirmatory biopsy) and prior to the inception of SRL therapy, the mean serum creatinine value was 195% greater than the baseline value just prior to the acute episode. Among the 13 patients (70%) with functioning grafts at one year, the mean serum creatinine value after inception of SRL therapy was 2.15 mg/dl (range 1.4 - 4.0). Among this cohort, five patients were weaned from steroids. SRL may thus represent a therapeutic alternative for the treatment of allograft rejection episodes refractory to both MMF and anti-lymphocyte antibodies.

Prevention and/or treatment of chronic nephropathy. Chronic nephropathy is the major cause of long-term renal allograft loss. Four observations suggest that SRL may be beneficial to avert this condition [40]. First, SRL inhibits growth factor-driven proliferation of smooth muscle and endothelial cells, in six different *in vitro* models, which are thought to reflect the processes producing the immuno-obliterative vascular endothelial and smooth muscle lesions that provide histopathologic hallmarks of chronic rejection. Second, SRL exerts a beneficial effect to mitigate vascular injury responses *in vivo*, namely, the balloon catheter arterial injury [41] or restenosis response following angioplasty [42]. Third, SRL dampens chronic rejection processes in mouse [43], rat [12, 44], and pig [12] models. The degree of donor-recipient histoincompatibility and the SRL dose over the range of 0.5-2.0 mg/kg/day were identified as the major determinants of benefit in a model of transplant vasculopathy [45]. However, even the lowest dose of SRL given to rats (0.5 mg/kg/day), which effectively produced a reduction in the incidence of vasculopathy from $62\pm13\%$ to $25\pm15\%$ ($p<0.005$), would translate to a dose of approximately 35 mg/kg/day in man. This dose is more than double the largest amount utilized chronically in renal transplant trials (15 mg/kg/day) [25]. Therefore, to exploit the potency of SRL in chronic as opposed to acute rejection settings, higher doses of the drug may be required. Fourth, when used in combination with CsA in humans, SRL reduces the incidence of acute rejection episodes, which are widely believed to forecast an increased risk of chronic rejection [46,47]. Further, during the early post-operative period, the administration of SRL at doses of 2-10 mg/day permits minimization of CsA dosing, thereby possibly mitigating renal dysfunction, a disorder that may exacerbate other processes leading to chronic graft failure.

Toxic Side Effects

Infections

Based on the results of the treatment of quiescent renal transplant recipients with a short course of ascending doses in the Phase I study [29], the addition of SRL to a CsA-based regimen only modestly increased the overall incidence of viral, bacterial, or fungal infections. In the Phase II study of *de novo* treatment of living-related kidney recipients, this impression was confirmed [25]. In contrast, a high infection rate, particularly with *Pneumocystis carinii* pneumonia (PCP), was observed in the multi-center Phase IIB trial upon addition of SRL to a CsA-Pred regimen. This increase was attributed to the policy of one center to not administer prophylactic agents for PCP [30], since this center encountered six cases of the disease. Thus, prophylactic treatment with trimethoprim-sulfamethoxazole is now mandatory for all patients receiving SRL. SRL significantly increased only one other infectious process, oral apthous ulcers, presumably due to herpes simplex. Despite the lack of routine anti-viral prophylaxis in either the Phase II or Phase III trials, SRL treatment did not increase the rate of occurrence or the severity of cytomegalovirus (CMV) disease compared to Aza- or placebo-treated controls. Furthermore, SRL did not increase the incidence of malignancies. Among the 400 patients treated with SRL at our institution for periods of at least one and up to five years, only three cases of post-transplant lymphoproliferative disease (PTLD) have occurred. All three cases of PTLD occurred within 90 days post-transplant and were associated with excessive immunosuppression: one woman had persistent renal allograft rejection refractory to murine OKT3, equine anti-human thymocyte globulin, and rabbit thymo-globulin; one second transplant recipient was treated by a physician parent with a regimen that produced extremely high concentrations of SRL and CsA; and one elderly man received OKT3 to provide a CsA holiday to permit renal allograft recovery from drug-induced nephro-toxicity. The rates of malignancy associated with SRL are similar to those generally encountered among patients treated with CsA-Pred.

Lack of Nephrotoxicity

Our Phase I study of 40 stable renal transplant recipients revealed that CsA and SRL have few overlapping toxicities. In particular, SRL did not exacerbate the hypertension or increase the degree of renal dys-function during a two-week treatment course [29]. However, in the pivotal trials, patients treated with SRL-CsA-Pred showed a slightly, but significantly, reduced renal function compared with patients treated with CsA-Aza-Pred or CsA-Pred. We believe that the adverse effect of SRL on renal function likely relates to a pharmacokinetic interaction between SRL and CsA that increases renal tissue CsA levels [48]. In salt-deprived rat models, the reduction in renal function associated with the drug combination, could be shown to be due to the augmented CsA kidney tissue concentrations [49].

Cytopenias

During the Phase I study, including a two-week treatment course in stable patients [29], and the Phase I/II long-term study in *de novo* transplant recipients [11], we observed that SRL reduces the production of platelets, of erythroid and of myeloid elements. These changes generally occur during the first month, are modest in degree, and resolve spontaneously. Though rarely required, drug dose reductions typically produce a reversal of the toxic effect beginning within five days, with full recovery by day 14. During the Phase I/II trial, an increased incidence of cytopenic events was associated with SRL C_0 >15 ng/mL. In comparison to the potency of the immunosuppressive effects of SRL, the severity of these adverse events seemed mild.

In the Phase III pivotal trials, platelet counts below 100,000/mm^3 or peripheral white blood cell counts below 3,500/mm^3 prior to transplant represented absolute contra-indications to study entry, and, post-transplant, they triggered a protocol of more intensive laboratory monitoring (**Table 1**). When compared with patients in the blinded Aza-treated control arm, renal transplant recipients treated with SRL showed less evidence of leukopenia.

SRL doses were reduced when platelet counts fell below 75,000/mm^3, and were suspended altogether when counts fell below 50,000/mm^3. Patients treated with SRL showed a greater incidence of thrombocytopenia than the Aza cohort. Although no patient was removed from drug treatment for this reason, platelet counts below 50,000/mm^3 required drug treatment suspension. When confrontedwith a or the need to continue SRL therapy in the face of cytopenia(s), we have delivered the non-immunostimulatory cytokines— erythropoietin, IL-11, or granulocyte colony stimulating factor (G-CSF)—to counter drug-induced effects on erythrocytes, platelets, or granulocytes, respectively (**Table 1**). Our strategy is based on the hypothesis that the myelodepression is the result of SRL-mediated inhibition of signal transduction via hematologic growth factor receptors that employ similar gp130/β chains, which are widely distributed among cytokine receptors, including hematologic, as well as lymphokine, receptor signal cascades, which are the pharmacologic target of drug action.

Hyperlipidemias

SRL appears to exacerbate steroid-induced hypertriglyceridemia and CsA-induced hypercholesterolemia in dose-dependent fashion [29]. Although the molecular mechanism of the effect of SRL to produce hyperlipidemia remains unclear, the drug appears to interfere with lipid clearance from low-density lipoproteins, possibly by inhibiting lipoprotein-lipase-mediated lipolysis and/or by disrupting signal transduction by insulin or insulin-like growth factors that are necessary for fatty acid uptake by adipocytes.

Although a significant fraction of renal transplant recipients exper-ience the toxic effect beginning usually in the second post-transplant month, the majority of patients display only modest elevations with spontaneous resolution of the hyperlipidemia. These elevations are well

Table 1. Clinical management of the adverse effects of sirolimus therapy.

Effect	Threshold for action	Countermeasure therapy
Thrombocyto-penia	$<100,000/mm^3$	Dose reduction
	$<50,000$	Drug suspension
	$<25,000$	Neumega® (50 µg/kg/d)
Absolute granulocyto-penia	$<2000/mm^3$	Dose reduction
	<1500	Drug suspension
	<750	Neupogen 5 µg/kg/d (s.c. or i.v.)
Anemia	Hematocrit <32%	Epogen (6000 U, 3 times/week)
	Hematocrit <25%	Epogen (10,000 U, 3 times/week)
Hypertrigly-ceridemia	>300 ng/dl	Gemfibrozil 600 mg QD
	>500 ng/dl	Gemfibrozil 600 mg b.i.d Fish Oil 2 tabs t.i.d.
	>1000 ng/dl	Drug dose reduction
	>1500 ng/dl	Drug suspension
Hypercholes-terolemia	With hypertriglyceridemia	Pravastatin: dose proportionate to increase
	Without hypertriglyceridemia	Atorvastatin: dose proportionate to increase

below the thresholds of 240 mg/dl cholesterol and 300 mg/dl triglycerides, which the National Cholesterol Education Program proposed as constituting cardiovascular risk factors. The spontaneous resolution of hyperlipidemia may be attributed to several factors, including improved dietary compliance, decreased CsA and steroid doses, and/or increased exercise associated with the recovery from end stage renal disease.

Patients with serum triglyceride values greater than 400 mg/dl and/or cholesterol values greater than 300 mg/dl should receive counter-measure therapy (**Table 1**). Since pravastatin has no interactions with the cytochrome P450 3A4 system, patients with isolated elevations of serum cholesterol (not triglyceride) levels are effectively managed by administration of the drug. In addition, pravastatin produces only modest rhabdomyolysis (as detected by increases in creatine phosphokinase levels). When there is a concomitant mild increase in serum triglyceride concentrations, atorvastatin may be used in place of pravastatin. However, the management of moderate to severe hypertriglyceridemia presents a more difficult situation, owing to the only modest activity of the combination of fish oil and fibrates. Nonetheless, SRL-treated patients rarely display serum triglyceride values above 1,000 mg/dl, the threshold at which patients exhibit a propensity for the occurrence of pancreatitis, a complication that has not occurred with increased frequency in this population.

Hypercholesterolemia has been implicated as a cause of cardiovascular complications (now the leading cause of mortality for patients under dual- or triple-drug regimens) and possibly, an increased incidence of chronic rejection [50, 51]; however, the significance of SRL-induced hypertriglyceridemia to increase the incidence or severity of cardiovascular complications is as yet unclear. At one year, the two large Phase III multicenter trials do not indicate a heightened incidence of cardiovascular complications among *de novo* treated transplant patients.

Miscellaneous toxicities. Gastrointestinal intolerance with diarrhea is the most prominent toxicity associated with macrocyclic lactones. Ototoxicity, hepatotoxicity, and dermatologic effects represent less commonly reported reactions, and incidences of pancreatitis, hemolytic anemia, and psychotic reactions are extremely rare [52]. Of great interest, macrocyclic lactones may share their apparently idiosyncratic, adverse cardiac toxicities with the somewhat related macrolides. The electrocardiographic sign of lengthening of the rate-correlated QT interval has been associated with intravenous administration of either tacrolimus (TRL, FK506, Prograf, Fujisawa, JP; [53, 54], or erythromycin, particularly in women [55-57]. This alteration may lead to the *torsades de pointes* ventricular arrhythmia in a similar fashion to potassium channel blockers, such as amiodarone and quinidine. Further, co-administration of cisapride, astemizole, terfenadine, or pimozide may augment the proclivity of macrocyclic lactones to produce cardiac side effects.

SRL displays little tendency to produce hepatotoxicity; in randomized trials, only modest increases in serum glutamic-oxalic acid transaminase have been observed. Anecdotal observations have noted an increased incidence of delayed wound healing, of lymphocele formation, of Achilles and plantar tendinitis, and of arthropathy, particularly in the heel. Clarification of the incidence and significance of these side effects is expected upon further analysis of the Phase III data through comparison of the long-term clinical courses of SRL- versus Aza-treated (United States Trial) and SRL- versus placebo-treated (Global Trial) patients.

SDZ-RAD: A SRL Analogue

In our recent Phase I, randomized, blinded, placebo-controlled study, we evaluated the pharmacokinetics and safety profile of a four-week course of once-daily, sequential ascending doses (0.75, 2.5, or 7.5 mg/day) of SDZ-RAD (RAD) capsules in renal transplant recipients on a stable regimen of CsA Neoral® and Pred [58]. RAD displayed a spectrum of side effects similar to that observed with SRL: namely, an heightened incidence of infections associated with increased immunosuppression and a dose-related occurrence of hypercholes-terolemia, thrombocytopenia, and hypertriglyceridemia, particularly at the 7.5 mg dose. The pharmacokinetic parameters of RAD displayed dose proportionality, with a good correlation between C_0 and AUC concentrations, but a moderate degree of drug accumulation (2.5-fold) at the 0.75 mg dose. The drug was absorbed rapidly, reaching a C_{max} within two hours. In contradistinction to SRL, which exhibits an average terminal half-life of between 57 and 62 hours, RAD displayed a significantly shorter 16- to 19-hour half-life, necessitating twice daily dosing. RAD concentrations reached a steady state by day four. Preliminary kinetic-dynamic correlations indicate correlations between thrombocytopenia (but not hyperlipidemia) and AUC, C_{max}, as well as weight-adjusted dose. At the end of a four-week course of simultan-eous dosing, no evidence indicated a pharmacokinetic interaction between CsA and RAD. Currently, controlled, multicenter Phase II/III pivotal trials are underway to determine the impact of the shorter half-life and increased hydrophilicity of RAD on the clinical outcomes of the drug as compared with MMF.

Macrocyclic Lactone Agents in the Matrix of New Immuno-suppressives

Interactions with Anti-IL-2R mAb

We have proffered a novel immunosuppressive strategy—the cytokine paradigm—for induction immunosuppressive therapy [59]. In addition to CsA and SRL, the paradigm includes the administration of either the humanized (daclizumab) or the chimeric (basiliximab) anti-IL-2R mAb. Both daclizumab and basiliximab bind to the α chain (CD25) of the IL-2R. Because CD25 does not bear an intracytoplasmic signaling mechanism, these mAb do not evoke the cytokine release syndrome. Furthermore, they only rarely elicit the production of neutralizing antibodies. When administered in combination with CsA and steroid therapy during pivotal trials, mAb were shown to decrease the incidence of acute rejection episodes from 40-50% to approximately 30%, as well as to produce minimal side effects. Since the chimeric form is 10-fold more potent than the humanized form, it only has to be administered as two 20 mg doses (day 0 and day 4). In contrast, the humanized form is prescribed as five biweekly intervals doses of daclizumab (1 mg/kg). Induction immunosuppression with SRL and anti-IL-2R mAb has now been used in 24 patients to permit extended periods of freedom from the administration of CsA. Upon resolution of the impaired function, we subsequently re-introduced CsA at low 50-100 mg twice-daily doses.

Interactions Between SRL and TRL or MMF

Once introduced into clinical practice, SRL will likely be widely utilized in drug combinations. Owing to the potency of the interaction of SRL with CsA, it has been suggested that another calcineurin inhibitor, TRL, might act synergistically with SRL [60]. Extensive investigation of this combination was not conducted during the development of SRL because *in vitro* assays indicated that SRL and TRL antagonize each other's effects when either drug is used in molecular excess [61]. However, *in vivo* studies assert that combinations of SRL and TRL display more than additive interactions to prolong the survival of rat or mouse heart tissue allografts [62, 63]. Unfortunately, these studies did not include simultaneous measurements of patient drug concentrations to assess the contribution of pharmacokinetic interactions to the apparent pro-longation of graft survival. Certainly, a final assessment can not be rendered without clinical trials comparing a TRL-SRL with a CsA Neoral®-SRL combination. Although these trials might be performed in a concentration-controlled fashion, it is unfortunately difficult to imagine them being performed in a blinded fashion. In addition, before undertaking such a trial, it should be observed that there may be a danger to conducting clinical trials based upon the results of experimental animal studies performed in a less than a rigorous fashion. This danger is exemplified by the recent claim of synergy between MMF and SRL based upon rat allograft survival [64]; in a subsequent European multicenter randomized trial, the effect of a SRL-MMF-Pred combination was inferior to that of a SRL-Aza-Pred combination.

Summary

SRL is a novel, promising immunosuppressive agent with a unique mechanism of action to disrupt co-stimulatory and cytokine-stimulated *T cell* activation via inhibition of a multifunctional kinase—mTOR. The drug has undergone development culminating in two large pivotal trials including almost 1,300 patients. These trials show that SRL reduces the incidence, time to onset, and severity of acute rejection episodes. In addition, a parallel series of studies documented the capacity of SRL-Aza-Pred or SRL-MMF-Pred to achieve similar 40% acute rejection rates as a CsA-Aza-Pred regimen, but with somewhat improved renal function. Although the incidence and severity of infectious diseases was similar between SRL and control study groups, SRL does display both myelodepressive and hyperlipidemic side effects. While the former toxicities are generally rapidly reversible, hyperlipidemia, albeit generally at levels *below* the threshold definition of predisposition to arteriosclerotic complications (cholesterol >240 mg/dl and triglyceride >400 mg/dl), leads to uncertainty about the long-term prognosis of patients for cardiovascular complications. As we enter the new millennium, SRL will certainly be used in a variety of drug combination regimens, both sequentially and simultaneously, to minimize early post-retrieval ischemia/reperfusion renal injury, to avert acute rejection episodes, to control refractory rejection, and to forestall chronic nephropathic processes.

References

1. Kuo CJ, Chung J, Fiorentino DF, et al. Rapamycin selectively inhibits interleukin-2 activation of p70 S6 kinase. Nature 1992; 358: 70-73.
2. June CH, Ledbetter JA, Gilespie MM, et al. *T cell* proliferation involving the CD28 pathway is associated with cyclosporine-resistant interleukin 2 gene expression. Mol Cell Biol 1987; 7: 4472-4481.
3. Graves LM, Bornfeldt KE, Argast GM, et al. cAMP- and rapamycin-sensitive regulation of the association of eukaryotic initiation factor 4E and the translational regulator PHAS-I in aortic smooth muscle cells. Proc Natl Acad Sci U S A 1995; 92: 7222-7226.
4. Brown EJ, Albers MW, Shin TB, et al. A mammalian protein targeted by G1-arresting-rapamycin-receptor complex. Nature 1994; 369: 756-758.
5. Brown EJ, Beal PA, Keith CT, et al. Control of p70 s6 kinase by kinase activity of FRAP *in vivo*. Nature 1995; 377: 441-446.
6. Simm A, Nestler M, Hoppe V. PDGF-AA, a potent mitogen for cardiac fibroblasts from adult rats. J Mol Cell Cardiol 1997; 29: 357-368.
7. Akselband Y, Harding MW, Nelson PA. Rapamycin inhibits spontaneous and fibroblast growth factor beta-stimulated proliferation of endothelial cells and fibroblasts. Transplant Proc 1991; 23: 2833-2836.
8. Marx SO, Jayaraman T, Go LO, et al. Rapamycin-FKBP inhibits cell cycle regulators of proliferation in vascular smooth muscle cells. Circ Res 1995; 76: 412-417.
9. Scott PH, Belham CM, al-Hafidh J, et al. A regulatory role for cAMP in phosphatidylinositol 3-kinase/p70 ribosomal S6 kinase-mediated DNA synthesis in platelet-derived-growth-factor-stimulated bovine airway smooth-muscle cells. Biochem J 1996; 318 (Pt 3): 965-971.
10. Obata T, Kashiwagi A, Maegawa H, et al. Insulin signaling and its regulation of system A amino acid uptake in cultured rat vascular smooth muscle cells. Circ Res 1996; 79: 1167-1176.
11. Kahan BD. Rapamycin: personal algorithms for use based on 250 treated renal allograft recipients. Transplant Proc 1998; 30: 2185-2188.
12. Calne RY, Collier DS, Lim S, et al. Rapamycin for immunosuppression in organ allografting. Lancet 1989; 2: 227.
13. Stepkowski SM, Chen H, Daloze P, et al. Prolongation by rapamycin of heart, kidney, pancreas, and small bowel allograft survival in rats. Transplant Proc 1991; 23: 507-508.
14. Knight R, Ferraresso M, Serino F, et al. Brief communication: Low-dose rapamycin potentiates the effects of subtherapeutic doses of cyclosporine to prolong renal allograft survival in the mongrel canine model. Transplantation 1993; 55: 947-949.
15. Kahan BD, Gibbons S, Tejpal N, et al. Synergistic interactions of cyclosporine and rapamycin to inhibit immune performances of normal human peripheral blood lymphocytes *in vitro*. Transplantation 1991; 51: 232-239.
16. Stepkowski SM, Napoli KL, Wang ME, et al. Effects of the pharmacokinetic interaction between orally administered sirolimus and cyclosporine on the synergistic prolongation of heart allograft survival in rats. Transplantation 1996; 62: 986-994.
17. Lown KS, Mayo RR, Leichtman AB, et al. Role of intestinal P-glycoprotein (mdr1) in interpatient variation in the oral bioavailability of cyclosporine. Clin Pharmacol Ther 1997; 62: 248-260.
18. Hebert MF, Roberts JP, Prueksaritanont T, et al. Bioavailability of cyclosporine with concomitant rifampin administration is markedly less than predicted by hepatic enzyme induction. Clin Pharmacol Ther 1992; 52: 453-457.

19. Wacher VJ, Wu CY, Benet LZ. Overlapping substrate specificities and tissue distribution of cytochrome P450 3A and P-glycoprotein: implications for drug delivery and activity in cancer chemotherapy. Mol Carcinog 1995; 13: 129-134.
20. Kaplan B, Meier-Kriesche HU, Napoli KL, et al. The effects of relative timing of sirolimus and cyclosporine microemulsion formulation coadministration on the pharmacokinetics of each agent. Clin Pharmacol Ther 1998; 63: 48-53.
21. Yatscoff RW, Wang P, Chan K, et al. Rapamycin: distribution, pharmacokinetics, and therapeutic range investigations. Ther Drug Monit 1995; 17: 666-671.
22. Zimmerman JJ, Kahan BD. Pharmacokinetics of sirolimus in stable renal transplant patients after multiple oral dose administration. J Clin Pharmacol 1997; 37: 405-415.
23. Kahan BD, Grevel J. Overview: Optimization of cyclosporine therapy in renal transplantation by a pharmacokinetic strategy. Transplantation 1988; 46: 631-644.
24. Napoli KL, Kahan BD. Routine clinical monitoring of sirolimus (rapamycin) whole-blood concentrations by HPLC with ultraviolet detection. Clin Chem 1996; 42: 1943-1948.
25. Kahan BD, Podbielski J, Napoli KL, et al. Immunosuppressive effects and safety of a sirolimus/cyclosporine combination regimen for renal transplantation. Transplantation 1998; 66: 1040-1046.
26. Lindholm A, Kahan BD. Influence of cyclosporine pharmacokinetics, trough concentrations, and AUC monitoring on outcome after kidney transplantation. Clin Pharmacol Ther 1993; 54: 205-218.
27. Kelly PA, Napoli KL, Dunne C, et al. Conversion from liquid to solid sirolimus formulations in stable renal allograft transplant recipients. Biopharm Drug Dispos (in press).
28. Kahan BD, for the Rapamune U.S. Study Group. A phase III comparative efficacy trial of Rapamune in renal allograft recipients [Abstract 198]. XVII World Congress, Montreal, Canada, 1998.
29. Murgia MG, Jordan S, Kahan BD. The side effect profile of sirolimus: a phase I study in quiescent cyclosporine-prednisone-treated renal transplant patients. Kidney Int 1996; 49: 209-216.
30. Kahan BD, Julian BA, Pescovitz MD, et al. Sirolimus reduces the incidence of acute rejection episodes despite lower cyclosporine doses in caucasian recipients of mismatched primary renal allografts: a phase II trial. Transplantation (in press).
31. Groth CG, Backman L, Morales JM, et al. Sirolimus (rapamycin)-based therapy in human renal transplantation: similar efficacy and different toxicity compared with cyclosporine. Sirolimus European Renal Transplant Study Group. Transplantation 1999; 67: 1036-1042.
32. MacDonald AS for the Rapamune Global Study Group. A randomized, placebo-controlled trial of Rapamune in primary renal allograft recipients [Abstract 426]. Abstracts of the Transplantation Society XXVII World Congress, Montreal, 1998.
33. DiJoseph JF, Sharma RN, Chang JY. The effect of rapamycin on kidney function in the Sprague-Dawley rat. Transplantation 1992; 53: 507-513.
34. Hong JC, Kahan BD. Use of anti-CD25 monoclonal antibody in combination with rapamycin to eliminate cyclosporine treatment during the induction phase of immunosuppression [Brief Communication]. Transplantation 1999; 68: 701-704.
35. Vincenti F, Kirkman R, Light S, et al. Interleukin-2 receptor blockade with daclizumab to prevent acute rejection in renal transplantation. Daclizumab Triple Therapy Study Group. N Engl J Med 1998; 338: 161-165.
36. Kahan, B.D., Rajagopalan, P.R., and Hall, M., for the United States Simulect® Renal Study Group. Reduction of the occurrence of acute cellular rejection among renal allograft recipients treated with basiliximab, a chimeric anti-interleukin-2-receptor monoclonal antibody. Transplantation 1999; 67: 276-284.

37. Pescovitz MD, Kahan BD, Julian B, et al. Sirolimus (SRL) permits early steroid withdrawal from a triple therapy renal prophylaxis regimen. XVI Annual Meeting of the American Society for Transplant Physicians, 1997.
38. Slaton JW, Kahan BD. Case report—sirolimus rescue therapy for refractory renal allograft rejection. Transplantation 1996; 61: 977-979.
39. Kahan BD, Podbielski J, Van Buren CT. Rapamycin for refractory renal allograft rejection [Abstract #711]. XVII Annual Meeting of the American Society of Transplant Physicians, 1998.
40. Kahan BD. The role of rapamycin in chronic rejection prophylaxis: a theoretical consideration. Graft 1998; 1 (2 Suppl II): 93-96.
41. Gregory CR, Huang X, Pratt RE, et al. Treatment with rapamycin and mycophenolic acid reduces arterial intimal thickening produced by mechanical injury and allows endothelial replacement. Transplantation 1995; 59: 655-661.
42. Gallo R, Padurean A, Jayaraman T, et al. Inhibition of intimal thickening after balloon angioplasty in porcine coronary arteries by targeting regulators of the cell cycle. Circulation 1999; 99: 2164-2170.
43. Morris RE, Huang X, Gregory CR, et al. Studies in experimental models of chronic rejection: use of rapamycin (sirolimus) and isoxazole derivatives (leflunomide and its analogue) for the suppression of graft vascular disease and obliterative bronchiolitis. Transplant Proc 1995; 27: 2068-2069.
44. Meiser BM, Billingham ME, Morris RE. Effects of cyclosporin, FK506, and rapamycin on graft-vessel disease. Lancet 1991; 338: 1297.
45. Schmid C, Heemann U, Tilney NL. Factors contributing to the development of chronic rejection in heterotopic rat heart transplantation. Transplantation 1997; 64: 222-228.
46. Kahan BD, Mickey R, Flechner SM, et al. Multivariate analysis of risk factors impacting on immediate and eventual cadaver allograft survival in cyclosporine-treated recipients. Transplantation 1987; 43(1): 65-70.
47. Almond PS, Matas A, Gillingham K, et al. Risk factors for chronic rejection in renal allograft recipients. Transplantation 1993; 55: 752-756.
48. Napoli KL, Wang ME, Stepkowski SM, et al. Relative tissue distributions of cyclosporine and sirolimus after concomitant peroral administration to the rat: evidence for pharmacokinetic interactions. Ther Drug Monit 1998; 20: 123-133.
49. Podder H, Stepkowski SM, Napoli KL, et al. Sirolimus exacerbates CsA-induced nephrotoxicity by raising CsA blood trough levels, but does not impair renal function by a pharmacodynamic interaction [Abstract #206]. XVIII Annual Scientific Meeting of the American Society of Transplant Physicians, 1999.
50. Dimeny E, Fellstrom B, Larsson E, et al. Hyperlipoproteinemia in renal transplant recipients: is there a linkage with chronic vascular rejection? Transplant Proc 1993; 25: 2065-2066.
51. Dimeny E, Tufveson G, Lithell H, et al. The influence of pretransplant lipoprotein abnormalities on the early results of renal transplantation. Eur J Clin Invest 1993; 23: 572-579.
52. Eichenwald HF. Adverse reactions to erythromycin. Pediatr Infect Dis 1986; 5: 147-150.
53. Hodak SP, Moubarak JB, Rodriquez I, et al. QT prolongation and near fatal cardiac arrhythmia after intravenous tacrolimus administration: a case report. Transplantation 1998; 66: 535-537.
54. Johnson MC, So S, Marsh JW, et al. QT prolongation and Torsades de Pointes after administration of FK506. Transplantation 1992; 53: 929-930.
55. Antzelevitch C, Sun ZQ, Zhang ZQ, et al. Cellular and ionic mechanisms underlying erythromycin-induced long QT intervals and torsade de pointes. J Am Coll Cardiol 1996; 28: 1836-1848.
56. Drici MD, Knollmann BC, Wang WX, et al. Cardiac actions of erythromycin: influence of female sex. JAMA 1998; 280: 1774-1776.

57. Guelon D, Bedock B, Chartier C, et al. QT prolongation and recurrent "torsades de pointes" during erythromycin lactobionate infusion. Am J Cardio 1986; 58: 666.
58. Kahan BD, Wong RL, Carter C, et al. A phase I study of a four-week course of the rapamycin analogue SDZ-RAD (RAD) in quiescent cyclosporine-prednisone-treated renal transplant recipients. Transplantation (in press).
59. Hong JC, Kahan BD. Two paradigms for new immunosuppressive strategies in organ transplantation. Curr Opin Organ Transplant 1998; 3: 175-182.
60. Mahalati K, McAlister V, Peltikian K, et al. A clinical pharmacokinetic study of tacrolimus and sirolimus combination immunosuppression [Abstract #105]. 18th Annual Scientific Meeting of the American Society of Transplantation, 1999.
61. Dumont FJ, Melino MR, Staruch MJ, et al. The immunosuppressive macrolides FK-506 and rapamycin act as reciprocal antagonists in murine *T cells*. J Immunol 1990; 144: 1418-1424.
62. Chen H, Qi S, Xu D, et al. Combined effect of rapamycin and FK 506 in prolongation of small bowel graft survival in the mouse. Transplant Proc 1998; 30: 2579-2581.
63. Vu MD, Qi S, Xu D, et al. Tacrolimus (FK506) and sirolimus (rapamycin) in combination are not antagonistic but produce extended graft survival in cardiac transplantation in the rat. Transplantation 1997; 64: 1853-1856.
64. Vu MD, Qi S, Xu D, et al. Synergistic effects of mycophenolate mofetil and sirolimus in prevention of acute heart, pancreas, and kidney allograft rejection and in reversal of ongoing heart allograft rejection in the rat. Transplantation 1998; 66: 1575-1580.

NEW AGENTS ON THE HORIZON

Jochen Klupp and Randall E. Morris

Introduction

Today, many new small and large molecular weight molecules are being developed for use as immunosuppressive agents. As the understanding of mechanisms of immune function improves, immunosuppressive drug discovery and development is able to more specifically target activation pathways that predominate in immune rather than nonimmune cells, thus decreasing nonspecific toxicity.

Advances in structure-based drug design enables newer versions of current drugs to show improved absorption, distribution and metabolism and is a technology that is being exploited to design entirely new molecules for several molecular targets that are important for the rejection response. For many years the primary objective in the development of immunosuppressants has been to separate the suppression of rejection from the toxic side effects of these drugs. For example, it might be possible to avoid nephrotoxic and neurotoxic side effects of calcineurin inhibitors by targeting enzymes distal to calcineurin in the activation cascade.

Since there are so many new drugs currently in development and it is impossible to predict which of them will be of clinical use (either new primary or adjunctive therapy), we have organized this chapter based on the known mechanisms of action of these new non biologic immunosuppressants.

Mohamed Sayegh and Giuseppe Remuzzi (editors), Current and Future Immunosuppressive Therapies Following Transplantation, 165-183.
© 2001 Kluwer Academic Publishers. Printed in the Netherlands.

New Inhibitors of Signal I Pathway

Potassium Channel Blockers

During T –cell activation, sustained elevated Ca^{2+} levels are needed to activate gene expression. After T cell receptor complex stimulation, IP_3 formation causes Ca^{2+} release from intracellular calcium stores. Emptying of the stores triggers Ca^{2+} influx through Ca^{2+}-release activated Ca^{2+}-channels [1], which is maintained by potassium efflux channels keeping T cell membrane polarized.

Blocking potassium channels in T lymphocytes *in vitro* has effects similar to calcineurin inhibitors. Ionomycin + PMA, CD2 or CD3 stimulated T cells can be inhibited as measured by ^{3}H-thymidine proliferation and IL-2 production [2]. This effect can be reversed by addition of exogenous IL-2 [1]. Nonselective potassium channel blockers like tetraethylammonium (TEA) and 4-aminopyridine (4-AP) show these effects in a very high, millimolar range [2].

Nonspecific inhibition of potassium channels, however would cause severe toxicity in clinical application. Further investigations showed that there are different subsets of potassium channels. For example, Kv1.3 a voltage-gated channel, is of special interest because it is expressed abundantly in lymphocytes, compared to lower levels in fibroblasts, brain and kidney cells [3] and dominates the membrane potential only in T lymphocytes [4].

Polypeptides isolated from scorpion venoms are able to block potassium channels in the pico-molar range. Charybdotoxin inhibits Ca^{2+} activated and voltage gated potassium channels and is able to inhibit T cell activation dose dependently [2]. Margatoxin is more specific than charybdotoxin, since margatoxin only inhibits voltage gated channels [5]. However, margatoxin is not specific for lymphocytes since it also inhibits Kv1.1 and Kv1.2 channels, which are expressed in brain, peripheral nerves and the heart [4]. *In vivo* studies of these toxins are complicated by the fact that, Kv1.3 is not expressed by rat cells nor cells in many other experimental animals. One study in minipigs showed that margatoxin after i.v. administration of 8μg/kg/day inhibits delayed-type hypersensitivity to tuberculin, as well as an antibody response to alloantigen as effectively as 1 mg/kg/day of tacrolimus [5]. As expected, higher doses showed neurological side effects. CP-339,818, a 1,4-dihydroquinoline compound blocks both Kv1.3 and Kv1.4, so it is not being developed for clinical use [6].

Structural changes of the sea anemone toxin, ShK, generated ShK-Dap^{22} which is a highly selective and potent blocker of Kv1.3 (IC_{50} of 102 pmol) [4]. ShK-Dap^{22} inhibits ^{3}H-thymidine incorporation in peripheral human T cells after mitogen stimulation, with an IC_{50} below 500 pmol. When injected into mice, ShK-Dap^{22} showed only minimal toxicity: paralytic doses were reached at 200mg/kg body weight.

Although further studies are required on potassium channel blockers, this group of substances have the potential to inhibit signal 1 pathway specifically and may have the potential to suppress graft rejection. Promising substances like ShK-Dap[22] need still more development to increase its oral bioavailability and its reduce toxicity before it can be used in large animal studies or human phase I trials.

SP100030

SP100030, 2-Chloro-4-(trifluoromethyl)-5-N-phenyl-pyrimidine-carbox-amide, is an agent which is able to inhibit NF-κB and AP-1 [7], both known to be crucial for Signal–1 transduction to induce IL-1, Il-2, IL-6, IL-8, TNF-α and cell adhesion molecule transcription. SP100030 was identified by its ability to block cytokine promoter activity in cells transfected with cytokine promoter-luciferase gene constructs. SP100030 concentration – dependently inhibits immune cells proliferation with IC_{50} values of 30 nmol/l. Also, in Jurkat T cells it blocks induced production of Il-2 and IL-8 at the same IC_{50}. This effect is observed in all (including human) T cells, but not in non–T cell lines (monocytes, epithelial cells, fibroblasts, synoviocytes, osteoblasts and endothelial cells) [8,9].

In a popliteal lymph node study (BALB/c - C3H mice) SP100030 dose-dependently suppresses the alloantigen-induced PLN weight: 10 mg/kg caused 52% inhibition, compared to 12 mg/kg cyclosporine which caused only 35% inhibition. In a murine ear–heart transplant model, 15 to 20 mg/kg SP100030 administered intraperitoneally pro-longs graft survival significantly for more than 30 days. Also adjuvant arthritis is reduced effectively in Lewis rats (20 – 30 mg/kg i.p.). No body weight changes or other toxicological side effects have been observed in these studies.

Although experience with SP100030 is limited to rodent models, results obtained show that, focusing on key enzymes of Signal 1 path-way should be able to produce significant immunosuppression with a good safety profile.

Tepoxalin

Another potent inhibitor of NF-κB activation is Tepoxalin (5-[4-chlorophenyl]-N-hydroxy-[4-methoxyphenyl]-N-methyl-1-H-pyrazole-3-propanamide; molecular weight:385). It was first discovered as a dual inhibitor of 5-lipoxygenase (LO) and cyclooxygenase (CO) and is effective in preventing inflammation and synovitis in several animal models [10]. Due to inability to inhibit gastric prostaglandin synthesis, Tepoxalin does not cause gastric mucosa damage at anti-inflammatory doses [11]. Further investigations showed that naproxen and other CO inhibitors, as well as zileuton (a LO inhibitor), do not show the same antiproliferative effects as tepoxalin [10,12].

Later it was shown that tepoxalin inhibits NF-κB activation in a dose related manor [13]. Tepoxalin inhibits OKT3 (IC_{50}: 5.9), PMA + ionomycin (IC_{50}: 1.6) and Il-2 induced (IC_{50}: 2.75) T cell stimulation. The antiproliferative effect is more pronounced on activated PBLs than on spontaneous proliferating cell lines [14]. It also blockes PMA + ionomycin induced IL-2R production and IL-2 induced cell proliferation and signal transduction [14]. Together with cyclosporine in suboptimal concentrations, tepoxalin suppresses T cell proliferation synergistically. Furthermore it was shown that tepoxalin suppresses Il-6, IL-8 and IFN-γ production [15, 16].

By its inhibition of NF-κB tepoxalin also suppresses expression of the cell adhesion molecules CD62E (E-selectin), CD11b/CD18 (Mac-1) and CD106 (VCAM-1), but not CD11a/CD18 (LFA-1) and CD54 (ICAM – 1) [16]. Since CD11b/CD18 and CD106 are effective in monocyte adhesion processes, tepoxalin is expected to modulate atherosclerosis and inflammation [16] as well as neutrophil migration [15]. MLR was suppressed with an IC_{50} of 1.3 μMol.

In vivo, tepoxalin suppresses local graft-versus-host responses by about 40% in mice. In skin transplantation (BALBB/cByJ (H-2^d) to C3H/HeJ (H-2^k) mice), tepoxalin prolongs median survival time to 15 days with a 50 mg/kg dose, compared to 8 days in the control group [12]. Coadministration of suboptimal doses of tepoxalin (12.5 mg/kg) and cyclosporine (50 mg/kg) prolongs skin graft survival for more than 40 days [12], suggesting synergism between both drugs.

The toxicological and pharmacological profiles of tepoxalin are showing promising results. In mice and rats LD_{50} is more than 10-fold higher than immunosuppressive doses (>400 mg/kg) [12]. In healthy human volunteers [17], oral doses from 35 to 300 mg were absorbed rapidly and reached t_{max} after 2 to 3 hours of administration. Except at the 300 mg dose, tepoxalin was not detected 24 hours after dosing ($t_{1/2}$ 1.3 to 8 hours). Tepoxalin is converted to RWJ20142, an active metabolite ($t_{1/2}$ 7 to 24 hours), which also blocks cyclooxygenase and lipooxygenase. Inhibition of NF-κB was not determined in this study. No major adverse events have been recorded. Five out of 20 healthy participants reported abdominal discomfort, diarrhea or lightheadness.

In summary, by blocking NF-κB, tepoxalin is mechanistically different from cyclosporine and tacrolimus and acts synergistically with cyclosporine. With only minor toxicity and a good pharmacological profile, transplantation studies in larger animals could be promising.

Dithiocarbamates

Dithiocarbamates are defined by possession of a $(R_1)(R_2)N-C(S)-S-R_3$ functional group [18]. They are known as anti-oxidants and they have agricultural (fungicides and insecticides, Tetramethylthiuram disulphide) and clinical (alcohol aversion therapy, Disulphiran DSF) applications. Especially Diethyldithiocarbamate (DDTC) and Pyrrolidine Dithiocarbamate (PDTC) are used for cell biology investigations. Like other antioxidants used as anti-inflammatory agents or radical scavengers (Acetylsalicylate ASS, Sulfasalazine 5-ASA, N-Acetylcystein NAC), PDTC and DDTC are able to inhibit activation of the NF-κB transcription factor [18-22] by preventing IκBα phosphorylation [23].

Similar to NAC, PDTC not only inhibits NF-κB, but also activates AP-1 [19]. Furthermore DTCs strongly inhibit NFAT and are able to inhibit T cell activation, CD25 expression in response to costimualtion with CD28 and CD2 antibodies, as well as IL-2 secretion by costimulation with antibodies against CD3 and CD28 [19]. Due to the AP-1 stimulation, CD69 expression is not completely blocked by DTCs after PMA and ionophore activation in T cells and ICAM-1 expression is activated in endothelial cells by PDTC. However, DTCs lead to blockade of IL-2 and thereby to inhibition of T cell activation.

Since NF-κB also promotes HIV-1 replication, all the drugs mentioned above have been investigated for antiviral therapy [20, 21]. The role of DTCs in preventing apoptotic cell death is still controversial: in doses which are able to block NF-κB (50 – 500 μM) PDTC is able to prevent apoptosis in human promyelocytic leukemia (HL-60) cells [24] but stimulates apoptosis of rabbit osteoclasts [25]. When thymocytes are incubated with PDTC or DDTC for incubation periods longer than six hours, cells show typical signs of apoptosis [18]. It is suggested that toxicity of PDTC is related to its ability to chelate metal in a lipophilic membrane-permeable complex [18]. PDTC has also been reported to induce apoptosis in vascular smooth muscle cells [26]. Another member of this family of metal chelators, DSF, enhances *in vivo* accumulation of copper in the cerebellum and hippocampus of treated rats [18].

Due to this potentially toxic profile, it is doubtful if PDTC or DDTC will ever enter larger animal trials. However, these substances will remain excellent instruments to investigate gene transcription in activated T cells furthermore.

Protein Tyrosine Kinase Inhibitors

Genistein (5,7,4'-trihydroxyflavone), an isoflavanoid compound, has been shown to specifically inhibit protein tyrosine kinases (PTK) [27]. Genistein is able to reduce activated killer T lymphocyte mediated lysis of tumor cells by 50% in a 100 micromolar solution [28]. Other PTK inhibitors like herbimycin A showed a higher potency in the same experimental setting (93% inhibition by 2 μMol). Genistein (180 μMol) inhibits the induction of Fas-based cytotoxicity [29] and is also able to inhibit PMA or PHA / anti-CD28 stimulated T cell proliferation in a 40 μMol solution [30]. Also IL2-R and IL2 production are inhibited by genistein at the same concentrations needed for inhibition of proliferation [30].

PT I, a synthetic derivative of genistein was further evaluated in an *in vivo* study with pancreatic islet allograft transplantation: Lewis rats treated with 3 mg/kg *PT I* for 15 days accepted Wistar-Furth islet allografts for almost 100 days. [31]

Others

Other signal 1 inhibitors are listed in (**Table 1**). Reports of these drugs are only anecdotal and their future importance remains to be seen.

Table 1. Only anecdotally cited signal I inhibitors under development.

Hydroquinone	Inhibits NF-κB reversibly. Pausible cause of toxicity of cigarettes	[97]
Momordins	Reduces Jan/Fos binding to Ap-1	[98]
Ro 09-2210	Small molecule isolated from fungus FC2506. Able to block CD3 and Cd25 induced T cell proliferation; inhibits AP-1 and selectively MEK1	[99]
YM-53792	Inhibitor of NF-AT activation but not of AP-1 or NFκB. Inhibits IL-2, IL-4, IL-5 in peripheral blood	[100]
Lymphostatin	Inhibits protein-tyrosine kinase p56lck dose dependently. Suppresses IL-2 production in vitro and MLR	[101,102]

New Inhibitors of Signal II Pathway

Methylxanthine Derivatives

Methylxanthine derivatives are known to have some immuno-modulatory effects. However, the IC_{50}'s of theophylline (>400 μmol) and pentoxifylline (113 μmol) are higher than plasma levels which can be achieved in clinical settings [32]. By inhibition of cAMP phosphodiesterase activity methylxanthine derivatives are able to suppress T cell proliferation to alloantigens and mitogens, inhibit generation of cytotoxic T lymphocytes and natural killer cell-mediated cytolysis [33]. These effects are mainly due to suppression of TH_1 function by reducing production of inflammatory cytokines, including TNF-α, IFN-γ and IL-2 [34]. Due to high plasma levels required, pentoxifylline showed no effect on the incidence of rejection episodes in renal transplant patients [35].

A802715, 7-propyl-1-(5-hydroxy-5 methylhexyl)-3 methylxanthin, was further developed due to its lower IC_{50} (41 μmol) in suppressing TNF-α and IFN-γ production after LPS stimulation [32]. Additionally A802715 enhances TH_2 driven cytokines like IL-6 and IL-10. [36]. In contrast to other methylxanthine derivatives, A802715 is able to suppress not only CD3 stimulated human T cells, but also CD28 stimulated human T cells [37]. *In vitro*, a synergistic effect between A802715 and cyclosporine was shown with a high combination index (1/CI=9, where 1/CI > 1 is synergistic) in MLR and cell-mediated lympholysis assays [37]. Whereas signal 1 inhibition can be ascribed to cAMP elevation, the mechanism of additional signal 2 inhibition of A802715 is not known.

In vivo, this effect could also be proven [38]: Minimally effective oral doses of A802715 (100mg/kg/day) in combination with cyclosporine (7.5 mg/kg/day) for 30 days led to long term survival of cardiac allografts in rats. In an MHC compatible model (Wag/Rij – R/A), this combination results in donor specific tolerance by suppressing cytotoxic T cells and persisting TH_2 cells. Tolerance could not be achieved in a MHC incompatible model (WKAH – PVG).

Methylxanthines may also be beneficial by decreasing cyclosporine side effects: cyclosporine induced nephrotoxicity may be caused by decreased cAMP levels [39] and pentoxifylline was effective in decreasing cyclosporine induced toxicity, probably related to an effect on endothelin release and vasoconstriction [40].

The combination of methylxanthine derivatives with an additional inhibitory effect on signal 2, like A802715, with cyclosporine is promising not only because of its synergistic effect in immunosuppression, but also by its potential reversal of cyclosporine nephropathy.

New Inhibitors of Nucleotide Synthesis

VX-497

Based on the three dimensional crystal structure of IMPDH, VX-497 was rationally designed. VX-497 belongs to a new class of phenyl oxazole inhibitors of IMPDH [41] and is structurally unrelated to other IMPDH inhibitors (**Figure 1**) like MPA or ribavirin. *In vitro* this uncompetitive and reversible inhibitor of IMPDH down regulates proliferation of human lymphocytes dose dependently. *In vivo* VX-497 prolongs skin graft survival in mice and prolongs heterotopic heart graft survival in a Brown Norway to Lewis heart transplant model [41]. In this study, graft survival was prolonged to 28 days with 75 mg/kg BID dosing.

The main difference between VX497 and MPA is the absence of enterohepatic circulation for VX-497. Since this enterohepatic recirculation is thought to be the main reason for gastrointestinal

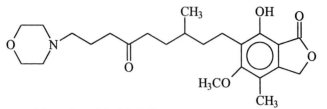

Mycophenolate Mofetil

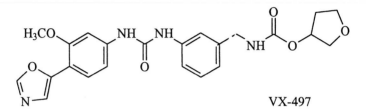

VX-497

Figure 1. Comparison of the chemical structures of the IMPDH inhibitors MMF and VX-497.

toxicity from treatment with mycophenolate mofetil, this aspect of VX-497 may lead to an improved tolerability. In effective doses (75 mg/kg BID) VX-497 caused no enteritis in histopathological studies.

Although only limited data are available for VX-497, this drug offers a new perspective in drug development: using structure based drug design to create a new molecule that inhibits a validated target (IMPDH) while simultaneous increasing safety by altering its route of excretion [42]. Future work will be needed to determine whether VX-497 is as effective as mycophenolate mofetil and to determine whether this new chemical entity can be used safely.

Malononitrilamides

Leflunomide (HWA 486) was first reported as a new chemical entity in 1976, but its ability to suppress immune function was not reported till 1985 [43]. Since then, the clinical, pharmacological and pharmaco-kinetic profiles of the drug itself and the active metabolite A77 1726 have become better understood [44]. The active metabolite of lefluno-mide (A77 1726) has a long plasma half-life of 11 to 16 days [45]. Therefore, changes in dose are not rapidly translated into changes in levels. This is not a problem in the treatment of rheumatoid arthritis since patients are on a fixed dose, but if leflunomide were to be used in transplant patients and if it were to require constant dose adjustment to maintain a narrow range of plasma levels, its long half-life would be

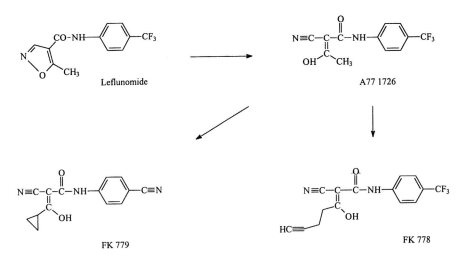

Figure 2. The MNA's Leflunomide, A77 1726, Fk778 and Fk779.

a liability. There are no plans to develop leflunomide for transplantation since it is at the end of its patent life. Since nothing is known about the doses and levels needed to suppress rejection in man and since drug-drug interactions between leflunomide and other medications used in transplant patients have not be investigated, use of leflunomide off-label does incur a risk.

In the last decade more than 80 derivatives of the MNA, A77 1726 have been created, by systematically exchanging molecular side groups [46]. Two compounds, MNA279 and MNA715, have been selected for further development. These are now known as FK779 and FK778. FK779 is 2-cyano-N-(4-cynaophenyl)-3-cyclopropyl-3-hydroxy-propen-oic acid amid ($C_{14}H_{11}N_3O_2$) and has a molecular weight of 253,26 Da; FK778 is chemically named 2-cyano-3-hydroxy-N-[4-(trifluoromethyl)-phenyl]-2-hepten-6-ynoic acid ($C_{15}H_{11}F_3N_2O_2$) and has a molecular weight of 308,26 Da (**Figure 2**). In contrast to leflunomide, FK778 and especially FK779 have a shorter half-life in rodents. Both have a very good oral bioavailability [47]. Like A77 1726 [48,49], both are able to bind specifically to dihydro-orotate-dehydrogenase (DHODH) and inhibit dose dependently de novo pyrimidine biosynthesis [44,47,50]. DHODH is the fourth enzyme in the de novo pathway for pyrimidine biosynthesis (**Figure 3**) and is located on the inner membrane of the mitochondria [51]. Pyrimidine nucleotides are essential for RNA and DNA synthesis and for membrane lipid biosynthesis and protein glycosylation. Activated T and B cells rely primarily on the de novo pathway for both purine and pyrimidine biosynthesis, whereas other cell types and resting T and B cells are able to synthesize purines and pyrimidines using the salvage pathway [52].

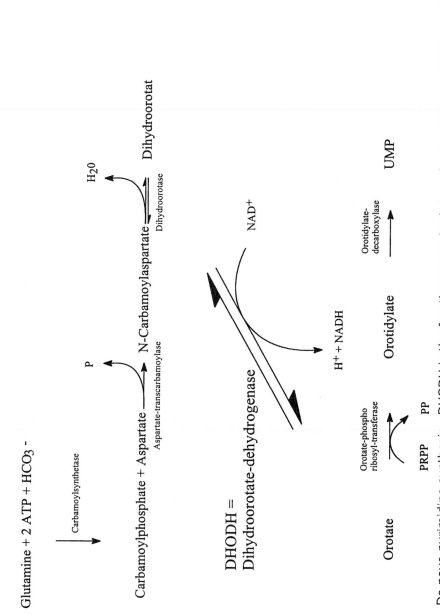

Figure 3. De novo pyrimidine synthesis. DHODH is the fourth enzyme in the synthesis, which is inhibited by the MNA's.

Mechanism of action. Leflunomide and its active metabolite A77 1726 are able to inhibit T cell activation directly, T cell independent B cell activation, IgG and IgM antibody production, and smooth muscle cell proliferation *in vitro* [44, 53]. Thus it was expected that the MNA's would have the same mechanism of action. Data showed that FK 778 inhibited human T cell activation (IC_{50} < 10 umol/L), with a potency that is independent of type of mode of stimulation of T cells by mitogen or of a combination of TCR signal and CD28-mediated activation [54]. In a culture of purified human B cells, activated by presence of BHK_{CD40L} cells, FK 778 effectively inhibit the proliferative response and also IgG and IgM synthesis [54]. FK 779 and 778 show also an effect on monocyte function and are able to reduce oxygen radical formation [55].

Comparing different MNA's with A77 1726 in different species, it was shown, that the antiproliferative potency of FK778 is equal to the active metabolite and more potent than FK779 in cultures of human and baboon immune cells [56]. In whole blood lymphocyte stimulation FK778 was more effective than FK779 in rhesus monkeys, dogs and cats and the rat T-cells were highly resistant to the effect of both analogues when compared with A77 1726 [57]. Both MNA's also inhibit growth-factor stimulated rat smooth muscle cells [58].

The primary mechanism by which MNA's inhibit cell proliferation is believed by some to be inhibition of membrane receptor-associated protein tyrosine kinase [59]. However, later studies showed that concentrations required for inhibiting tyrosine kinase far exceed the concentration [60] required for antiproliferative effects. It is possible that concentrations of MNA's *in vivo* could be high enough that inhibition of tyrosine kinase activity contributes to the antiproliferative effect of these drugs.

Preclinical animal studies. So far, all published *in vivo* studies for FK 778 and 779 have been in rodents. After single and multiple oral dose studies in rats, the AUC increases dose-dependently [44]. In contrast to A77 1726, FK778 and 779 show decreased clearance after multiple dosing compared to single dosing. For a given dose of MNA or leflunomide, the exposure (AUC) differs (FK778 > FK779 > A77 1726). The pharmacokinetics show high interindividual variability at a given dose.

Prompted by their ability to suppress T and B cell proliferation, including IgG and IgM response, FK778 and 779 were examined for treatment of graft-versus-host-disease (GvHD) [47]. In an acute life-threatening GvHD model involving injection of $1x10^8$ parenteral C57B1/6 splenocytes into B6C3F1 hybrid recipient mice, both MNA's were able to prolong survival in a dose-dependent manner (2.5 to 20 mg/kg). With high concentrations mortality was prevented completely [61-64].

In different rodent models (Lewis to Fisher (F344), Dark Agouti to Lewis) FK778 and 779 were able to prolong skin allograft survival in a dose dependent manner after oral gavage. The minimum effective dose (2.5mg/kg) prolonged graft survival for 5 to 10 days. Both MNA's showed similar dose response curves and an efficacy equal to cyclosporine in preventing acute skin graft rejection [65]. For reversal of acute rejection, again both MNA's were effective at a dose of 10/mg/kg, whereas a delayed treatment with cyclosporine (20mg/kg) failed to rescue the skin grafts [65]. Potentiation of efficacy was also shown between tacrolimus and MNAs for prevention and treatment of skin allograft rejection. Using a combination of ineffective doses of tacrolimus dose (0.2 mg/kg) and FK778 or FK779 (20mg/kg), tolerance induction (survival > 75 days) was achieved after withdrawal of immunosuppression at day 20.

After heterotopic heart transplantation between different strains of rats, oral treatment of 10mg/kg FK778 resulted in indefinite graft survival. Even after stopping immunosuppression more than half of the grafts survived more than 3 months [66]. Delayed treatment from postoperative day 4 on, prolonged graft survival from 38 to more than 100 days [67]. Furthermore, the MNA's potentiated the immunosuppressive effect of cyclosporine in the rat heart model [47, 50].

In a life dependent kidney transplantation trial (DA to PVG), 10 days of FK779 treatment (10 mg/kg) prolongs animal survival to 36.5 ± 34.0 days versus 9 days in the control group [47]. In a dose evaluation study 50% of the treated rats died after dosing with 15 mg/kg FK779 due to gastrointestinal side effects. At 7.5mg/kg, no toxicity was observed and kidney allograft survival was prolonged for up to 34 days, with only slight increases in urea and creatinine [47].

The ability of MNA's to prevent smooth muscle cell proliferation led to studies preventing and treating graft vascular disease and chronic rejection. It could be demonstrated that in BN femoral allograft segments transplanted orthotopically into LEW rats, intimal thickening was reduced by MNA's at a dose of 10/mg/kg [68].

Blocking T cell independent B cell activation and antibody formation is a promising mode of action for suppressing responses to xenografts. In the mouse to rat skin xenograft model, FK778 and 779 prolong skin graft survival dose dependently (10 – 20 mg/kg). Also, delayed therapy increases graft survival significantly. Xenoantibody formation was reduced at a dose of 20 mg/kg [47,69]. Both cyclosporine and tacrolimus, potentiate the efficacy of the MNAs, whereas single therapy with an ineffective dose of cyclosporine (10 mg/kg) or tacrolimus (0.2 mg/kg) is not able to prolong xenograft survival [70,71]□.

In the hamster to rat cardiac xenotransplantation model, a combination of cyclosporine and MNA's results in a long-term xenograft survival [66]. After administration of 10 mg/kg cyclosporine and 10 mg/kg of FK778 graft survival is prolonged for over 30 days.

In summary these studies demonstrate that the MNA's are promising new immunosuppressive agents. Blocking T- and B-cell proliferation and potentiation of the efficacy of cyclosporine or tacro-limus support ongoing development of these MNAs and other members of this class for suppression of after allo- and xenograft rejection. Ongoing preclinical efficacy studies in nonhuman primates and human Phase I trials will provide the pharmacokinetic, efficacy, and safety data that will determine which of the MNA's enters Phase II trials.

Deazaguanine analogues

Purine nucleoside phosphorylase (PNP) is an essential enzyme of the purine salvage pathway. It has been shown that humans with an inherited deficiency of PNP have a relatively selective depletion of T cells, while B-cell immunity remains intact [72]. Most likely, this selective inhibition of T cells is secondary to an accumulation of deoxy-guanosine-triphosphate (dGTP), which apparently suppresses ribonu-cleotide reductase activity and hence, DNA synthesis [73].

8-amino-guanosine and 8-amino-9-benzyl-guanine derivatives have been developed to inhibit PNP. However, they showed high toxicity in doses required for T cell suppression [72]. Applying crystallographic methods and structure-based design, new PNP-inhibitors (9-deaza-guanine derivatives) were developed for treatment of T cell-mediated inflammatory response, T cell-leukemia and prevention of organ rejection [74]. BCX-34 (2-amino-1,5-dihydro-7-(3-pyridinylmethyl)-4H-pyrrolo[3,2-d]pyrimidin-4-one) (**Figure 4**) is a potent 9-deazaguanine derivative, which is not only able to increase intracellular dGTP in human cells, but also to decrease intracellular guano-sine-triphosphate (GTP) [73]. Decreased pools of GTP caused by mycophenolic acid are, known to suppress T cell proliferation [75].

In vitro BCX-34 inhibits human, mouse and rat red blood cell PNP with IC50's of 36, 32 and 5 nMol, respectively. In a T cell culture of human leukemia cells (CCRF-CEM) BCX-34 inhibits cell proliferation in the presence, but not in the absence of deoxyguanine (dGuo).Deoxycytidine reverses the inhibition caused by BCX-34 and dGuo [73]. The maximum inhibitory effect on human PNP and T cell proliferation is

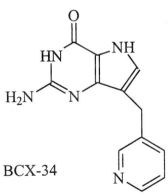

BCX-34

Figure 4. BCX-34 (2-amino-1,5-dihydro-7-(3-pyridinylmethyl)-4H-pyrrolo [3,2-d]pyrimidin-4-one) is a potent 9-deazaguanine derivative.

about 80%, whereas BCX-34 is not able to inhibit rat or mouse T cell proliferation. Since PNP in rodent T cells is inhibited, the reason for its lack of efficacy is explained by the fact that rodent T cells do not accumulate dGTP, but the mechanism responsible for the failure of rodent cells to accumulate dGTP is not understood. Additional *in vitro* studies [76] showed that BCX-34 is not only acting in malignant human T cell-lines, but also in peripheral blood mononuclear cells. After OKT3, tetanus toxoid and IL-2 induced proliferation, BCX-34 showed IC_{50}'s of 4 µMol, 0.7 µMol and 14.6 µMol. BCX-34 does not inhibit tetanus toxoid induced IL-2 release, which confirms the hypothesis that this drug arrests cells late in their cell cycle. The human mixed lymphocyte reaction is also inhibited by BCX-34 dose dependently [77].

The pharmacokinetics of BCX-34 showed a rapid disappearance after iv injection (within 3 hours; 1mg/kg in rats) and a good oral bioavailability of 76%. Half-lives were not calculated in these studies, but detectable plasma levels were observed 12 hours after a 10 mg/kg oral dose of BCX-34 [73]. Toxicological data have not been published and only neurological disorders of PNP deficient patients suggest what the adverse effects of this drug maybe.

Since BCX-34 is not able to inhibit rodent T cell proliferation, no *in vivo* efficacy data are available yet. Clinical trials are testing BCX-34 in dermal applications for psoriasis and T cell lymphoma [73]. Based on its mechanism of action, its high bioavailability, and its capability to potentiate the efficacies of cyclosporine and tacriolimus, BCX-34 may be used for use in transplantation. Further toxicological trials and efficacy studies in non-human primates would have to be done to better predict its future for use in transplant patients.

Others

FTY720

Myriocin (ISP-1) was isolated from the ascomycete Isaria sinclairii, which is parasitic in insects and plants. Extracts from this fungi imperfecti, have been used widely in traditional Chinese medicine. However ISP-1 produced fatal side effects in experimental animals during drug evaluation and further development was stopped. FTY720, 2-amino-2-(2-[4-octylphenyl]ethyl)-1,3-propanediol hydrochloride ($C_{19}H_{33}NO_2$−HCL - **Figure 5**) with a molecular weight of 343.94 Da is a synthetic structural analog of ISP-1. [78,79]

FTY720 has a completely new mechanism of action, which is not related to any other mechanism of action of any known immunosuppressive agents. It inhibits T cell dependent and independent immunity and suppresses T cell infiltration into grafted organs by depletion of peripheral lymphocytes to 3% of the original cell count within 3 hours

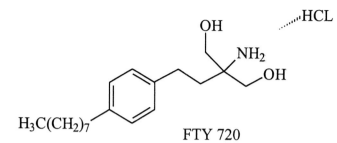

Figure 5. FTY 720 is acting by homing the lymphocytes into Payer Plaques and lymph nodes

after oral application [80]. FTY 720 does not effect T or B cell function *in vitro* in concentrations which are able to modulate immune response *in vivo*. Although the mechanism of action is not yet fully understood, it is likely that FTY720 acts by a combination of altered T cell traffic but probably not by inducing apoptosis as originally thought [81,82].

Mechanism of Action. ISP-1 and related compounds inhibit allogenic mixed lymphocyte reactions (MLR) and interleukin-2 dependent proliferation in a mouse cell line [80]. However, FTY720 in doses up to 1000 nmol/l does not inhibit MLR, Il-2 production, mRNA expression by antigen- or mitogen-stimulated T cells [83], cytokine-driven cell proliferation, or cytotoxic T cell generation or action [84]. High concentrations (4×10^{-6} M) added *in vitro* to rat lymphocytes induce chromatin condensation, formation of apoptotic bodies and DNA fragmentation [82,84,85]. Two lines of evidence led to the hypothesis that FTY720 leads to apoptotic cell death: First, FTY720 (10mg/kg) induces a marked reduction of peripheral lymphocytes in rats, and second, dead cell increased with time in spleen cells cultured with FTY720 [85].

More recent reports however indicate, that FTY720 acts by selectively depleting T and B cells from blood and sequesters lymphocytes into lymph nodes and Peyer's plaques [86-88]. The initial explanations for this mechanism of action were, that FTY720 increases adhesion of lymphocytes to high endothelial venules in the lymphoid tissues by up-regulating LFA-1, ICAM-1 and L-selectin [87,89]. Later analysis showed that FTY720 does not modulate selectins and adhesion molecule expression in lymphocytes and high endothelial venules. Since effect of FTY720 is blocked by pertussis toxin, it has been suggested that FTY720 functions through G-protein coupled receptors and that increased response of lymphocytes to chemokines may cause the homing into lymph nodes and Peyer's plaques (Brinkmann V. at al.; unpublished data). Supporting the hypothesis that FTY720 is acting by increasing the homing of lymphocytes rather than by inducing T cell death is that FTY720 does not alter the function of the resting memory

T cell pool. For example, mice immune to Lymphocytic Choriomeningitis Virus efficiently eliminate the virus from lung, kidney, liver spleen and blood after ending FTY720 treatment.

Toxicity and Pharmacokinetics. While ISP-1 induces severe digestive disorders at a dose of 1 mg/kg, resulting in death of the animals, the toxicologic profile of FTY720 is completely different: It was observed to have no toxic effects on rats (3 mg/kg) and monkeys (0.3 mg/kg) at doses that are immunosuppressive [80,85]. LD_{50} in rats is 300 to 600 mg/kg. No deaths were reported in dogs that received a single dose of less than 200 mg/kg [80]. Rats gained weight during 5 mg/kg treatment and showed only slightly increased levels of BUN , creatinine, and transaminase [90]. In other toxicologic studies (Brinkmann et al., not published) no renal, pancreatic or bone marrow toxicity was observed. At high concentrations adverse effects on lungs have been recorded.

Oral bioavailability in rats (80%), dogs (60%), and monkeys (40%) is good, with a half-life of 12 to 29 hours in a dose range between 0.1 and 3 mg/kg [80]. None of the identified metabolites is immunosuppressive. The metabolites are excreted in urine and feces at ratios between 20 to 50% in different species.

Preclinical animal studies.   In autoimmune and anti-inflammatory models FTY720 inhibited hypersensitivity responses in mice (0.03 mg/kg), joint destruction in an arthritis model in rats (0.1 mg/kg) and allergic encephalomyelitis [80]. In dose response studies, 0.1 to 10 mg/kg FTY720 prolongs skin, heart, liver and small bowel survival in rats [80,84,91]. Also in graft-versus-host disease in rats, FTY720 causes unresponsiveness (0.1–0.3 mg/kg) [92]. In canine kidney transplantation FTY720 given twice (5 mg/kg) at before and on the day of operation day results in a median graft survival of 21 days versus 9 days in the control group [85]. Posttransplant daily dosing (5 mg/kg) is not effective. However FTY 720 when combined with a subtherapeutic dose of cyclosporine (10 mg/kg) prolongs graft survival significantly [85]. Synergistic interaction with cyclosporine (CI=0.15–0.37) or sirolimus (CI=0.22–0.53) was also reported in heart, liver and small bowel transplantation in rats [84,93] and with tacrolimus in heart transplantation [94]. In a nonhuman primate kidney model, FTY720 and subtherapeutic cyclosporine prolongs graft survival in a supra-additive effect [80]. Furthermore, FTY720 (5 mg/kg) is able to reverse ongoing rejections after heterotopic heart [94] and orthotopic liver transplants [85] in rats and after kidney transplantation in dogs [95]. Together with allochimeric class I MHC antigen FTY720 induces tolerance in a Wistar Furth to ACI rat heart transplant model [96].

In summary, FTY720 shows promising results in different animal studies. Its different mode of action and acceptable safety profile in animals suggests this drug will have a role in clinical transplantation in combination with other drugs or as rescue therapy for ongoing rejections.

References

1. Terasaki PI, Cecka JM, Gjertson DW, Takemoto S, Cho YW, Yuge J. Risk rate and long-term kidney transplant survival. Los Angeles: UCLA Tissue Typing Laboratory; 1997.
2. Vella JP, Sayegh MH. Maintenance pharmacological immunosuppressive strategies in renal transplantation. Postgrad Med J 1997;73(861):386-90.
3. Vella JP, O'Neill D, Atkins N, Donohoe JF, Walshe JJ. Sensitization to human leukocyte antigen before and after the introduction of erythropoietin. Nephrol Dial Transplant 1998;13(8):2027-32.
4. Novick AC, Ho-Hsieh H, Steinmuller DS, et al. Detrimental effect of cyclosporine on initial function of cadaver renal allografts following extended preservation: results of randomized prospective trial. Transplantation 1986;42:154.
5. Kahan BD. Drug Therapy: Cyclosporine. N Engl J Med 1989;321(25):1725-38.
6. Matas AJ, Gillingham KJ, Payne WD, Najarian JS. The impact of an acute rejection episode on long-term renal allograft survival (t1/2). Transplantation 1994;57(6):857-9.
7. Basadonna GP, Matas AJ, Gillingham KJ, Payne WD, Dunn DL, Sutherland DE, et al. Early versus late acute renal allograft rejection: impact on chronic rejection. Transplantation 1993;55(5):993-5.
8. Zhou YC, Cecka JM. Sensitization in renal transplantation. Clin Transpl 1991;1991:313-23.
9. Katznelson S, Cecka JM. Immunosuppressive regimens and their effects on renal allograft outcome. Clin Transpl 1996:361-71.
10. Katznelson S, Gjertson DW, Cecka JM. The effect of race and ethnicity on kidney allograft outcome. Clin Transpl 1995;1995(379):379-94.
11. Neylan JF. Immunosuppressive therapy in high-risk transplant patients: dose-dependent efficacy of mycophenolate mofetil in African-American renal allograft recipients. U.S. Renal Transplant Mycophenolate Mofetil Study Group. Transplantation 1997;64(9):1277-82.
12. Neylan JF. Racial differences in renal transplantation after immunosuppression with tacrolimus versus cyclosporine. FK506 Kidney Transplant Study Group. Transplantation 1998;65(4):515-23.
13. Tejani A, Sullivan EK. Factors that impact on the outcome of second renal transplants in children. Transplantation 1996;62(5):606-11.
14. Gjertson DW. Multifactorial analysis of renal transplants reported to the United Network for Organ Sharing Registry: a 1994 update. Clin Transpl 1994:519-39.
15. Cecka JM. The UNOS Scientific Renal Transplant Registry--ten years of kidney transplants. Clin Transpl 1997:1-14.
16. Thorogood J, Houwelingen JC, Persijn GG, Zantvoort FA, Schreuder GM, van RJ. Prognostic indices to predict survival of first and second renal allografts. Transplantation 1991;52(5):831-6.
17. Zandvoort FA, D'Amaro J, Persijn GG, Cohen B, Schreuder GM, van Rood JJ, et al. The impact of HLA-A matching on long-term survival of renal allografts. Transplantation 1996;61(5):841-4.
18 Mytilineous J, Lempert M, Middleton D, Williams F, Cullen C, Scherer S, et al. HLA class I of 215 "HLA-A, -B, -DR zero mismatched" kidney transplants. Tissue Antigens 1997;50:355-8.
19. Opelz G. Correlation of HLA matching with kidney graft survival in patients with or without cyclosporine treatment. Transplant. 1985;40:240-43.
20. Hata Y, Ozawa M, Takemoto S, Cecka JM. HLA Matching. In: Terasaki PI, editor. Clinical Transpl. Los Angeles: UCLA Tissue Typing Laboratory; 1997. p. 381-96.

21. Terasaki PI, Cecka JM, Gjertson DW, Takemoto S. High survival rates of kidney transplants from spousal and living unrelated donors. N Engl J Med 1995;333(6):333-6.
22. Goes N, Urmson J, Ramassar V, Halloran PF. Ischemic acute tubular necrosis induces an extensive local cytokine response. Evidence for induction of interferon-gamma, transforming growth factor-beta 1, granulocyte-macrophage colony-stimulating factor, interleukin-2, and interleukin-10. Transplantation 1995;59(4):565-72.
23. Takada M, Chandraker A, Nadeau KC, Sayegh MH, Tilney NL. The role of the B7 costimulatory pathway in experimental cold ischemia/reperfusion injury. J Clin Invest 1997;100(5):1199-203.
24. Tullius SG, Heemann U, Hancock WW, Azuma H, Tilney NL. Long-term kidney isografts develop functional and morphological changes which mimic those of chronic allograft dysfunction. Ann Surg 1994;220:425-32.
25. Troppmann C, Gillingham KJ, Benedetti E, Almond PS, Gruessner RW, Najarian JS, et al. Delayed graft function, acute rejection, and outcome after cadaver renal transplantation. The multivariate analysis. Transplantation 1995;59(7):962-8.
26. Alegre ML, Lenschow DJ, Bluestone JA. Immunomodulation of transplant rejection using monoclonal antibodies and soluble receptors. Dig Dis Sci 1995;40(1):58-64.
27. Attavar P, Budhai L, Kim BH, Roy-Chowdhury N, Roy-Chowdhury J, Davidson A. Mechanisms of intrathymic tolerance induction to isolated rat hepatocyte allografts. Hepatology 1997;26(5):1287-95.
28. Monaco AP, Wood ML. Studies on heterologous antilymphocyte serum in mice: Optimal cellular antigen for induction of immunological tolerance with ALS. Tran Proc 1970;2:489.
29. Sayegh MH, Turka LA. T cell costimulatory pathways: promising novel targets for immunosuppression and tolerance induction. J Am Soc Nephrol 1995;6(4):1143-50.
30. Denton MD, Reul RM, Dharnidharka VR, Fang JC, Ganz P, Briscoe DM. Central role for CD40/CD40L interactions in transplant rejection. Pediatric Nephrology 1998;2(1):6-15.
31. Kirk AD, Harlan DM, Armstrong NN, Davis TA, Dong Y, Gray GS, et al. CTLA4-Ig and anti-CD40 ligand prevent renal allograft rejection in primates. Proc Natl Acad Sci U S A 1997;94(16):8789-94.
32. Sayegh MH, Fine NA, Smith JL, Rennke HG, Milford EL, Tilney NL. Immunologic tolerance to renal allografts after bone marrow transplants from the same donors [see comments]. Ann Intern Med 1991;114(11):954-5.
33. Spitzer TR, Delmonico F, Tolkoff-Rubin N, McAfee S, Sacktein R, Saidman S, et al. Combined HLA-matched donor bone marrow and renal transplantation for multiple myeloma with ESRD: induction of allograft tolerance through mixed lymphohematopoietic chimerism. Transplantation 1999;68:480.
34. Hricik DE, Almawi WY, Strom TB. Trends in the use of glucocorticoids in renal transplantation. Transplantation 1994;57(7):979-89.
35. Ratcliffe PJ, Dudley CR, Higgins RM, Firth JD, Smith B, Morris PJ. Randomised controlled trial of steroid withdrawal in renal transplant recipients receiving triple immunosuppression. LancetLancet 1996;348(9028):643-8.
36. Tran H, Acharya M, Auchincloss H, Carpenter CB, McKay D, Kirkman R, et al. Cyclosporine sparing effect of daclizumab in renal transplantation. J Am Soc Nephrol 1999;10:749.
37. Groth CG, Backman L, Morales JM, Calne R, Kreis H, Lang P, et al. Sirolimus (rapamycin)-based therapy in human renal transplantation: similar efficacy and different toxicity compared with cyclosporine. Sirolimus European Renal Transplant Study Group [see comments]. Transplantation 1999;67(7):1036-42.

38. Michael HJ, Francos GC, Burke JF, Besarab A, Moritz M, Gillum D, et al. Comparison of the effects of cyclosporine versus antilymphocyte globulin on delayed graft function in cadaver renal transplant recipients. Transplantation 1989;48:805.

39. Belitsky P, MacDonald AS, Cohen AD, Crocker J, Hirsch D, Jindal K, et al. Comparison of antilymphocyte globulin and continuous iv cyclosporine as induction immunosuppression for cadaver kidney transplants. Transplant Proc 1991;23:999.

40. Gaston RS, Hudson SL, Deierhoi MH, Barber WH, Laskow DA, Julian BA, et al. Improved survival of primary cadaveric renal allografts in blacks compared with quadruple immunosuppression. Transplantation 1992;53:103.

41. Tesi RJ, Henry ML, Elkhammas EA, Ferguson RM. Predictors of long-term primary cadaveric renal transplant survival. Clin Transplants 1993;7:345.

42. Katznelson S, Cecka JM. Immunosuppressive regimens and their effect on renal allograft outcome. In: Terasaki PI, editor. Clin Transpl. Los Angeles: UCLA Tissue Typing Lab; 1997. p. 379-94.

43. Brennan DC, Flavin K, Lowell JA, Howard TK, Shenoy S, Burgess S, et al. A randomized, double-blinded comparison of Thymoglobulin versus Atgam for induction immunosuppressive therapy in adult renal transplant recipients. Transplantation 1999;67(7):1011-8.

44. Rubin RH, Tolkoff RN, Oliver D, Rota TR, Hamilton J, Betts RF, et al. Multicenter seroepidemiologic study of the impact of cytomegalovirus infection on renal transplantation. Transplantation 1985;40(3):243-9.

45. Cockfield SM, Preiksaitis JK, Jewell LD, Parfrey NA. Post-transplant lymphoproliferative disorder in renal allograft recipients. Clinical experience and risk factor analysis in a single center. Transplantation 1993;56(1):88-96.

PART THREE: BIOLOGICALS

WHY TO WE NEED INDUCTION THERAPY?

John Vella and John Neylan

Introduction

The natural history of organ transplantation across the MHC barrier in the absence of immunosuppression is that of rejection. There are clearly defined periods at which a graft is at risk [1]. Registry data indicate that the period of greatest risk for acute rejection is within the first 3-6 months post-transplantation. Beyond the first post-transplant year, the risk of acute rejection diminishes substantially, although the risk never diminishes to zero (**Figure 1**). The introduction of newer and more potent immunosuppressive therapies combined with effective anti-microbial prophylaxis has resulted in a significant decline in the incidence of acute rejection and graft loss over the last 25 years [1,2]. Currently available immunosuppressive agents effectively prevent rejection in most, although not all, transplant recipients. It is apparent that there is a degree of interpatient variability in the requirements for immunotherapy. For example, the risk of acute rejection is greater in children, African-Americans and in recipients who are sensitized to HLA [3]. Taken together, these observations have provided the rationale for the development of induction immunosuppressive strategies that minimize the risk of rejection for a given individual. However, there is no consensus on what constitutes the optimal prophylactic induction immunosuppressive therapy to prevent renal allograft rejection. One of the controversies was triggered by the observation that cyclosporine is associated with an increased incidence and duration of delayed allograft function. Historically, such risks were greatest when

Mohamed Sayegh and Giuseppe Remuzzi (editors), Current and Future Immunosuppressive Therapies Following Transplantation, 187-204.

IMPROVEMENTS IN EARLY GRAFT SURVIVAL POST TRANSPLANTATION

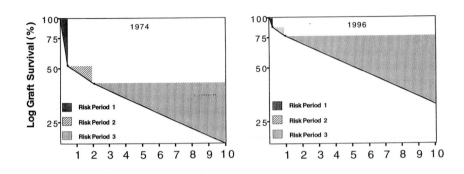

Years Post Transplant

Figure 1. Comparative Renal allograft survival: 1974-1996   The figure shows at least 2 periods when allograft recipients were at greatest risk of graft loss. There is an early period of high risk (divided here into an early period of highest risk [period 1] followed by a period of intermediate risk [period 2]). After this early period, there ensues a period of constant low risk, characterized by a progressive decline in the number of functioning grafts (risk period 3). The current success rates of transplantation are largely based on improvements in short-term allograft survival rates.

the starting dose of cyclosporine exceeded 12 to 14 mg/kg per day (doses which are currently rarely used), and when the cold ischemia time prior to transplantation is greater than 24 hours [4]. It is presumed that cyclosporine-induced renal vasoconstriction exacerbates ischemic injury in this setting [5]. Lowering the initial dose of cyclosporine to below 10 mg/kg per day may diminish the incidence of primary nonfunction or delayed function although perhaps at the price of increased risk of acute rejection.

Post-transplant induction immunosuppressive strategies may be divided into 2 categories (see **Table 1**). The first relies upon relatively high doses of conventional immunosuppressive agents. The second utilizes antibodies directed against T cell antigens in combination with lower doses of conventional agents. In general, the rationale underlying the use of anti-T cell antibody therapies include the following:
- Augmented immunosuppression
- Delayed introduction of calcineurin inhibitors
- Immunological conditioning

This chapter will focus on risk factors for acute rejection, the underlying mechanisms by which they operate and some general principals of management as they pertain to induction immunotherapy.

Table 1. Currently licensed induction therapies

Triple Therapy	Quadruple Therapy/Sequential Therapy

1. Calcineurin inhibitor:
    Cyclosporine
    Tacrolimus
	1. Antibody
	    Polyclonal
	        ALG
	        ALS
	        Thymoglobulin
	    Monoclonal
	        OKT3
	    Anti-Interleuin-2 receptor:
	        Daclizumab
	        Basiliximab

2. Steroid	*2. Steroid*

3. Antimetabolite
    Mycophenolate
    Azathioprine
 	
    or
	3. Antimetabolite(±lower dose):
	    Mycophenolate
	    Azathioprine
	
	    or

4. Sirolimus	*4. Sirolimus*

	5. Calcineurin inhibitor
	(lower dose or delayed introduction):
	    Cyclosporine
	    Tacrolimus

The ensuing chapters will provide a detailed account of the individual agents that are used, and the data that has accumulated from preclinical and clinical trials regarding their therapeutic efficacy in the clinic.

Augmented Immunosuppression

A number of alloantigen-specific and alloantigen non-specific mechanisms have been shown to impact on the risk of acute rejection which in turn impacts on both short and long-term allograft survival rates. Summarized below are some of the principal determinants of acute rejection that have been used to support the use of intensified prophylactic immunotherapy under various circumstances.

Effect of Acute Rejection on Graft Survival

The presence or absence of acute rejection is the dominant immunological factor that predisposes to chronic graft loss [6,7]. For living donor transplant recipients, the incidence of chronic rejection was found to be 0.8% in those who had no acute rejection, 20% in those with an acute rejection within 60 days of transplantation and 43% in those with acute rejection more than 60 days after transplantation [7].

Table 2. Risk factors for rejection

1.	HLA matching *HLA-DR: early determinant (<6 months)* *HLA-B: intermediate determinant (>6<18 months)* *HLA-A: late determinant (>24 months*
2.	Sensitization to HLA
3.	Ethnicity Increase risk in African-Americans>Caucasians/Hispanics>Asians
4.	Previous transplant lost to rejection
1.	Recipient Age (greatest risk in children < 5 years)
2.	Donor Source: Cadaver –v- Living
7.	Allograft Injury *Brain death* *Ischemia/Reperfusion*

For cadaver transplant recipients, the incidence of chronic rejection was 0% in those who had no acute rejection, 36% in those with acute rejection within 60 days of transplantation and 63% in those with acute rejection more than 60 days after transplantation. For both LRD and CAD recipients, no grafts were lost to chronic rejection among those who did not first have at least 1 acute rejection episode. The registry data also indicates that such acute rejection episodes are strongly predictive of chronic allograft dysfunction and graft loss. Rejection episodes during the first hospitalization resulted in an 8% lower 10 year graft survival [1]. The factors that contribute to an increased risk of acute rejection are summarized in **Table 2**. The identification of such risk factors permits the stratification of patients into groups at low, intermediate or high risk of rejection. Most transplant centers currently use either double or triple therapy for "low risk" patients (i.e. living donor recipients, well matched kidneys, no delayed graft function). Conversely, most centers use quadruple or sequential therapy (i.e. antibody induction with the introduction of a calcineurin inhibitor delayed for the first week or so post-transplant) in "high risk" patients. Factors impacting on the risk of rejection that are frequently used as the rationale to intensify immunosuppressive therapy are described in detail below.

Sensitization to HLA

Cytotoxic antibodies against HLA class I (A,B,C) or class II (DR,DQ) are found in subjects who have been immunized to these glycoproteins by pregnancy and childbirth, blood transfusion, or a prior HLA mismatched allograft. Such antibodies virtually exclude successful transplantation if they are detected in the recipient at the time of transplantation. Hyperacute rejection occurs in up to 80-90 percent of recipients who have a positive pretransplant crossmatch to donor T cells. In the event that such a graft is transplanted, host immuno-globulin binds to the accessible endothelial structures of the graft vasculature resulting in the secondary fixation of complement and activation of clotting cascades. Fibrinoid necrosis of blood vessel walls rapidly ensues with the subsequent formation of platelet and fibrin thrombi, attraction of mononuclear cells and polymorphonuclear leukocytes into the glomeruli. Ischemic necrosis of the renal cortex occurs within minutes to hours after implantation.

Highly sensitized patients have a decreased statistical chance of being transplanted because of their high likelihood of a positive pretransplant crossmatch [3]. In addition, such antibodies place patients awaiting transplantation at a significant disadvantage, as their waiting time is markedly prolonged and they are at increased risk of both delayed graft function and rejection in the perioperative period in spite of a negative pretransplant cross-match [8]. Taken together, these effects explain why the development of antibodies to HLA results in a selective accumulation of sensitized patients on the transplant lists of transplant programs. Current registry data indicate that increasing recipient PRA has a detrimental, although weak, effect on short and long-term primary allograft survival rates. A stepwise reduction in both one and three year graft survival of 1-2% was seen under different cyclosporine based immunosuppressive regimens as PRA increased from 0-10% to 11-50% to 51-10% although tacrolimus may be protective to such highly sensitized individuals [9].

Ethnicity

There are racial differences in the risk of graft loss: African-American recipients have a significantly higher risk of graft loss due to rejection compared with Caucasians [10]. In addition, it has been found that African-Americans require 50% more mycophenolate [11] and require higher tacrolimus levels in order to prevent rejection compared with Caucasians in order to enjoy the same reduction in the rate of rejec-tion with these novel agents [12]. The precise reason underlying this clinical observation is poorly understood, although it has been sugges-ted people of African descent may have cytokine gene polymorphisms leading to enhanced immune response for a given antigenic stimulus.

Recipient Age

Acute rejection is an extremely frequent event in pediatric transplantation. In one study, acute rejection data collected over a 10 year period in a cohort of over 5000 children was analyzed [13]. In 2,520 living donor recipients there were 2,540 rejection episodes (rejection rate 110%), and in 2,579 cadaver donor (CD) transplants 3,653 episodes were observed (rejection rate 132%). For living donor recipients the first rejection occurred sooner when there was at least one HLA-DR mismatch and prophylactic T cell antibody was not used. For cadaver allograft recipients, the absence of prophylactic T cell antibody and donor age below five years were the major risk factors. In addition to this startling incidence of early acute rejection, late acute rejections were seen in 22% patients who were rejection free at one year. For living donor transplant recipients in the age range of 0-5 years, irreversible rejection was observed in 8.7% compared to 4.1% for older children. Similar results for cadaver donor transplants were 12.6% versus 6.6%. The precise reason for this greatly increased risk of both early and late rejection remains unclear; however, it is likely that children have a more robust immune response, which is inadequately controlled by conventional triple therapy immunosuppression.

The Impact of HLA Matching

The association of HLA antigen mismatching with increased risk of both acute and chronic graft loss is the result of specific immunological injury. Registry data indicate that HLA-B, DR mismatching still accounts for up to 6.4% of the variance in 1 year graft survival [14]. In addition, registry data show a graded result in terms of half-lives amongst cadaveric grafts, based upon numbers of mismatches for HLA-A, -B, and -DR added together. Since 1991, the 3 year graft survival differential between recipients of HLA identical grafts versus recipients that receive 6 antigen mismatched grafts is 12% [15]. When the effect of A, B and DR matching are analyzed separately, it is apparent that each antigen exerts an effect at different time points post-transplantation. The maximal effect of DR mismatching is seen within the first 6 months post-transplantation (corresponding to risk period 1 in **Figure 1**). Mismatching for B antigens exerts the greatest detrimental effect in the first 2 years (corresponding to risk period 2 in **Figure 1**) [16]. The adverse outcome associated with mismatching for the A antigen is only seen after 3 years post-transplantation (corresponding to risk period 3 in **Figure 1**) [17]. The HLA effect is not absolute, as 5% of HLA identicals may lose their grafts from early rejection, the result of immunity directed to other antigen systems (for example, minor HLA antigens). Conversely, 6 HLA antigen mismatched grafts on occasion escape all clinical signs of rejection, indicating that some patients are well protected by current immunosuppressive agents.

It is important to note that serology based tissue typing techniques are subject to a degree of error. Such errors can occur when a rare antigen is not detected due to the lack of a relevant antiserum or alternatively, the reaction pattern of clusters of antisera may be misinterpreted. Other problems may arise due to variation in reagent lots or other technical factors. Taken together, various studies have shown that serologic class I typing can vary by as much as 15-30%. It has recently been shown by genomic typing that zero antigen mismatched recipients enjoy a superior long-term graft survival compared with recipients who receive serologically defined zero antigen mismatched kidneys which are subsequently shown to be mismatched by the molecular techniques [18]. When organ allocation is based on HLA typing, the effect of cold ischemia time on long-term survival is of concern (see below). Opelz et al have previously shown that the beneficial effect of HLA matching outweighs the detrimental effect of prolonging the cold ischemia time in kidneys that are transported [19]. The current data indicate that no difference in graft survival at 5 years was seen when recipients of 6 antigen matched kidneys underwent between 3-36 hours of cold ischemia time. The effect of prolonged cold ischemia time was evident, however, in recipients of mismatched grafts. A stepwise reduction of 1-2% in survival was seen when cold ischemia time was incrementally increased every 12 hours in the mismatched patients [20].

Recent reports of graft survival of living unrelated kidneys donated by a spouse show results which are very close to those with 1 haplotype mismatched (3 HLA mismatches) family member donors, with an average half life of 12 years [21]. If HLA mismatching were the only factor, such grafts should have poorer results, in the range of randomly matched cadaver grafts which generally have about 3-4 HLA mismatches and an average half life of 8.4 years. Since the number of HLA mismatches is similar for spousal donors and the 3-4 HLA mismatched cadaveric donors, the better results with living donors is best explained by less ischemic injury. In addition, as the absence of an HLA barrier (zero mismatches) in cadaveric cases yields an average half life of 13 years, one can also conclude that ischemic injury has a minimal effect in the absence of HLA incompatibility. The only recipients who do not benefit from a zero HLA-A, B, DR mismatched kidney are those who receive a graft from a donor greater than 60 years of age. The half life of kidneys from donors age less than 60 years ranges from 7-8 years, contrasting with 4.6 years for kidneys from mismatched donors greater than 60 years. Because such miserable graft survival occurs also with zero HLA mismatches, it has been proposed that UNOS should no longer support a policy of 6 antigen matching on kidneys retrieved from donors over the age of 60. In summary, the HLA barrier is quantitatively most important in patients who receive an injured organ, or who start a rejection in spite of baseline immunosuppression.

Delayed Introduction of Calcineurin Inhibitor

The use of "sequential" antibody followed by cyclosporine or tacrolimus therapy has been advocated by a number of groups in order to circumvent the nephrotoxic potential of the latter agents in the early post-transplant period at a time when the kidney is particularly sensitive to ischemic insults. Such protocols are based on observations that tissue injury has an adverse outcome on both short-term and long-term graft outcomes. The major determinants of tissue injury include:
- Brain death
- Ischemia/Reperfusion

Effect of Tissue Injury on Graft Outcome

Tissue injury plays a major role in both short and long-term allograft function. Such injury is induced by a number of different stressors of which the most important are brain death and ischemia/reperfusion. Taken together, these processes lead to acute tubular necrosis, which is identified clinically by the failure of the allograft to function promptly in the early post-transplant period. Such a delay in graft function impacts on the risk of rejection at 2 levels. First, the absence of renal function negates the use of the serum creatinine as an indicator of graft well being. Thus, acute rejection may go undetected. Second, the process that led to the acute tubular necrosis may prime the graft to alloimmunity. This occurs *because injury by whatever process promotes a pro-inflammatory milieu* in which endothelial MHC class II is upregulated and messenger RNA for both cytokines and chemokines is also produced in greater amounts [22]. Thus, recipient T cell recognition of donor alloantigen in the presence of the necessary co-stimulatory signals is more likely to occur. This in turn leads to the effector mechanisms of rejection which include DTH, alloantibody responses and cell-mediated cytotoxicity.

Impact of Brain Death. The primary source for solid organ transplants are cadavers who have suffered irreversible central nervous system damage. The clinical observations that organs from living donors, regardless of their relationship to the recipient, are superior to those of cadavers suggest an impact of brain death itself on their quality. Although knowledge of the systemic changes that occur following massive central nervous system injury remains limited, interest is growing in the pathophysiology of this condition. The effect of brain death on the function of peripheral organs have led to an increasing number of experimental and clinical studies designed to elucidate the complex of hemodynamic, neurohormonal and immunological alterations which occur.

Brain death involves a syndrome, which includes rapid swings in blood pressure, hypotension, coagulopathy, pulmonary changes, hypothermia and electrolyte abnormalities. It has been suggested that organs experiencing warm ischemia due to hemodynamic instability in brain dead donors express higher levels of cytokines than those from ideal living donors. Experimentally, kidneys and hearts from brain dead donor animals experience accelerated acute rejection compared with controls, which emphasizes clinical data showing a greater incidence and severity of acute rejection in cadaveric organs over those from living related sources [21]. In a rat model of brain death, peripheral organs demonstrated increased mRNA expression of both lymphocyte- and macrophage-associated products as well as upregulation of MHC class I and II antigens and the costimulatory molecule B7 suggesting increased immunogenicity in the peripheral organs of these animals [23].

The Role of Ischemia/Reperfusion

Although extensively examined in other contexts, ischemia/ reperfusion injury has been relatively underappreciated in organ transplantation as an alloantigen-independent event which may contribute not only to early delayed graft function but also to late allograft dysfunction. Total ischemia of an allograft is the sum of the transient warm ischemic interval before or during actual removal from the donor, cold ischemia associated with preservation and storage, and that ischemia occurring during the period of revascularization. Both the ischemic insult and the events of postischemic reperfusion contribute to tissue injury. Although the mechanisms by which these insults may contribute to ultimate graft demise are still unclear, evidence is growing that the events surrounding organ removal, storage, and engraftment may increase graft immunogenicity by upregulating MHC antigens and triggering the cytokine adhesion molecule cascade to influence the eventual development of rejection.

Following primary ischemia, reperfusion dependent events contribute to the aggravation of ischemia-induced parenchymal injury through prolongation of focal ischemia (no-reflow) or through the action of leukocyte derived cytotoxic mediators (reflow paradox) with leukocyte slowing and sticking to vascular endothelial cells. These initial interactions cause the so-called rolling effect, which leads to progressive slowing of leukocyte traffic along the vascular wall, adherance of these circulating cells to the endothelium and their ultimate infiltration into graft tissue. Selectin, one of a series of adhesion molecules responsible for such leukocyte endothelial interactions, appears to trigger subsequent events. Selectins are not expressed under resting conditions but are upregulated rapidly after injury, initiating neutrophil binding, leukocyte sticking and cellular infiltration. Takada et al studied the role of these molecules during cold ischemia of native kidneys in uninephrectomized rats and demonstrated peak mRNA expression of E-selectin within 6 hours, in parallel to PMN infiltration [23]. T cells and macrophages entered the injured kidney by 2-5 days, and T_h1 products (IL-2, TNFα, IFNγ) and macrophage-associated products (IL-1, IL-6, TGFβ) remained highly expressed after 2 days. MHC class II antigen expression was upregulated, suggesting increased immunogenicity of the organ. When a soluble P-selectin glycoprotein ligand was administered 3 hours after reperfusion, expression of E-selectin mRNA remained at baseline. Leukocytes did not infiltrate the organ during the 7 day period, and their associated products were markedly inhibited. MHC class II expression also remained at near baseline.

Prolonged ischemia may be a risk factor for chronic rejection. In an experimental rat model, Munger et al demonstrated that reduced ischemic time significantly ameliorated later vascular and glomerular changes. Conversely, creatinine levels increased steadily over time in rat recipients of kidney allografts subjected to prolonged ischemia. Tullius et al studied the late functional consequences of ischemia/ reperfusion injury in an ischemic kidney model in uninephrectomized rats with the single native kidney subjected to ischemic insults similar to those occurring during engraftment [24]. Serum creatinine levels and proteinuria, initially elevated, returned transiently to baseline, then increased progressively after 12 weeks. Glomerular filtration rate (GFR) slowly diminished over time. Functional impairment was associated with tubular atrophy and glomerulosclerosis. These and other experimental observations suggest that significant initial ischemia/reperfusion injury around the time of transplantation may contribute to late changes in graft structure and function.

Since the number of acute rejection episodes correlates well with ultimate graft survival, as mentioned in previous sections [15] it would seem likely that DGF would predispose to chronic rejection. In one report, the 5-year survival rate of cadaveric grafts experiencing neither DGF nor acute rejection was 85%, while that of grafts sustaining both injuries was 60%. However, most studies addressing the role of DGF in ultimate graft survival are often retrospective and do not control for acute rejection episodes. In one multivariate analysis, DGF without acute rejection was found to have no impact on long-term graft survival [25]. Until better designed prospective trials are performed, debate will continue as to what extent DGF initiates a programmed process in graft which ultimately leads to chronic dysfunction.

Immunologic Conditioning

The third proposed use for anti-T cell antibody therapy is the induction of "immunological conditioning", either by inducing tolerance or alternatively the minimization of immunosuppressive drugs.

Tolerance is a state of immunological unresponsiveness to an allograft in the presence of an intact immune system. Animal models of tolerance induction have relied upon one of 2 basic mechanisms:

T cell depletion/anergy regimens. One of the most obvious ways to interrupt an immune response is to interfere with antigen-recognition. A variety of monoclonal antibodies directed at T cell surface antigens have been developed and tested for their ability to achieve this goal. Of these, two are particularly noteworthy: Anti-CD3/TCR and anti-CD4. OKT3 is a murine monoclonal antibody against CD3, an invariant portion of the TCR complex present on the surface of all T cells. Administration of OKT3 leads to transient T lymphopenia followed by the appearance of T cells without surface TCRs. The potential mechanisms of action of OKT3 therefore are multiple, including complement-mediated lysis of antibody-coated T cells, antibody-dependent cellular cytotoxicity, opsonization for phagocytosis, and modulation of the TCR off the surface of the T cell, leaving it unable to recognize antigen. Anti-CD4 monoclonal antibodies are targeted against CD4, the molecule which defines MHC class II restricted T cells and which participates in TCR-mediated activation of these cells. These antibodies target a more restricted subset of T cells, and either result in killing of these cells (depleting antibodies) or functional inactivation (non-depleting antibodies). Transient treatment in animal studies can lead to longstanding immunosuppression or tolerance [26,27]. Polyclonal antibodies such as ALS have also been used under similar circumstances which resulted in sometimes indefinite graft survival [28].

Costimulation blockade. The relatively recent discoveries that T cells require costimulatory signals, identification of major costimulatory pathways, and development of reagents to inhibit those pathways, have enabled investigators to test the hypothesis that blockade of costimulatory signals *in vivo* could induce tolerance. Using CTLA4Ig, a soluble fusion protein which is a CD28 homolog and which preferentially binds to CD28-ligands B7-1 and B7-2, several groups have shown greatly prolonged organ allograft and tissue xenograft survival in experimental animals [29]. Recent studies blocking another costimulatory pathway, CD40, CD40-ligand, suggest that targeting this pathway also may prove useful in inducing tolerance [30]. In addition, combination therapy targeting CD28 and CD40 pathways has resulted in long-term engraftment in primate models of transplantation [31].

In spite of the fact that a large number of anti-T cell antibodies have been used in humans as both prophylactic and rescue therapies for rejection, in general such patients have clearly not been rendered tolerant. In fact, true tolerance in humans is a decidedly rare event having been achieved only under some unusual circumstances. For example, Sayegh et al. reported that bone marrow recipients who subsequently develop ESRD may safely receive a living donor kidney from the same individual who donated the bone marrow without immunosuppression [32]. In a more recent example, Spitzer et al. reported a case of a patient rendered tolerant after a combined bone marrow and renal transplant for multiple myeloma. The patient received a lethal dose of irradiation with cyclophosphamide combined with OKT3 before being reconstituted. The patient was subsequently weaned off all immunosuppression within 3 months of transplantation and more importantly, did not suffer any rejection episodes [33].

Minimization of Immunosuppression: The significant renal and extrarenal toxicity associated with conventional immunosuppressive drugs that are in routine clinical use has provided the rationale for the utilization of an antibody induction agent while omitting one of the components of the "convential triple therapy" regimen. The agents most disfavored and consequently most likely to be dropped depend on one's point of view. Alternate approaches have been omission of corticosteroids along with their well-known plethora of side effects or the else calcineurin inhibitors with their nephrotoxic potential. Unfortunately, although some patients benefit from steroid withdrawal, the risk of acute or chronic rejection is so significant that most transplant centers advise against such an approach unless the individual is suffering severe adverse reactions in response to the prednisone [34,35]. More recently, it had been hoped that concurrent use of mycophenolate may permit early steroid withdrawal. The recently performed NIH study examining this hypothesis concluded otherwise however.

The other approach that has been studied recently is omission of the calcineurin inhibitor. One such protocol recently reported involved the use of anti-CD25 antibodies in conjunction with high dose mycophenolate and prednisone but without the use of cyclosporine. Preliminary data indicate that while up to 40% of patients suffer an episode of acute rejection, no grafts were lost to rejection. Furthermore, patients who did not reject had excellent renal function [36]. An alternate approach to the avoidance of cyclosporine is the use of rapamycin. In a recently published trial, sirolimus was equally effective in preventing rejection in place of cyclosporine in the presence of azathiprine and prednisone [37]. Interestingly, the creatinine clearance in the rapamycin group was 10mls/min higher than the cyclosporine group at the end of the first year. These patients did not receive antibody induction however and rejection rates were as high as 41%, an unacceptable level in today's climate of 20% rejection rates. Conceivably, the addition of an antibody induction limb to such a protocol could significantly reduce the risk of at least early rejection.

Efficacy of Antibody Therapy

While the arguments presented above have been utilized by proponents of antibody induction therapy, the published data are less clear that such an approach is associated with a clearly beneficial outcome.

Table 3. Graft survival rates according to PRA status and immunosuppressive protocol.

Regimen	PRA 0-10%		PRA 11-50%		PRA 51-100%	
	1-Year	3-Year	1-Year	3-Year	1-Year	3-Year
CAP	88	76	87	74	85	73
Ind-CAP	88	75	87	73	84	73
CP	88	74	87	74	84	66
Ind-CP	90	76	84	74	82	65
FAP+FP *	90	-	94	-	92	-

CAP- triple therapy with Cyclosporine, Azathioprine and Prednisone; Ind-CAP- induction therapy with ATG, OKT3 or ALG plus CAP; CP- cyclosporine, prednisone; Ind-CP- Antibody induction therapy plus cyclosporine, prednisone; FAP- FK506+Azathioprine, Prednisone; FP- FK506+Prednisone.

* $p < 0.01$ for PRA 11-50% and 51-100% groups.

Data adapted from Katznelson S, Cecka JM. Immunosuppressive regimens and their effect on renal allograft outcome. In: Terasaki PI, ed. Clin Transpl. Los Angeles: UCLA Tissue Typing Lab, 1997:364. vol 1996.

For example, registry data depicted in **Table 3** show that for highly sensitized patients, 1 and 3 year allograft survival rates were only substantially better in those who received tacrolimus based immuno- suppression as compared with these who received cyclosporine. *More importantly, this effect was seen irrespective of antibody induction therapy.*

Proponents of sequential induction therapy in the setting of delayed graft function point out that recipients who avoid early cyclosporine recover renal function more rapidly than those who do not [38]. However, in one randomized prospective study in which cyclosporine and ALG were compared, although creatinine fell more rapidly in the group that did not receive cyclosporine, renal function by day 10 was no different. Rejection frequency and 2 year allograft survival rates were similar [39]. On a cautionary note, the frequency of post- transplant lymphoproliferative disease was significantly higher in the ALG group. Taking a different approach, Troppman and coworkers reviewed a cohort of 457 recipients of primary cadaver allografts from a single center who received sequential ALG with CyA/Aza/Pred.They found a DGF rate of 23% which correlated with the duration of cold ischemia. Patients experiencing DGF had a higher incidence of rejection (57%) and all patients with rejection had a decreased actuarial graft survival rate. However, patients with DGF but without rejection had similar graft survival to patients with immediate function and no rejection [25]. These important data indicate that ATN in the setting of transplantation is a pro-inflammatory state and as such increases the risk of rejection. These 2 "hits" when seen together may have a major impact although ATN in the absence of rejection has little or no effect on long-term graft survival.

A number of studies have been performed to evaluate the hypothesis that certain racial groups may benefit from antibody induction therapy. An early retrospective report by Gaston et al. indicated that ALG induction therapy conferred an improvement in clinical outcome in blacks though not whites [40]. However, these observations were not confirmed by analysis of the registry data [41,42].

More recent data has accumulated about a newer rabbit anti-T cell polyclonal antibody preparation, Thymoglobulin® (Sangstat, Menlo Park, CA) currently licensed for use in renal transplantation by the FDA. Preliminary studies suggest that short courses of this agent used post-transplant can profoundly reduce the risk of rejection short- and long-term and may also enhance 1-year graft survival [43]. There are no data on graft survival beyond the first post-transplant year with Thymoglobulin as yet.

Safety of Antibody Induction Therapy

One of the chief concerns that arises surrounding the use of antibody induction is an increase in the risk of side effects due to suppression of the immune system. Two specific entities that are more commonly encountered are CMV disease and post-transplant lymphoproliferative disease.

CMV: One of the principal risk factors for the development of CMV disease in recipients previously exposed to CMV is the presence of an antibody induction regimen. In one old study, those at risk for primary CMV had a worse outcome (53.1% alive at 6 months with a functioning allograft vs. 70.8%) or patients at risk for reactivation CMV (53.1% vs. 71.1%)[44]. As a consequence of such data, most transplant centers routinely provide prophylactic anti-CMV therapy in recipients receiving anti-lymphocyte therapy.

PTLD: In addition to the increased risk of CMV, the risk of lymphoma is increased by antibody induction. For example, in one single center study, the risk of PTLD was as high as 23% for patients at risk for primary EBV infection who received ALG and subsequently OKT3 rescue [45].

Conclusion

Transplantation today remains a safe and effective method of treating end stage organ failure. However, our current success rates are based on the use of drugs that are associated with a significant toxicity. The optimal "cocktail" for the individual depends on a variety of both donor and recipient specific factors summarized in **Table 4**. It is unlikely

Table 4. Considerations in the Choice of Induction Strategy

Effect on the Graft:
Delayed Graft Function
Acute Rejection
Long-term Allograft Survival
Effect on the Recipient:
Morbidity and Mortality
Infection
Myelosuppression
Malignancy
HAMA
Cytokine Release Syndrome
Route of Administration (Central –v- Peripheral)
Cost

that there will ever be a global consensus on what constitutes the optimal regimen. However, the increasing variety and efficacy of agents that are becoming available should hopefully provide us with a sufficiently diverse arsenal in order to individualize therapy to suit the needs of the patient. While it is not clear that any one regimen is better than any other regimen, maintaining a flexible approach and an open mind is most likely to translate into good outcomes. Finally, while a lot of data has accumulated about some of the older induction agents, newer agents such as thymoglobulin and the anti-CD25 antibodies are yet in their infancy. Only time will tell whether the preliminary data collected thus far will be confirmed.

References

1. Terasaki PI, Cecka JM, Gjertson DW, Takemoto S, Cho YW, Yuge J. Risk rate and long-term kidney transplant survival. Los Angeles: UCLA Tissue Typing Laboratory; 1997.
2. Vella JP, Sayegh MH. Maintenance pharmacological immunosuppressive strategies in renal transplantation. Postgrad Med J 1997;73(861):386-90.
3. Vella JP, O'Neill D, Atkins N, Donohoe JF, Walshe JJ. Sensitization to human leukocyte antigen before and after the introduction of erythropoietin. Nephrol Dial Transplant 1998;13(8):2027-32.
4. Novick AC, Ho-Hsieh H, Steinmuller DS, et al. Detrimental effect of cyclosporine on initial function of cadaver renal allografts following extended preservation: results of randomized prospective trial. Transplantation 1986;42:154.
5. Kahan BD. Drug Therapy: Cyclosporine. N Engl J Med 1989;321(25):1725-38.
6. Matas AJ, Gillingham KJ, Payne WD, Najarian JS. The impact of an acute rejection episode on long-term renal allograft survival (t1/2). Transplantation 1994;57(6):857-9.
7. Basadonna GP, Matas AJ, Gillingham KJ, Payne WD, Dunn DL, Sutherland DE, et al. Early versus late acute renal allograft rejection: impact on chronic rejection. Transplantation 1993;55(5):993-5.
8. Zhou YC, Cecka JM. Sensitization in renal transplantation. Clin Transpl 1991;1991:313-23.
9. Katznelson S, Cecka JM. Immunosuppressive regimens and their effects on renal allograft outcome. Clin Transpl 1996:361-71.
10. Katznelson S, Gjertson DW, Cecka JM. The effect of race and ethnicity on kidney allograft outcome. Clin Transpl 1995;1995(379):379-94.
11. Neylan JF. Immunosuppressive therapy in high-risk transplant patients: dose-dependent efficacy of mycophenolate mofetil in African-American renal allograft recipients. U.S. Renal Transplant Mycophenolate Mofetil Study Group. Transplantation 1997;64(9):1277-82.
12. Neylan JF. Racial differences in renal transplantation after immunosuppression with tacrolimus versus cyclosporine. FK506 Kidney Transplant Study Group. Transplantation 1998;65(4):515-23.
13. Tejani A, Sullivan EK. Factors that impact on the outcome of second renal transplants in children. Transplantation 1996;62(5):606-11.
14. Gjertson DW. Multifactorial analysis of renal transplants reported to the United Network for Organ Sharing Registry: a 1994 update. Clin Transpl 1994:519-39.
15. Cecka JM. The UNOS Scientific Renal Transplant Registry--ten years of kidney transplants. Clin Transpl 1997:1-14.
16. Thorogood J, Houwelingen JC, Persijn GG, Zantvoort FA, Schreuder GM, van RJ. Prognostic indices to predict survival of first and second renal allografts. Transplantation 1991;52(5):831-6.
17. Zandvoort FA, D'Amaro J, Persijn GG, Cohen B, Schreuder GM, van Rood JJ, et al. The impact of HLA-A matching on long-term survival of renal allografts. Transplantation 1996;61(5):841-4.
18. Mytilineous J, Lempert M, Middleton D, Williams F, Cullen C, Scherer S, et al. HLA class I of 215 "HLA-A, -B, -DR zero mismatched" kidney transplants. Tissue Antigens 1997;50:355-8.
19. Opelz G. Correlation of HLA matching with kidney graft survival in patients with or without cyclosporine treatment. Transplant. 1985;40:240-43.
20. Hata Y, Ozawa M, Takemoto S, Cecka JM. HLA Matching. In: Terasaki PI, editor. Clinical Transpl. Los Angeles: UCLA Tissue Typing Laboratory; 1997. p. 381-96.

21. Terasaki PI, Cecka JM, Gjertson DW, Takemoto S. High survival rates of kidney transplants from spousal and living unrelated donors. N Engl J Med 1995;333(6):333-6.
22. Goes N, Urmson J, Ramassar V, Halloran PF. Ischemic acute tubular necrosis induces an extensive local cytokine response. Evidence for induction of interferon-gamma, transforming growth factor-beta 1, granulocyte-macrophage colony-stimulating factor, interleukin-2, and interleukin-10. Transplantation 1995;59(4):565-72.
23. Takada M, Chandraker A, Nadeau KC, Sayegh MH, Tilney NL. The role of the B7 costimulatory pathway in experimental cold ischemia/reperfusion injury. J Clin Invest 1997;100(5):1199-203.
24. Tullius SG, Heemann U, Hancock WW, Azuma H, Tilney NL. Long-term kidney isografts develop functional and morphological changes which mimic those of chronic allograft dysfunction. Ann Surg 1994;220:425-32.
25. Troppmann C, Gillingham KJ, Benedetti E, Almond PS, Gruessner RW, Najarian JS, et al. Delayed graft function, acute rejection, and outcome after cadaver renal transplantation. The multivariate analysis. Transplantation 1995;59(7):962-8.
26. Alegre ML, Lenschow DJ, Bluestone JA. Immunomodulation of transplant rejection using monoclonal antibodies and soluble receptors. Dig Dis Sci 1995;40(1):58-64.
27. Attavar P, Budhai L, Kim BH, Roy-Chowdhury N, Roy-Chowdhury J, Davidson A. Mechanisms of intrathymic tolerance induction to isolated rat hepatocyte allografts. Hepatology 1997;26(5):1287-95.
28. Monaco AP, Wood ML. Studies on heterologous antilymphocyte serum in mice: Optimal cellular antigen for induction of immunological tolerance with ALS. Tran Proc 1970;2:489.
29. Sayegh MH, Turka LA. T cell costimulatory pathways: promising novel targets for immunosuppression and tolerance induction. J Am Soc Nephrol 1995;6(4):1143-50.
30. Denton MD, Reul RM, Dharnidharka VR, Fang JC, Ganz P, Briscoe DM. Central role for CD40/CD40L interactions in transplant rejection. Pediatric Nephrology 1998;2(1):6-15.
31. Kirk AD, Harlan DM, Armstrong NN, Davis TA, Dong Y, Gray GS, et al. CTLA4-Ig and anti-CD40 ligand prevent renal allograft rejection in primates. Proc Natl Acad Sci U S A 1997;94(16):8789-94.
32. Sayegh MH, Fine NA, Smith JL, Rennke HG, Milford EL, Tilney NL. Immunologic tolerance to renal allografts after bone marrow transplants from the same donors [see comments]. Ann Intern Med 1991;114(11):954-5.
33. Spitzer TR, Delmonico F, Tolkoff-Rubin N, McAfee S, Sackstein R, Saidman S, et al. Combined HLA-matched donor bone marrow and renal transplantation for multiple myeloma with ESRD: induction of allograft tolerance through mixed lymphohematopoietic chimerism. Transplantation 1999;68:480.
34. Hricik DE, Almawi WY, Strom TB. Trends in the use of glucocorticoids in renal transplantation. Transplantation 1994;57(7):979-89.
35. Ratcliffe PJ, Dudley CR, Higgins RM, Firth JD, Smith B, Morris PJ. Randomised controlled trial of steroid withdrawal in renal transplant recipients receiving triple immunosuppression. LancetLancet 1996;348(9028):643-8.
36. Tran H, Acharya M, Auchincloss H, Carpenter CB, McKay D, Kirkman R, et al. Cyclosporine sparing effect of daclizumab in renal transplantation. J Am Soc Nephrol 1999;10:749.
37. Groth CG, Backman L, Morales JM, Calne R, Kreis H, Lang P, et al. Sirolimus (rapamycin)-based therapy in human renal transplantation: similar efficacy and different toxicity compared with cyclosporine. Sirolimus European Renal Transplant Study Group [see comments]. Transplantation 1999;67(7):1036-42.

38. Michael HJ, Francos GC, Burke JF, Besarab A, Moritz M, Gillum D, et al. Comparison of the effects of cyclosporine versus antilymphocyte globulin on delayed graft function in cadaver renal transplant recipients. Transplantation 1989;48:805.
39. Belitsky P, MacDonald AS, Cohen AD, Crocker J, Hirsch D, Jindal K, et al. Comparison of antilymphocyte globulin and continuous iv cyclosporine as induction immunosuppression for cadaver kidney transplants. Transplant Proc 1991;23:999.
40. Gaston RS, Hudson SL, Deierhoi MH, Barber WH, Laskow DA, Julian BA, et al. Improved survival of primary cadaveric renal allografts in blacks compared with quadruple immunosuppression. Transplantation 1992;53:103.
41. Tesi RJ, Henry ML, Elkhammas EA, Ferguson RM. Predictors of long-term primary cadaveric renal transplant survival. Clin Transplants 1993;7:345.
42. Katznelson S, Cecka JM. Immunosuppressive regimens and their effect on renal allograft outcome. In: Terasaki PI, editor. Clin Transpl. Los Angeles: UCLA Tissue Typing Lab; 1997. p. 379-94.
43. Brennan DC, Flavin K, Lowell JA, Howard TK, Shenoy S, Burgess S, et al. A randomized, double-blinded comparison of Thymoglobulin versus Atgam for induction immunosuppressive therapy in adult renal transplant recipients. Transplantation 1999;67(7):1011-8.
44. Rubin RH, Tolkoff RN, Oliver D, Rota TR, Hamilton J, Betts RF, et al. Multicenter seroepidemiologic study of the impact of cytomegalovirus infection on renal transplantation. Transplantation 1985;40(3):243-9.
45. Cockfield SM, Preiksaitis JK, Jewell LD, Parfrey NA. Post-transplant lymphoproliferative disorder in renal allograft recipients. Clinical experience and risk factor analysis in a single center. Transplantation 1993;56(1):88-96.

PONYCLONAL ANTILYMPHOCYTE ANTIBODIES

Paul Morrissey and Anthony P. Monaco

Introduction

Polyclonal antilymphocyte antibodies (henceforth ALS/ALG or ATS/ATG) was the first biological immunosuppressive agent introduced into clinical transplantation with the exception of ionizing radiation. Indeed, ALS was the first heterologous antibody used for immunosuppressive effects in man. There now exist over thirty years experience in the clinical use of antilymphocyte antibodies in solid organ transplantation and in selected autoimmune disorders. An enormous literature exists which has established clear-cut and widely accepted indications for the use of ALS in man. A number of commercially manufactured antilymphocyte (ALS/ALG) and antithymocyte (ATS/ ATG) preparations are currently available. In addition, many large transplant programs still manufacture their own preparations for use in their own programs. It is conservatively estimated that between 300,000 and 400,00 transplant patients have been treated with various forms of ALG or ATG. Thus polyclonal antilymphocyte preparations have had and continue to have a significant impact in clinical transplantation.

Historical Development of Experimental and Clinical Antilymphocyte Antibodies

Leslie Brent has written a detailed and complete history of the discovery and development of antilymphocyte antibodies for experimental and clinical use [1]. The biological effects of antisera

Mohamed Sayegh and Giuseppe Remuzzi (editors), Current and Future Immunosuppressive Therapies Following Transplantation, 205-220.
© 2001 Kluwer Academic Publishers. Printed in the Netherlands.

prepared against white cells, especially lymphocytes, have been known for many years since the first description by Metchnikoff [2] and others [1] at the beginning of the 20th century. These early studies described essentially anti-inflammatory effects. The modern era of the experimental study of ALS started with Woodruff and Forman [3] in 1951. They demonstrated that ALS administered *in vivo* induced profound lymphopenia and tissue lymphocyte depletion which was associated with *in vivo* suppression of delayed type hypersensitivity, the first demonstration of the potential immunosuppressive effects of ALS. Additional immunosuppressive activity was shown by Interbitzen [4] and by Waksman and colleagues [5]. The real potential for the use of ALS to modify allograft rejection was clearly established in the early 1960's. Waksman's group [6], Woodruff and Anderson [7,8], Monaco and colleagues (9), and Hume and colleagues [10] showed that ALS suppressed skin allograft rejection in rodents. Subsequently, Monaco et al. [11,12] showed that adjuvant based ALS preparations were extremely immunosuppressive and could prolong primary, secondary and even xenograft skin graft rejection – a remarkable observation. Shortly thereafter, Monaco et al. [13] showed that ALS prepared against canine lymphocytes induced prolonged survival of canine renal allografts without any additional immunosuppression. The demonstration by these same authors that rabbit anti-human ALS suppressed delayed sensitivity reactions and skin allograft rejection in man [14] provided the final major impetus for the large scale development of ALS preparations to be used in man.

Examples of Commercially Available Polyclonal Antilymphocyte Antibodies

Polyclonal ALS/ATS is usually produced by immunization of heterologous large animal species such as horse or rabbits with purified suspensions of lymphocytes or thymocytes derived from human tissue obtained from surgical operations or autopsies. Immunization protocols vary, but usually incorporate adjuvants. Stringent screening of donors of lymphocytes/thymocytes is employed to insure against possible transmission of virus. Donors are screened negative for HbsAg, HCV, HIV I and II antigens, HIV antibody, and HTLV I and II antibody. The purified gamma globulin is obtained by standard techniques. A number of *in vitro* laboratory assays and *in vivo* animal testing techniques are utilized to ensure consistent immunosuppressive potency. A common *in vivo* immunosuppressive assay includes administration to macaque monkeys in a skin allograft model. At the present time, there are two commercially available polyclonal antilymphocyte antibody preparations used in the United States, ATGam (Pharmacia-Upjohn Company) and Thymoglobulin (SangStat). Minnesota ALG (MALG), a horse antihuman lymphoblast polyclonal antibody preparation, was extensively used for years, but is currently no longer available.

ATGam is an immunoglobulin G (IgG) prepared from hyperimmune serum of horses immunized with human thymic lymphocytes. The usual dose for treatment of rejection is up to 15 mg/kg/day for 10-14 days with an option of 7 additional doses on an every other day schedule if needed. For induction or rejection prophylaxis, a dose of 15 to 30 mg/kg/day for 14 days has been recommended or a fixed dose of 15 mg/kg/day for 14 days with an additional 15 mg/kg every other day for a further 14 days. It has been standard recommended practice to administer the ATGam through a vascular shunt, A-V fistula, or a high-flow central vein through an in-line filter (0.2 to 1 micron) over a four hour period. However, note should be made that Rahman et al [23] reported that ATGam was routinely administered through a vein without significant problems or complications. These authors added low doses of heparin and Solucortef to the ATGam solution. ATGam is a potent immunosuppressive agent and there is a general tendency to use less than the recommended doses. Nevertheless, the largest recorded dose given to a patient is 7000 mg in a single daily dose without signs of toxicity. Other patients have received up to 50 doses in a four month period and others have received as many as four 28-day courses of 21 doses without significant toxicity. Note should be made that peripheral administration of polyclonal ALG (ATGam) has been regularly performed by Hardy's group [23]. These authors added low dose heparin into the infusion solution and noted excellent patient tolerance and minimal local reactions.

It is standard recommended procedure to administer a test dose before the administration of the first infusion of ATGam. This is usually done by an intradermal injection of 0.1 milliliter of a 1:1000 dilution (5 micrograms of horse IgG) of ATGam along with a contralateral normal saline control. The occurrence of a systemic reaction including a generalized rash, tachycardia, dyspnea, hypotension, or anaphylaxis precludes use of ATGam. If a significant wheal and flare (10 millimeters of more) and/or a marked local swelling occurs, subsequent infusion of ATGam should be undertaken cautiously. In over thirty years of experience using polyclonal ALS, one of us (APM) has never encountered a significant test reaction that precluded use of the ALS in a specific patient. Premedication with Solumedrol/Solucortef, aceta-minophen, and/or antihistamines is recommended. ATGam is generally well tolerated. A mild first-dose cytokine syndrome consisting of varying degrees of chills, fever, myalgia, and arthralgia can occur, but this symptom complex is unlike the severe cytokine syndrome associated with OKT3. Serum sickness symptoms are rare and mild if present. Hematological effects include possible thrombocytopenia, leukopenia, anemia and hemolysis in varying degrees, a consequence of contaminating antibodies to blood cell components. Severe thrombocytopenia, leukopenia, anemia, or hemolysis may require cessation or reduction of therapy.

Thymoglobulin (SangStat) is a purified, pasteurized gamma immune globulin, obtained by immunization of rabbits with human thymocytes. The reconstituted preparation contains 5 mg/ml of Thymoglobulin of which >90% is rabbit gamma immune globulin (IgG). As with ATGam, human red cells (obtained from US registered or FDA licensed blood banks) are used in the manufacturing process to deplete cross-reacting antibodies to non-T cell antigens. A viral inactivation step (Pasteurization, i.e. heat treatment of active ingredients at 60 C/10 hours) is performed for each lot. Extensive testing is done on all Thymoglobulin lots for potency (lympho-agglutination, E-rosette inhibition assays) and cross-reactive antibodies (hemagglutinins, platelet agglutinins, anti-human serum protein antibodies, anti-glomerular basement membrane antibodies and fibroblast toxicity assays).

The usual dose of Thymoglobulin is 1.5 mg/kg/day for 10-14 days. Recommended administration is via a high-flow vein using an in-line 0.22 micron filter over a minimum 6 hour period after premedication with corticosteroids, acetaminophen, and/or antihistamine). As with ATGam, Thymoglobulin is well tolerated, but a mild first dose cytokine syndrome of fever, chills, arthralgia and myalgia frequently occurs. Thrombocytopenia, leukopenia, and anemia also occur with Thymoglobulin. The Thymoglobulin dose should be reduced by one-half if the WBC count is between 2,000 and 3,000 cells/mm^3 or if the platelet count is between 50,00 and 75,000 cells/ mm^3. Termination of Thymoglobulin therapy is recommended if WBC falls below 2,000 cells/mm^3 or if platelet count falls below 50,000 cells/mm^3.

The majority of transplant centers administer ALS/ATG preparations in empirical fashion according to recommended fixed-dose regiments. Forsythe [24] has emphasized that different polyclonal agents have established differences which must be taken into account for patient therapy. He studied lymphocyte binding and lymphocytotoxicity of various polyclonal preparations from different companies and various batches within each preparation. His studies demonstrated that different polyclonal antibody products may produce different reactions in the same individuals while the same ALS/ATG may cause a variable effect on the immune systems of different individuals. He advocated monitoring of T cell counts during ATG therapy; he stated that administration of ATG at doses to keep the T cells <50/mm3 resulted in less total ATG utilization than when administered at fixed recommended doses. Furthermore, T cell monitored patients had equal efficacy in the treatment of steroid resistant rejection but with less viral and other infectious complications. Similar results were obtained when ATG was administered using T cell monitoring for induction therapy in high risk patients. Forsythe [24] has emphasized that generally patient variability is not considered when ATG is administered according to a fixed dose protocol so that over-immunosuppression or under-immuno-suppression can occur. He strongly recommends the use of daily T cell monitoring be used to govern the daily dose of antilymphocyte agents. In his clinic, this technique has brought about a reduction in the total dose of ATG utilized with no loss of efficacy of the agent and a concomitant reduction in serious viral infections.

Revillard and colleagues [17] have emphasized that the antibody response to ATG is not very profound, but can be clinically significant. The antibody response to polyclonal agents is probably decreased due to concomitant immunosuppression. They state that anti-ATG IgM responses can occur in patients eight days or so after initiation of treatment followed by an IgG response a few days later. ATG-anti-ATG immune complex formation can cause mild fever, malaise, headache, transient arthritis (knees, cervical column, temporal-maxillary joint) plus occasional skin rash and thrombocytopenia. These symptoms usually disappear within a few days of ATG cessation. These authors state that an anti-ATG response can result in neutralization of ATG immunosuppression therapy and even subsequent acute rejection. The antibody response can be characterized by a serial fall in circulating ATG levels assessed by ELISA studies or measurement of antilymph-ocytic antibodies by flow cytometry, followed by appearance of IgM or IgG antilymphocyte antibodies detected by ELISA methods. They advise cessation of ATG administration in patients who manifest symptoms compatible with immune-complex disease between day 8 and 12 of the treatment regimen and to increase the concurrent immunosuppressive treatment.

Immunomodulatory Antibody Specificities in Polyclonal Antilymphocyte Sera

In the original description of experimental polyclonal ALS, it was established that the actual amount of immunoglobulin directed against lymphocytes was less than 2% of the total immunoglobulin extracted. During the three decades since the experimental and clinical usefulness of ALS has been identified, our understanding of the complexity of the immune response has grown dramatically. We now know that the immune response involves many steps, the interruption of one or more of which could lead to varying degrees of immunosuppression. Also, this modern understanding of the immune response has provided the reagents to analyze the specific antibody content of potent ALS/ALG preparations and thereby suggest explanations for the mechanism(s) of action. Indeed, it is remarkable that subsequent analysis of ALS preparations has identified multiple specific antibodies that could mediate all of the potential mechanisms of action that were suggested in the early experimental studies with ALS (see below). Bonnefoy-

Berard et al. [15] first provided specific analysis that showed potent ALS preparations contained antibodies against numerous functional leukocyte surface molecules. They showed that antibodies to CD45, CD3, CD5, CD11a, and CD18 were present at high titer and that additional antibodies to CD2, CD4, CD8, CD25, HLA-DR and β_2 microglobulin were also present. In a subsequent study, Rebellato et al [16] provided a comprehensive identification of the major antibodies in polyclonal rabbit ALG. They identified at least 23 antigenic specificities. The highest titer antibodies (>1:4000) were anti-CD6, CD16, CD18, CD28, CD38, CD40, and CD58 (mostly non-T cell specific antibodies). In addition, these authors observed that the rabbit ATG antibodies that persisted longest *in vivo* in Rhesus monkeys are antibodies to CD3, CD4, CD8, CD11a, CD40, CD45, CD54, and MHC Class I (antibodies directed to signal transduction and adhesion molecules). These authors suggested that the persistence of antibodies *in vivo* may be directly related to prolonged anergy of circulating T cells observed in recipients after rabbit ATG treatment.

Mechanism of Action of ALS/ATS

Brent [1] has elegantly summarized the early history of ALS particularly in regard to the early concepts of the mechanism(s) of action of ALS. The first thought was that the selective depletion of circulating and tissue lymphocytes mediated by direct lymphocytotoxicity and/or opsonization accounted for the immunosuppressive effect of ALS. Persistent immunosuppression after recovery from lymphopenia suggested that some other mechanism (s) were also operative. In addition, the concept of "blindfolding" was also introduced, i.e., interaction of ALS antibodies with the lymphocytes prevented in some way their recognition of graft antigen(s). Another idea was that ALS antibodies caused sterile activation, i.e., lymphocytes recognized graft antigens and were activated, but for some reason could not exert cytopathic effects. A fourth idea was that ALS, by producing widespread (tissue) lymphopenia, produced a unique state of immunological incompetence similar to the developing neonatal immune system which fostered tolerance induction in some unexplained way. It is extraordinary that the availability of appropriate modern immunological reagents has permitted identification of various antibody specificities that could explain the immunological mechanisms suggested by these early experimental observations.

Within the first day after administration of a potent antilymphocyte globulin, peripheral blood lymphocyte counts drop drastically, usually to below 200/μl. Indeed, many investigators adjust ATG dosage by daily monitoring of E-rosette forming cells or counts of CD3+ or CD2+ lymphocytes. Following administration of a potent ALS, CD4+, CD8+ and

CD56+ lymphocytes drop to the 10-20/μl range and B cell counts increase. A population of null cells lacking T and B cell markers then accounts for 30-40% of peripheral blood lymphocytes. This population consists of T cells that have modulated surface antigens. Elegant studies by Revillard et al [17] and others [18] have shown that the mechanisms of lymphocyte depletion after ATS involves complement-dependent opsonization and lysis and Fc-dependent opsonization. These authors have studied Fc-dependent mechanisms of *in vivo* lymphocyte depletion. Both horse and rabbit ATGs can bind human C1q and activate the human complement cascade. They found that the density of ATG molecules required for C1q binding is only achieved with horse ATG treatments, usually when high ATG doses are given with horse ATG therapy (0.1 to 0.5 mg/ml). In contrast, only rabbit-produced ATG (not horse) efficiently interacts with human Fcγ receptors on phagocytes. Thus, Fc-dependent opsonization occurs predominantly during rabbit ATG therapy (0.1mg/ml). Their studies have shown that complement-dependent lysis and Fc-dependent opsonization are controlled by the density of ATG molecules at the cell surface and the structure of the Fc receptor of the IgG molecules (horse or rabbit). As noted above, most potent ATG/ALG preparations have numerous other antibody specificities that recognize numerous lymphocyte surface molecules. These antibodies do not contribute to complement dependent lysis or Fc-dependent opsonization and are probably irrelevant to these activities. However, they probably interrupt various aspects of the immune response and therefore contribute to the net immunosuppressive effect.

Revillard's group [19] has also established that ATG also induces surface Fas (Apo-1, CD95) expression in naïve T cells and Fas-ligand gene and protein expression in both naïve and primed T cells, resulting in Fas/Fas-L interaction mediated cell death. Interestingly, ATG-induced apoptosis and Fas-L expression were not observed with ATG preparations lacking CD2 and CD3 antibodies. Most importantly, susceptibility to ATG induced apoptosis was restricted to activated cells, was dependent on IL-2, and was prevented by cyclosporine A, FK506, or rapamycin. These authors suggested that low dose ATG could be evaluated clinically in treatment protocols aimed at selective depletion of *in vivo* activated T cells in order to avoid massive lymphocyte depletion and over immunosuppression. Merion et al [20] focused on another outcome of the multiple specific antibodies contained in polyclonal ALS preparations. These authors showed that certain ATG preparations (ATGam) recognize and cross-link multiple cell surface receptors and co-stimulator molecules on human T cells. They suggested that engagement of multiple specificities in the context of allogeneic or mitogenic stimulation could lead to partial T cell activation and anergy. This mechanism obviously could contribute to facilitating tolerance.

Several potent ATS preparations have been shown to induce certain functional effects which contribute to overall immunosuppression. These preparations are mitogenic for peripheral T cells *in vitro* at concentrations achieved in the patient's serum during treatment (0.1 µg/ml). Activation of T cells is accomplished within a narrow range of ATG concentrations. Bonnefoy-Berard et al [18] have demonstrated that in contrast to OKT3, the T cell activating properties of ATGs can be demonstrated *in vitro* in the absence of cross-linking by receptors since ATG F(ab)$_2$ fragments are potent activators. T cell activation is associated with proinflammatory type I cytokines (IL-2, IFN-γ, and TNF-α) and may account for the first-dose cytokine syndrome with fever, chills, headache, and occasionally dyspnea. The syndrome is usually milder than that associated with OKT3 and probably reflects the combined effects of activation, co-activations, and multiple antibody specificities in ATG. In addition, potent ATG preparations induce modulation,, i.e. measurable decrease in cell surface expression of a number of molecules which control T cell activation and/or adhesion, including CD3/TCR, CD4, CD8, CD2, and CD5. These effects are achieved at lower ATG concentrations (1 to 10 µg/ml) and are likely to account in part for the T cell functional impairment that occurs after ATG administration. Modulation of TCR/CD3 by ATG is associated with T cell unresponsiveness to antigens and allogeneic cells as has been shown with OKT3. *In vitro*, ATGs induce a TH-dependent transient activation of B cells [21] followed by apoptosis of activated B cells. ATGs can induce apoptosis of some hematopoietic cell lines and that of lymphoblastoid B cells obtained by infection with Epstein–Barr virus.

More recent studies have provided additional information on possible mechanisms of action of polyclonal ALS and/or ATG. Muller et al [22] identified long-term changes induced *in vivo* by polyclonal ALS. These authors showed that polyclonal ALS induced dose dependent, long-term changes in T lymphocyte subsets which persisted over a period of years. They showed that five years after ATG administration and clinical transplantation, ATG recipients had reversed CD4 to CD8 ratios which were not present in transplant recipients treated with OKT3. The altered ratio was due to a persistent depletion of the CD4+ cells and to increased regeneration of CD8+ cells, in particular of the CD8+ bright, CD57+ subpopulation. The Cd8+CD57+ subset appears to be a regulatory cell population. Alterations in the lymphocyte subsets are likely to have significant long-term functional consequences. A crucial question is whether this new homeostasis reflects a beneficial immunomodulation (such as long-term graft survival and remission of auto-immune diseases) or an impairment of immune responses (such as that associated with infections and malignancies). This question is still open despite the clinical use of these agents for nearly 30 years and is due to the lack of long-term studies. Further studies are necessary to determine whether these cells have an important immunoregulatory (suppressive) function and a beneficial effect for graft function.

Indications for Polyclonal Antilymphocyte Therapy

The over thirty years of clinical experience with polyclonal antilymphocyte antibodies has established an enormous literature which defines clear-cut and widely accepted indications for their use. In solid organ transplantation, ALS is indicated for **induction therapy.** Induction therapy refers to a course of immunosuppression given in the pre-, peri- and/or immediately post-transplant period for a finite period of time. The immunosuppression given as induction therapy is over and above the drug protocol given for continued maintenance immunosuppression. Polyclonal ALS was the first biological immunosuppressive therapy used for induction therapy (with the exception of total body irradiation). Induction therapy by ALS is used to suppress the T cell response and prevent or delay the onset of acute rejection. Induction therapy with ALS is indicated for high-risk kidney and non-renal transplants, i.e. sensitized (high PRA) recipients, secondary transplants, African-American recipients, delayed graft function, etc. Induction therapy with ALS is also indicated when delay in institution of nephrotoxic immunosuppressive drugs (calcineurin inhibitors) is desired, i.e. to prevent rejection before therapeutic levels of other drugs are achieved. In addition, induction therapy with ALS has been used as a basic strategy in protocols aimed at **steroid avoidance, sparing or elimination.** ALS is also indicated in the treatment **of established acute rejection**. However, since most initial or secondary acute rejection reactions are reversed with simple steroid treatment, ALS treatment is usually reserved for **steroid-resistant rejection**. Polyclonal ALS is an established therapy for **graft-versus-host-disease** in clinical bone marrow transplantation. Also, polyclonal ALS has an established primary indication for **aplastic anemia.**

Clinical Efficacy of Polyclonal ALS in the Cyclosporine and Post-Cyclosporine Era

Prior to the cyclosporine era, the routine addition of polyclonal ALS to the existing azathioprine-prednisone regimens was obvious and intuitive. Similarly, the use of ALS to treat steroid-resistant rejection became the most effective available treatment in these situations prior to the availability of monoclonal antibodies against lymphocytes. With the advent of more effective immunosuppression in the cyclosporine era, the need for antilymphocyte therapy, particularly for induction, has been questioned. In the cyclosporine era, many programs continued to use some type of antilymphocyte antibody (polyclonal or monoclonal) in the presence of delayed graft function (because of cyclosporine nephrotoxicity) or high-risk recipient status (sensitization, retransplantation). However, in the absence of delayed graft function or categorical high-risk, routine antilymphocyte antibody for induction continues to be questioned in the era of potent immunosuppressive drugs such as cyclosporine, tacrolimus, sirolimus, etc.. In this regard, support for induction therapy is found in a recent meta-analysis of the effect of antilymphocyte induction therapy on renal allograft survival in patients treated with cyclosporine based triple therapy (cyclosporine, prednisone, azathioprine) [25]. This study showed a 9% improvement in long-term survival (1-3 years) in patients who had received some type of antilymphocyte antibody therapy. The case remains fairly strong for induction antibody therapy in high risk patients. A recent randomized prospective study comparing induction with and without polyclonal ATG in high risk sensitized kidney allograft recipients treated with cyclosporine, prednisone and azathioprine showed a definite survival advantage for patients given ATG induction [26]. Even addition of ATG induction to low risk living donor kidney recipients treated with cyclosporine based therapy showed an advantage for ATG induction which lowered the incidence of acute rejection [27]. It is clear that even in the modern era of potent immunosuppressive agents, antilymphocyte therapy (monoclonal or polyclonal) continues to play a significant role. As newer immunosuppressive agents are introduced, the role of antilymphocyte therapy will continue to require review. The use of newer immunosuppressive agents, such as mycophenolate mofetil in maintenance immunosuppressive programs suggests the logical question of a continued role for inductive antilymphocyte therapy. Very little information is available on this subject, but it is of interest that a recent study by Florence et al [28] showed a favorable effect of polyclonal ATG induction in reducing acute rejection after 18 months in kidney recipients given cyclosporine, prednisone, and mycophenolate mofetil. Also, the excellent efficacy of polyclonal ATG in reversing acute rejection in the cyclosporine era was recently confirmed again and the superiority of rabbit-based ATG over horse-based ATG was emphasized [29]. Furthermore, Birkeland [30] has recently demonstrated that induction therapy with polyclonal antibody incorporated into standard immunosuppression with cyclosporine and azathioprine or mycophenolate mofetil facilitated total avoidance of steroid use with excellent short and long term patient and graft survival.

The question as to whether a horse or rabbit produced polyclonal antilymphocyte antibody preparation offers any advantage or superiority in efficacy was studied by Brennan et al. [31]. They performed a prospective, randomized study of Thymoglobulin and ATGam for induction in renal transplantation. These authors found that patients treated with Thymoglobulin had remarkable freedom from acute and recurrent rejection and superior patient and graft survival at

12 and 18 months. In this study, Thymoglobulin-treated patients exhibited more prolonged and sustained lymphopenia. Nevertheless, Thymoglobulin-treated patients had less CMV infection and similar overall incidence of infections. Also, Thymoglobulin had been shown to be superior to ATGam in treatment of acute rejection in the first six months post-transplant [29]. Woodle et al [32] reported that this beneficial effect extended to beyond 1 year in that patients successfully treated for rejection with Thymoglobulin had a significantly increased duration of subsequent rejection-free graft survival compared to ATGam-treated patients.

In addition to the role of polyclonal antibody therapy in relation to the newer chemical immunosuppressive agents is the question of what role polyclonal ALS will play versus existing and newer monoclonal antibodies. Burk and Maturszewski [33] recently reviewed published studies of the use of polyclonal ATG and OKT3 in renal transplantation. Although various individual centers demonstrate advantages for ATG or OKT3 over each other in varying situations, the authors concluded that the current literature contained no prospective, randomized, controlled comparisons of OKT3 and ATG used in conjunction with standardized regimens of conventional immunosuppressive agents and anti-rejection protocols. Thus far, the same observations apply to the newer mono-clonal antibodies. The lack of toxicity, particularly the absence of the cytokine release syndrome, and the ease of administration make the newer monoclonal anti-IL-2 receptor antibody preparations extremely attractive. These preparations have significantly (but not dramatically) reduced the incidence of acute rejection when used as inductive therapy [34,35]. Long-term effects are not established and they have not been proven effective in the treatment of acute rejection or steroid-resistant rejection. Also, their efficacy in high risk, sensitized or retransplanted patients is not established – areas of proven polyclonal ALS efficacy. No studies have been performed in which polyclonal ALS has been compared with the newer monoclonal (anti-IL-2 receptor) antibodies. These studies are critical for an accurate evaluation of the clinical role of newer monoclonals, particularly with the availability of extremely potent rabbit antithymocyte sera (29). Indeed, one legacy of polyclonal ALS is that it is the most widely used antilymphocyte preparation in clinical transplantation. The multiple specificities to lymphocyte surface molecules present in polyclonal ALS may constitute a distinct advantage which permits interruption of the allograft response at multiple stages. *Thus, effective polyclonal antilymphocyte sera are the standard against which all newer monoclonals should be evaluated. The concept that any new monoclonal would automatically be better than a polyclonal sera is unjustified and certainly not supported (thus far) by any experimental or clinical data.*

Polyclonal Antilymphocyte Serum and Tolerance

Polyclonal ALS has had a unique and important history in the study of experimental allograft tolerance. This has been reviewed by Brent [1]. Monaco et al [36] were the first to show that the non-specific immunosuppressive state induced by ALS could be converted to a state of specific tolerance by addition of replicating F1-hybrid lymphoid cells using a skin allograft model in rodents. This observation was confirmed and expanded by Lance and Medawar [37]. Subsequently, Monaco, Wood, and Gozzo [38,39] described a mouse skin graft model of tolerance using transient ALS immunosuppression and post-transplantation donor specific bone marrow infusion. Extensive and continuing studies of the ALS-bone marrow model have shown that the mechanism of tolerance is multifactorial. Initial treatment with ALS induces non-specific host derived suppressor cells [40] but addition of bone marrow produces a microchimeric state with persisting suppressor cells identifiable as of donor origin [41,42] reminiscent of the veto concept of Muraoka and Miller [43]. Recent studies have also shown a role for clonal reduction and anergy in addition to suppression and possible microchimerism [44,45] with the various mechanisms evolving in a sequential manner. The ALS-bone marrow model of Monaco and colleagues has been extended to renal allografts in dogs [46,47] and Rhesus monkeys [48,49], and to liver allografts in baboons [50]. Initial trials of polyclonal ALS and donor specific bone marrow in renal allografts in man have yielded equivocal results [51-55] but recent studies in liver transplantation [56,57] are extremely encouraging. Since donor specific bone marrow infusion with ALS pretreatment has yielded some degree of tolerance in every species tested thus far and with every type of allograft tested, it is highly likely that this effect will also be eventually obtained in man [58].

References

1. Brent, L, Immunoregulation: The Search for the Holy Grail (Chapter 6) In: A history of Transplantation Immunology, Academic Press, 1997
2. Metchnikoff, E. Etudes sur la resorption des cellules. Ann Inst Pasteur 13:737-743,1899
3. Woodruff, MFA and Forman, B. Effects of antilymphocyte serum on suspension of lymphocytes *in vitro*. Nature 168:36-38,1958
4. Interbitzen, T. Int Arch Allergy 4:150-153,1956
5. Waksman, B and Arboysm S. Antisera to lymphocytes. In: Mechanisms of Antibody Formation. Czech Acad Sci Prague 1960 pg 165-187.
6. Waksman, BH, Arboys, S, and Aronson, BG. The use of specific lymphocyte antisera to inhibit hypersensitivity reactions of the delayed type. J Exp Med 114:997-1001, 1961
7. Woodruff, MFA and Anderson, NE. Effects of lymphocyte depletion by thoracic duct fistula and administration of antilymphocyte serum on the survival of skin homografts in rats. Nature 200:702-704, 1963
8. Woodruff, MFA and Anderson, NE. Antilymphocyte serum and its mode of action. Ann NY Acad Sci 130:119-121, 1964
9. Gray, JG, Monaco, AP, and Russell, PS. Heterologous mouse antilymphocyte serum to prolong skin homografts. Surg Forum 15:142-143, 1964
10. Sach, JH, Fillipone, DR, and Hume, DM. Studies on the immune destruction of lymphoid tissue. I. Lymphocytotoxic effect of rabbit anti-rat lymphocyte sera. Transplantation 2:60-66, 1964
11. Gray, JG, Monaco, AP, and Wood, ML. Studies on heterologous antilymphocyte serum in mice. I. *In vitro* and *in vivo* properties. J Immunol 96(2):217-220, 1966
12. Monaco, AP, Wood, ML, Gray, JG et al. Studies on heterologous antilymphocyte serum in mice. II. Effect on the immune response. J Immunol 96(2):229-238, 1966
13. Monaco, AP, Abbott, WM, Otherson, HB et al. Antisera to lymphocytes: Prolonged survival of canine allografts. Science 153(741)1264-1267, 1966
14. Monaco, AP, Wood, ML, van der Werf, BA et al. Recent observations of antilymphocyte serum in mice, dogs, and man. In: GEW Wolstenholme and M O'Connor (eds). Ciba Foundation Study Group, No. 29, Antilymphocyte Serum, London,A. Churchill, 1967;111-123.
15. Bonnefoy-Berard, N, Vincent, C, and Revillard, JP. Antibodies against functional leukocyte surface molecules in polyclonal antilymphocyte and antithymocyte globulins. Transplantation 51(3): 669-673, 1991
16. Rebellato, LM, Gross, V, Verbanac, KM et al. A comprehensive definition of the major antibody specificities in polyclonal rabbit antithymocyte globulin. Transplantation 57(5):685-689, 1994
17. Revillard, JP, Bonnefoy-Berard, N, Preville, X et al. Immunopharmacology of Thymoglobulin. Grafts(Supplement) 2(1):6-9, 1999
18. Bonnefoy-Berard, N, Vincent, C, Verrier, B et al. Monocyte independent T cell activation by polyclonal antithymocyte globulin. Cell Immunol 143(2):272-283, 1992
19. Genestier, L, Fournell, S, Flacher, M et al. Induction of Fas (Apo-1, CD95)-mediated apoptosis of activated lymphocytes by polyclonal antilymphocyte globulin. Blood 91(7):2360-2368, 1998
20. Merion, RM, Howell, T, and Bromberg, JS. Partial T cell activation and anergy induction by polyclonal antithymocyte globulin. Transplantation 65(11):1481-1489, 1998

21. Bonnefoy-Berard, N, Genestier, L, Flacher, M et al.   Apoptosis induced by polyclonal antilymphocyte globulins in human B cell lines.   Blood   83(4):1051-1059, 1994
22. Miller, TF.   Long-term T cell dynamics following the use of polyclonal and monoclonal antibodies.   Graft(supplement)   2(1):15-20, 1999
23. Rahman, GF, Hardy, MA, and Cohen, DJ.   Administration of equine anti-thymocyte globulin via peripheral vein in renal transplant recipients.   Transplantation   69(9):1958-1960, 2000
24. Forsthe, JL.   ATG dosing;   Daily or less frequently?   Graft (supplement)   2(1):10-14, 1999
25. Szczech, LA, Berlin, JA, Aradhye, S et al.   Effect of antilymphocyte induction on renal allograft survival: a meta-analysis.   J Amer Soc Neph   8(11):1771-1777, 1997.
26. Thibauddin, D, Alamartine, E, De Fellippis, J et al.   Advantage of antilymphocyte induction in sensitized kidney recipients; a randomized prospective study comparing induction with and without antilymphocyte globulin.   Nephrol Dial Transplant   13(3):711*715, 1998
27. Cardella, CJ, Cattran, D, Fenton, SA et al.   Induction with rabbit antilymphocyte sera reduces rejection episodes in immunologically low risk renal transplant recipients.   Transplant Proc   29(7A):29S-31S, 1997
28. Florence, LS, Howard, DR, Chapman, PH et al.   Presentation at 23rd American Society of Transplant Surgeons, Chicago, May 1997
29. Gaber, AO, First, MR, Tesi, RJ et al.   Results of the double-blind, randomized, multicenter, phase III clinical trial of thymoglobulin versus ATGam in the treatment of acute graft rejection episodes after renal transplantation.   Transplantation   66(1):29-37, 1998
30. Birkeland, SA.   Steroid-free immunosuppression after kidney transplantation with antithymocyte globulin induction and cyclosporine and mycophenolate mofetil maintenance therapy.   Transplantation   66(9):1207-1210,1998
31. Brennan, DC, Flavin, K, Lowell, JA et al.   Comparison of Thymoglobuline and ATGam for induction in renal transplantation.   Graft (supplement)   2(1):21-23, 1999
32. Woodle, ES, First, MR, Gaber, AO et al.   12 month outcome of the double blind, randomized multicenter rejection trial of Thymoglobulin versus ATGam in renal transplants.   Graft (supplement)   2(1):24-27
33. Burk, ML and Natuszewski, RA.   Muromonab-3 and antithymocyte globulin in renal transplantation. Ann Pharmacother   32(11):1370-1378, 1977
34. Vincenti, F, Kirkman, R Light, S et al.   Interleukin-2 receptor blockade with diclizumab to prevent acute rejection in renal transplantation.   Diclizumab triple therapy study group.   N Engl J Med   338(3):161-165, 1998
35. Kahan, BD, Rajagopalan, PR, Hall, ML et al.   Basilixamab (simulect) is efficacious in reducing the incidence of acute rejection episodes in renal allograft patients; results at 12 months   Transplantation 65(12):S189-S194, 1998
36. Monaco, AP, Wood, ML, and Russel, PS.   Studies on antilymphocyte serum in mice.   III. Immunological tolerance and chimerism produced across the H-2 locus with adult thymectomy and antilymphocyte serum.   Ann NY Acad Sci   129:190-193, 1966
37. Lance, E and Medawar, PB.   Quantitative studies on tissue transplantation immunity.   IX. Induction of tolerance with antilymphocyte serum.   Proc R Soc Lond Biol Sci 173(33):447-473, 1969
38. Monaco, AP and Wood, ML.   Studies on heterologous antilymphocyte serum in mice.   Vii. Optimal cellular antigens for induction of immunological tolerance with antilymphocyte serum.   Transpl Proc   2(4):489-496, 1970

39. Gozzo, JJ, Wood, ML, and Monaco, AP. Use of allogeneic homozygous bone marrow cells for the induction of specific immunologic tolerance in mice treated with antilymphocyte serum. Surg. Forum 21:281-284, 1970

40. Simpson, MA and Gozzo, JJ. Studies on the mechanism of action of rabbit antithymocyte serum. I. Induction of suppressor cells. Transplantation 30(1):64-72, 1980

41. Maki, T, Simpson, MA, and Monaco, AP. Development of suppressor T cells by antilymphocyte serum treatment in mice. Transplantation 34(6):376-381, 1982

42. Maki, T, Gottschalk, R,, and Wood, ML. Specific unresponsiveness to skin allografts in ALS treated, marrow injected mice; Participation of donor marrow derived suppressor cells. J Immunol 127(4):1433-1438, 1981

43. Muraoka, S and Miller, RG. Cells in bone marrow and T cell colonies grown from bone marrow can suppress generation of cytotoxic T lymphocytes directed against their self antigen. J Exp Med 152(1):54-71, 1980

44. Hale, DA, Gottschalk, R, Maki, T et al. Determination of an improved sirolimus (rapamycin) based regimen for induction of allograft tolerance in mice treated with antilymphocyte serum and donor specific bone marrow. Transplantation 65(4):473-478, 1998

45. Hale, DA, Gottschalk R, Umemura A, Maki T, Monaco AP. Establishment of stable multilineage hematopoietic chimerism and donor-specific tolerance without irradiation. Transplantation 69(7):1242-51, 2000

46. Hartner, WC, DeFAzio, SR, Maki, T et al. Prolongation of renal allograft survival in antilymphocyte serum treated dogs by post-operative injection of density gradient fractionated donor bone marrow. Transplantation 42(6):593-597, 1986

47. Hartner, WC, Markees, TG, DeFazio, SR et al. The effect of antilymphocyte serum, fractionated donor bone marrow, and cyclosporine on renal allograft survival in mongrel dogs. Transplantation 52(5):784-789, 1991

48. Thomas, JM, Carver, FM, Cunningham, P et al. Kidney allograft tolerance in primates without chronic immunosuppression – the role of veto cells. Transplantation 51(1):198-207, 1991

49. Thomas, JM, Verbanac, KM and Thomas FT. The veto mechanism in transplant tolerance. Transplant Rev 5:209-214, 1997

50. Myburgh, JA, Smit, JA, Mieny, CJ et al. Hepatic allotransplantation in the baboon. 3. The effects of immunosuppression and administration of donor specific antigen after transplantation. Transplantation 12(3):202-210, 1971

51. Barber, WH, Mankinn, JA, Laskow, DA et al. Long term results of a controlled, prospective study with transfusion of donor specific bone marrow in 57 cadaveric renal allograft recipients. Transplantation 51(1):70-74,, 1991

52. Shapiro, R, Rao, AS, Fontes, P et al. Combined kidney/bone marrow transplantation – evidence of augmentation of chimerism. Transplantation 59(2):306-309, 1995

53. Garcia-Morales, R, Carreno, M. Mathew, J et al. The effects of chimeric cells following donor bone marrow infusion as detected by PCR-flow assays in kidney transplant recipients. J Clin Invest 99(5):1118-1129, 1997

54. Garcia-Morales, R, Esquenazi, V, Zucker, K et al. Assessment of the effects of cadaver bonemarrow on chimerism in kidney transplant recipients by the polymerase chain reaction-flow technique. Transplantation 62(8):1149-1161, 1996

55. Garcia-Morales, R, Carreno, M, Mathew, J et al. Continuing observation on the regulatory effect of donor specific bone marrow cell infusions and chimerism in kidney transplant recipients. Transplantation 65(7):956-965, 1998

56. Ricordi, C, Karatzas, T, Nery, J et al.   Human islet allografts in patients with type 2 diabetes undergoing liver transplantation.   Transplantation   63(3):473-475, 1997

57. Tsarouvha, AK, Rocordi, C, Noto, TA et al.   Donor peripheral blood stem cell infusion in recipients of living related liver allografts.   Transplantation 64(2):362-364, 1997

58. Monaco, AP.   A new look at polyclonal antilymphocyte antibodies in clinical transplantation.   Graft (supplement)   2(1):2-5, 1998

MONOCLONAL ANTIBODY TARGETING OF THE T CELL RECEPTOR COMPLEX

Lucienne Chatenoud

Introduction

OKT3 was the first murine monoclonal antibody to be introduced in clinical practice for both the treatment and the prevention of acute renal allograft rejection [1-3]. The initial rationale for these studies was the capacity of OKT3 to stain all mature peripheral T cells and to completely abolish both T cell proliferation and the generation of cytotoxic T cell effectors in *in vitro* mixed lymphocyte cultures [4]. Interestingly enough, this occurred in 1981, few years before it could be firmly established that the specific molecular target of OKT3 was one of the polypeptide chains included within the major T cell recognition element namely, the T cell antigen receptor (TCR)/CD3 complex.

In fact, the fine molecular structure of the TCR was first described in 1984. T cell receptors expressed by the vast majority of T lymphocytes are polypeptide heterodimers, termed ab, which share many structural similarities with B cell antigen receptors (immunoglobulins) since they include a variable and a constant portion. T cells bearing another form of TCR, the gd heterodimer, are less numerous (5-10% of peripheral T cells). Importantly, both ab and gd TCRs are expressed at the T cell surface in tight association with a set of five distinct non-polymorphic polypeptide chains constituting the TCR/CD3 complex. Further functional studies clearly established that the TCR ab and gd chains are the "antigen recognition" elements of the complex while CD3 chains, in particular the e and z chains, are the "signal-transducing" elements [5,6]. OKT3 as well as most of the other therapeutic CD3 antibodies that have

Mohamed Sayegh and Giuseppe Remuzzi (editors), Current and Future Immunosuppressive Therapies Following Transplantation, 221-234.
© 2001 Kluwer Academic Publishers. Printed in the Netherlands.

been studied in humans, rodents or monkeys are specific for the e chain of the TCR/ CD3 complex.

It is quite evident from both the clinical and the experimental data accumulated so far that CD3 antibodies are among the most potent immunosuppressive agents available. Moreover, quite interestingly and unexpectedly, recent experimental data, not only in rodents but also in non-human primates, and both in transplantation and autoimmunity, have suggested that CD3 anti-bodies may also promote long-term antigen specific unrespon-siveness namely, immune tolerance.

Our aim will be to review these results and to discuss why the future of clinically applicable immunointervention strategies using CD3 anti-bodies especially of humanized CD3 antibodies, that are not immuno-genic and do not provoke, as murine OKT3, the major cytokine-related "flu-like" acute syndrome, do hold great promise in clinical immunology.

The Molecular Structure of the TCR/CD3 Complex

T cells expressing ab TCRs bind through their variable regions pro-cessed antigenic peptides presented in the context of major histocom-patibility (MHC) class I or class II molecules. In contrast, data on the fine specificity of gd TCRs expressing T cells suggest that they behave more like immunoglobulins in that they seem to recognize antigens directly and do not require the presence of neither MHC nor other antigen presenting molecules for adequate antigen recognition. Just as immunoglobulin chains, ab and gd TCR chains are the products of distinct gene segments, encoding for variable (V), diversity (D) (for TCR b and d), joining (J) and constant regions, that rearrange in T lymphocytes [6]. Immunoprecipitation studies using clonotypic anti-bodies after solubilisation with gentle detergents, such as digitonin, revealed the presence of the five other polypeptide chains (e.g. the CD3 chains) that coprecipitated with the ab TCR and were termed CD3 g, d (although the nomenclature may be misleading these are non polymorphic CD3 chains distinct from gd TCR), e and z. The z chain is present in the complex as a disulfide-bonded homodimer (z-z) or heterodimer. This heterodimer associates the z chain to h (an alternate splicing product of the z gene) in mouse cells and to the g chain of the $F_c eRI$ and the $F_c gRIII$ (CD16) receptors in human cells [6]. There is compelling evidence to show that there are at least two ab hetero-dimers per TCR/ CD3 functional complex $[[ab]_2[g/de]_2[zz]_4]$ assembled at the T cell surface [6].

Clinical Use of CD3 Antibodies

The clinical use of CD3 antibodies essentially developed in solid organ transplantation. Between 1981 and 85 a first pilot trial, including few patients, immediately followed by a large randomized multicenter trial clearly established the efficacy of OKT3 to reverse early acute renal allograft rejection episodes [1,2,7], a use for which the antibody was rapidly licensed both in the USA and Europe. The dose regimen was based on the data from the pilot trial in which escalating doses were applied [1,2]. Thus, 5 mg/day were administered for 10 to 15 consecutive days. The general practice was also to decrease the dosages of other concurrent medications during OKT3 treatment.

The use of OKT3 rapidly expanded from the treatment of early acute rejection to that of rejection episodes unresponsive to conventional high-dose corticosteroids and polyclonal anti-lymphocyte globulins, also termed "rescue" treatment. Various studies, including large numbers of patients, have demonstrated the efficacy of the antibody also in this setting [8-10]. In addition, these interesting results obtained in renal transplantation also encouraged the use of the antibody for liver and heart transplant rejection. In both situations OKT3 essentially developed as a rescue treatment [11-14].

OKT3 has also been used in several centers as an "induction" therapy namely, as a first line treatment to prevent or delay the advent of acute rejection episodes and to improve long-term allograft survival. Moreover, particularly in renal transplantation, the use of OKT3 in the early post-transplant period was of interest to avoid complications linked to cyclosporin nephrotoxicity. Various controlled single-center studies demonstrated the efficacy of OKT3 in this setting when compared to control regimens some of which included polyclonal anti-T cell antibodies (i.e. Minnesota ALG) [15-17]. In this context OKT3 was administered for 10-14 consecutive days, starting on the day of transplant, in association to corti-costeroids, azathioprine and cyclosporin. In most cases cyclosporin was applied by the end of the antibody therapy. This is a clinically relevant issue since the data from the European registry suggest that long term allograft survival is significantly reduced when cyclosporin treatment is introduced concomitantly to OKT3 and not consecutively [18].

OKT3 induction therapy was also applied with success for induc-tion in liver transplantation [19-22]. Despite these results OKT3 was not generally adopted as a routine prophylactic treatment because of : first, the risk of sensitization, which could preclude the use of the antibody for a steroid-resistant rejection [20,23,24] and secondly, the occurrence of the "flu-like" syndrome that, as compared to ATG or conventional triple therapy with cyclosporin, could complicate the management of the patients [21,25-27].

It may be interesting to mention at this point that monoclonal antibodies recognizing other chains than CD3e within the TCR/ CD3 complex have also been tested in the clinic. Some beneficial effect was reported in open studies using the BMA 031 antibody, specific for the TCR constant portion, that were, however, not reproduced in controlled trials [28-30]. In contrast to OKT3, high doses of BMA-031 could be used safely since it was very well tolerated. In terms of cytokine release, like OKT3, BMA 031 induced TNF release but, at variance with OKT3, no other cytokines were detected [31]. Another mouse IgM antibody to human TCR, T10B9.1A-31, has also been tested which, despite encouraging initial results, was not developed [32].

Major Side Effects Observed with OKT3 Are Circumvented by Humanized Non-Mitogenic CD3 Antibodies

The immunization to the xenogeneic protein rapidly appeared as one major complication of the OKT3 use [3,25,33]. Especially, in the first protocols in which the antibody was administered either alone or combined to low doses of corticosteroids and azathioprine, more than 70% of treated patients mounted an antiglobulin res-ponse that could appear very rapidly, before the end of the first antibody course (i.e. by day 7-8 of treatment), and completely clear the monoclonal antibody from circulation thus neutralizing its therapeutic activity [3,25,33].

The characteristics of the OKT3-specific humoral response is identical to that observed with other cell binding xenogeneic monoclonal antibodies used either in the clinic or in experimental models. IgM and IgG antibodies are formed that are directed exclusively to isotypic or idiotypic determinants of the injected monoclonal [33]. In the case of the anti-OKT3 response, OKT3 being a mouse IgG2a, anti-isotypic antibodies reacted with all mouse IgG2 immunoglobulins [33,34]. Anti-idiotypic antibodies are directed to determinants only expressed by the OKT3 hypervariable regions and very effectively compete with the antigen for the monoclonal antibody binding [33]. Studies conducted in our laboratory on affinity chromatography purified anti-OKT3 antibody fractions clearly demonstrated that only IgG anti-idiotypic antibodies did neutralize OKT3 therapeutic activity [33,34]. Anti-isotypic antibodies are mostly non-neutralizing [34].

The antiglobulin response to OKT3 and also to other T cell binding monoclonal antibodies is oligoclonal [35]. This may explain that, at variance to polyclonal antisera, serum sickness was never described in patients immunized to OKT3. Immune complexes do form and are detectable in the circulation [L. Chatenoud, unpublished data] but are probably present in insufficient amounts to mediate tissue deposition. The potential risk of anaphylaxis, due to anti-OKT3 IgE antibodies, turned out to be a rare event [36]. Thus, from the clinical point of view, the abrogation of the therapeutic efficacy linked to IgG anti-idiotypic antibodies has been the sole important and deleterious consequence of the anti-OKT3 globulin response [33]. In practice, for many years, the only means to circumvent sensitization has been the addition of conventional immunosuppressants to OKT3. Adding corticosteroids, azathioprine and cyclosporin the rate of sensitization was reduced to 15-25% and, in most cases, antibodies did not affect efficacy since they appeared only by the end of OKT3 treatment [37]. Of course, the panorama will completely change with the advent of humanized CD3 antibodies. At present two humanized non mitogenic CD3 antibodies have been used in reported pilot clinical trials. One is a reshaped antibody derived from the rat YTH 12.5 antibody that expresses a g1 constant region lacking the CH2 domain glycosylation site [38,39]. All aglycosylated antibodies are unable to bind to Fc receptors or activate complement. The other antibody is one of the human reshaped versions of OKT3, gOKT3-5 [40]. It is also a human g1 whose Fc CH2 domain has been mutated HuOKT3g1(Ala-Ala) to express a 100-fold decreased affinity for human Fc receptors as compared to parental OKT3 [40].

Another major problem linked to OKT3 use was its mitogenic potential that caused, upon the first administration, a massive cytokine release and the acute "flu-like" syndrome [21,26,27]. Although, as the cytokine release, the syndrome is self-limited and resolves by the second to third day of treatment it may seriously complicate the patients' management. Main symptoms include high fever, chills, headache, repeated episodes of vomiting and diarrhea and, in few cases, severe and potentially life-threatening conditions, such as severe respiratory distress (i.e. pulmonary edema), neurotoxicity or hypotension [21,25-27].

All this is related to the massive though transient systemic release of various cytokines (TNF, IFN g, IL- 2, IL-3, IL-4, IL-6, IL-10 and GM-CSF) [21,27,41-46] essentially produced by activated T cells. In practice a single injection of high-dose corticosteroids, administered at least one hour prior to the first OKT3 injection, has been an effective palliative to significantly decrease the severity of the syndrome by diminishing the amount of cytokines released [26]. Another very effective approach was the administration of antibodies to TNF [47,48].

However, a more radical solution to this problem, as with the sensitization, is now accessible through the use of humanized non mitogenic antibodies. In fact, it has been well established that the mitogenic capacity of CD3 antibodies is monocyte dependent and mostly linked to the binding of the Fc antibody portion to Fc receptors, probably facilitating cross-linking. Thus, *in vitro* CD3 F(ab')2 fragments, which lack the Fc portion, are not mitogenic and the degree of CD3-induced T cell proliferation varies depending on the isotype of the antibody used which is known to impact on its affinity for human monocyte Fc receptors (IgG2a >> IgG1 >> IgG2b >> IgA) [49,50]. Similarly, and as expected, *in vivo*, murine CD3 antibodies of the IgA isotype, which are not mitogenic, are very well tolerated in transplanted patients [51]. Moreover, this is also the case for CD3 F(ab)'2 fragments administered to mice [50,52,53] or monkeys (J. Thomas, personal communication).

These results prompted the design of humanized "non mitogenic" CD3 antibodies engineered, as previously mentioned, to prevent the binding of constant Fc portion to human Fc receptors [38,40]. The aglycosylated human g1 YTH 12.5 antibody failed to induce T cell proliferation, in the presence of human serum and its ability to redirect T cell-mediated target killing was significantly reduced [38]. In addition, in transgenic mice expressing the human CD3-e chain, g1 YTH 12.5 did not induce a significant TNF release at variance with the parental YTH 12.5 CD3 antibody [38]. Similarly, the HuOKT3g1(Ala-Ala) antibody is not mitogenic *in vitro* and it did not show a significant *in vivo* cytokine releasing capacity in an experimental model in which human spleno-cytes from cadaveric organ donors were inoculated into severe com-bined immunodeficient mice (hu-SPL-SCID mice) [40]. Importantly, recent data from two pilot clinical trials using these antibodies show not only that they are well tolerated but also suggest that they are as effective as OKT3 in reversing acute allograft rejection [54,55]. This is well in keeping with all the experimental evidence showing that the immunosuppressive and tolerance promoting capacity are identical be-tween non-mitogenic and mitogenic CD3 antibodies [50,53,56-59].

One last important side effect, that is however not specific to OKT3 as compared to other immunosuppressive drugs, is that of overim-munosuppression. Reported data support the conclusion that the fre-quency of malignancies including Epstein Barr Virus-induced B cell lym-phomas tightly correlates with the potency of the overall immuno-suppressive regimen applied. CD3 antibodies being extremely potent one must be particularly cautious with the drug combinations used. Concerning OKT3, using well adapted regimens the risk of lymphoma was not higher than that observed in patients receiving anti-lymphocyte polyclonal antisera [21]. Thus, between 1985 and 1991 according the internal registry of Johnson & Johnson, the pharmaceutical company producing the antibody, the incidence of lymphomas was 0.48% (192/40,000). Moreover, and well in keeping with these conclusions, in the study by Swinneng et al., who reported on an exceedingly high incidence of B cell lymphomas in OKT3 treated heart transplant recipients [11.4% (9/79)] [60], the malignancies developed in the subgroup of patients who received a cumulated dose of OKT3 higher than 75mg (i.e., a treatment longer than the usually recommended 14 day period or patients who received more than one antibody course) or in those who also had ATG during their post-transplant course.

CD3 Antibody Treatment Promotes Immune Tolerance

Antibodies to human CD3 are tightly species-specific and do not cross-react with lymphocytes from non human primates except for chimpan-zees. This explains that antibodies such as OKT3 as well as the more recently available humanized non mitogenic anti-bodies have not been the subject of studies in such models.

However, there is compelling evidence obtained from meaningful preclinical experimental models, using equivalent antibodies specific for the e chain of the CD3 complex, showing that, at variance with what initially thought, CD3 antibodies may promote immune tolerance. Interestingly enough this has been shown to be the case not only in transplantation but also in autoimmunity.

Studies conducted by the group of B. Hall showed that treatment with an antibody to rat CD3 induced permanent engraftment of histoincompatible vascularized heart grafts linked to immune tolerance as assessed by the survival of donor skin grafts while third party grafts were normally rejected [61].

Studies in non human primates (i.e. rhesus monkeys) essentially involved the use of a CD3 immunotoxin, conjugating the FN18 monoclonal antibody to the mutant diphtheria toxin protein CRM9 [62,63]. The group of S. Knechtle investigated the use of the CD3 immunotoxin alone on renal allograft survival. Although the immunotoxin significantly prolonged allograft survival (35 to 1011 days in treated animals as compared to 5 to 9 in controls) true transplant tolerance did not develop [64]. Long term limitations were the development of anti-donor antibodies and the advent of chronic rejection [a pattern similar to that observed in long term renal allograft recipients treated with the CD40 Ligand antibody hu5C8 [65] and interstitial nephritis. The group of J. Thomas conducted similar studies and here again the CD3 immunotoxin alone, or combined with corticosteroids, was immunosuppressive but permanent engraftment was not observed [66]. At variance these authors obtained very interesting results by combining the CD3 immunotoxin donor bone marrow cells (in 4 out of 6 monkeys kidneys survived for more than 4 months, the longest survival exceeded 600 days (Thomas,1997#124)) or to deoxyspergualin (5 out of 8 monkeys kidneys survived long term, longest survival 550 days) [66]. In addition, in monkeys presenting with autoimmune diabetes a short course with the CD3 immunotoxin, supplemented with cyclosporine and steroids administered for only 4 days, allowed the long term survival of xenogeneic pancreatic islets. Thus, all three islet recipients have remained euglycemic at 410, 255, and 100 days of follow-up despite recovery of peripheral T cells to normal levels [67].

Working with non obese diabetic (NOD) mice, that spontaneously develop a form of autoimmune insulin-dependent diabetes mellitus which closely resembles the human disease [68,69], our group showed that CD3 could restore self-tolerance in overtly diabetic animals [52,53]. Thus, in mice presenting with full-blown diabetes (i.e. presence of glycosuria and glycemia $\geq$ 4g/l) a 5 consecutive days treatment with low doses (5 to 20mg) of the hamster CD3 antibody 145 2C11 (70) induced, within 2 to 4 weeks, complete disease remission in 60-80% of mice [52,53]. The effect was durable and specific for ß-cell-associated antigens since CD3-protected mice rejected histoincompatible skin grafts normally while, unlike control untreated overtly diabetic NOD females, they did not destroy syngeneic islet grafts [52].

One may, very schematically, distinguish three main not mutually exclusive modalities through which CD3 antibodies can mediate their immunosuppressive/ tolerance promoting activity that are : **1)** cell depletion **2)** the inhibition or blockade of TCR/ CD3 through antigenic modulation and/ or coating and **3)** the unique capacity to trigger cell-mediated immunoregulatory circuits that redirect destructive alloreactive responses towards a non-destructive type of alloreactivity. Although the fine cellular and molecular mechanisms mediating this last effect are still ill-defined it may represent one major pathway explaining the tolerogenic properties of various anti-T cell antibodies and in particular CD3.

The different CD3 antibodies we just discussed possess variable depleting potencies. For instance 1452 C11, at the usual regimen applied (5-20mg/ day for 5 days), induces approximately a 30-40% depletion of CD3+ cells (as assessed in the spleen and lymph nodes) [52,71]. Remnant cells undergo antigenic modulation i.e. the redistribution of TCR/ CD3 receptors followed by their internalization or shedding [71-73]. Modulated T cells (CD3-TCR-CD4+ or CD3-TCR-CD8+) reexpress the TCR/ CD3 complexes within 8 to 12hrs once the antibody is cleared from the surrounding medium. Cells undergoing CD3 antibody mediated antigenic modulation cells are unresponsive to antigen specific or mitogen stimulation [72,73].

A variety of mechanisms are probably involved in CD3 antibody-mediated cell destruction that include, antibody dependent cell-mediated cytotoxicity (ADCC), redirected T cell lysis [74] and, in particular for antibodies to CD3, the induction of apoptosis [75-77]. A certain degree of T cell depletion is observed in mice upon injection of F(ab')2 fragments of CD3 which may also be mediated by apoptosis.

As expected the CD3 immunotoxin used in monkeys was highly depleting despite the low doses administered (total doses of 133 to 300mg injected over 3 days starting at the time of transplantation). With this regimen peripheral blood and lymph node T cells decreased to 1% of pretreatment levels for two to three consecutive weeks [64,66,67,78].

CD3 antibody treatment can also elicit immunoregulation under the form of either Th1 / Th2 mediated immune deviation or transferable T cell-mediated active tolerance. *In vitro* studies performed by J. Smith et al. have indicated that in certain conditions CD3 antibodies could selectively stimulate Th2 cells and not Th1 [79,80]. It is particularly interesting to note that this effect was essentially noted with preactivated T cells and when a non-mitogenic CD3 antibody was used thus, suggesting the particular interest of applying non-mitogenic antibody once the immune response has already been engaged i.e. established autoimmunity as described above. These *in vitro* data are in keeping with recent *in vivo* studies showing a preferential Th2 cell stimulation upon non-mitogenic CD3 treatment in the rat [81] and in mice [82,83].

In the NOD model the data argue for the presence of immunoregulatory or dominant tolerance immune mechanisms that closely resemble those described in young prediabetic mice (52,53,69,84-87).

Just as prediabetic NOD mice anti-CD3 protected mice (20 to 40 weeks of age) present with an insulitis including CD3+aß+ CD4+ and CD8+ cells that remains confined to the periphery of the islets, i.e., peripheral insulitis [52,53], in great distinction to what is observed in untreated age-matched NOD mice that regularly exhibit an invasive / destructive type of insulitis. Moreover, co-transfer experiments evidenced in the spleen of CD3-protected mice the presence of CD3$^+$CD62L$^+$ cells that very effectively inhibit the transfer of diabetes by diabetogenic T lymphocytes (L. Chatenoud, unpublished results).

Conclusions

OKT3 has represented one of the most potent treatments to prevent or treat established rejection. Its more extensive usage has been refrained by the severe side effects linked to its mitogenic activity leading to the cytokine related "flu" like syndrome. The availability of several non mitogenic antibodies that are both effective and well tolerated opens totally new perspec-tives not only in transplantation but also for autoimmune diseases.

Additionally, more than immunosuppressants CD3 antibodies appear to be among the most potent inducers of "operational " tolerance to allo and autoantigens. Other biological agents including CD4 antibodies, CD40 Ligand antibodies, used alone or in combination to CTLA4-Ig, have also been shown to be active but their clinical application still poses a number of practical problems.

Among the immunological effects induced by CD3 antibodies that seem essential for their tolerogenic activity is the capacity to deliver "positive signals" via TCR/ CD3. The direct evidence obtained upon CD3 treatment for the activation of immunoregulatory cells, whether or the Th2 type or of T cells mediating transferable active or dominant tolerance argues in that direction. One should not minimize, though, the importance of the CD3-induced T cell depletion and/ or TCR/ CD3 blockade since these mechanisms could intervene first, by freezing down ongoing deleterious immune responses before they created irreversible lesions and secondly, by favoring the emergence of immunoregulatory T cells. It has indeed been suggested that T cell depletion, even when it involves selected T cell subsets, may favor the emergence of immunoregulatory T cells. This has notably been shown for total lymphoid irradiation and for depleting CD4 and CD8 antibodies [88,89]. One may hypothesize that TCR/ CD3 "blinding", either by coating or antigenic modulation, may, in this context, lead to the same effect as depletion. This issue may be particularly pertinent to the case of non mitogenic CD3 antibodies that are less depleting and were shown to mediate "partial" T cell signaling.

References

1. Cosimi AB, Colvin RB, Burton RC, et al. Use of monoclonal antibodies to T cell subsets for immunologic monitoring and treatment in recipients of renal allografts. N Engl J Med 1981;305:308-314.
2. Cosimi AB, Burton RC, Colvin RB, et al. Treatment of acute renal allograft rejection with OKT3 monoclonal antibody. Transplantation 1981;32:535-539.
3. Vigeral P, Chkoff N, Chatenoud L, et al. Prophylactic use of OKT3 monoclonal antibody in cadaver kidney recipients. Utilization of OKT3 as the sole immunosuppressive agent. Transplantation 1986;41:730-733.
4. Kung P, Goldstein G, Reinherz EL, Schlossman SF. Monoclonal antibodies defining distinctive human T cell surface antigens. Science 1979;206:347-349.
5. Clevers H, Alarcon B, Wileman T, Terhorst C. The T cell receptor/CD3 complex: a dynamic protein ensemble. Annu Rev Immunol 1988;6 :629-662.
6. Davis MM, Chien YH. T cell antigen receptors. In: Paul WE, editors. Fundamental Immunology. New York: Raven Press, 1999:341-366.
7. Ortho X. A randomized clinical trial of OKT3 monoclonal antibody for acute rejection of cadaveric renal transplants. Ortho Multicenter Transplant Study Group. N Engl J Med 1985;313:337-342.
8. Goldstein G. Overview of the development of Orthoclone OKT3: monoclonal antibody for therapeutic use in transplantation. Transplant Proc 1987;19:1-6.
9. Hricik DE, Zarconi J, Schulak JA. Influence of low-dose cyclosporine on the outcome of treatment with OKT3 for acute renal allograft rejection. Transplantation 1989;47:272-277.
10. Norman DJ, Barry JM, Bennett WM, et al. The use of OKT3 in cadaveric renal transplantation for rejection that is unresponsive to conventional anti-rejection therapy. Am J Kidney Dis 1988;11:90-93.
11. Colonna Jo 2D, Goldstein LI, Brems JJ, et al. A prospective study on the use of monoclonal anti-T3-cell antibody (OKT3) to treat steroid-resistant liver transplant rejection. Arch Surg 1987;122:1120-1123.
12. Woodle ES, Thistlethwaite Jr JR, Emond JC, et al. OKT3 therapy for hepatic allograft rejection. Differential response in adults and children. Transplantation 1991;51:1207-1212.
13. Goldstein G, Kremer AB, Barnes L, Hirsch RL. OKT3 monoclonal antibody reversal of renal and hepatic rejection in pediatric patients. J Pediatr 1987;111:1046-1050.
14. Gilbert EM, Dewitt CW, Eiswirth CC, et al. Treatment of refractory cardiac allograft rejection with OKT3 monoclonal antibody. Am J Med 1987;82:202-206.
15. Frey DJ, Matas AJ, Gillingham KJ, et al. Sequential therapy--a prospective randomized trial of MALG versus OKT3 for prophylactic immunosuppression in cadaver renal allograft recipients. Transplantation 1992;54:50-56.
16. Debure A, Chkoff N, Chatenoud L, et al. One-month prophylactic use of OKT3 in cadaver kidney transplant recipients. Transplantation 1988;45:546-553.
17. Abramowicz D, Goldman M, de Pauw L, Vanherweghem JL, Kinnaert P, Vereerstraeten P. The long-term effects of prophylactic OKT3 monoclonal antibody in cadaver kidney transplantation--a single-center, prospective, randomized study. Transplantation 1992;54:433-437.
18. Opelz G. Efficacy of rejection prophylaxis with OKT3 in renal transplantation. Collaborative Transplant Study. Transplantation 1995;60:1220-1224.
19. Farges O, Ericzon BG, Bresson-Hadni S, et al. A randomized trial of OKT3-based versus cyclosporine-based immunoprophylaxis after liver transplantation. Long-term results of a European and Australian multicenter study. Tansplantation 1994;58:891-898.

20. Millis JM, McDiarmid SV, Hiatt JR, et al. Randomized prospective trial of OKT3 for early prophylaxis of rejection after liver transplantation. Transplantation 1989;47:82-88.
21. Eason JD, Cosimi AB. Biologic immunosuppressive agents. In: Ginns LC, Cosimi AB, Morris PJ, editors. Transplantation. Malden, USA: Blackwell Science, 1999:196-224.
22. Robbins RC, Oyer PE, Stinson EB, Starnes VA. The use of monoclonal antibodies after heart transplantation. Transplantation Science 1992;2:22-27.
23. Farges O, Samuel D, Bismuth H. Orthoclone OKT3 in liver transplantation. Transplant Sci 1992;2:16-21.
24. Ericzon BG, Salmela K, Barkholt L, Hockerstedt K. OKT3 prophylaxis in liver transplantation: the Scandinavian experience. Transplant Proc 1990;22:223-224.
25. Cosimi AB. Clinical development of Orthoclone OKT3. Transplant Proc 1987;19:7-16.
26. Chatenoud L, Legendre C, Ferran C, Bach JF, Kreis H. Corticosteroid inhibition of the OKT3-induced cytokine-related syndrome--dosage and kinetics prerequisites. Transplantation 1991;51:334-338.
27. Abramowicz D, Schandene L, Goldman M, et al. Release of tumor necrosis factor, interleukin-2, and gamma-interferon in serum after injection of OKT3 monoclonal antibody in kidney transplant recipients. Transplantation 1989;47:606-608.
28. Schlitt HJ, Kurrle R, Wonigeit K. T cell activation by monoclonal antibodies directed to different epitopes on the human T cell receptor/CD3 complex: evidence for two different modes of activation. Eur J Immunol 1989;19:1649-1655.
29. Land W, Hillebrand G, Illner WD, et al. First clinical experience with a new TCR/CD3-monoclonal antibody (BMA 031) in kidney transplant patients. Transpl Int 1988;1:116-117.
30. Smely S, Weschka M, Hillebrand G, et al. Prophylactic use of the new monoclonal antibody BMA 031 in clinical kidney transplantation. Transplant Proc 1990;22:1785-1786.
31. Chatenoud L, Legendre C, Kurrle R, Kreis H, Bach JF. Absence of clinical symptoms following the first injection of anti-T cell receptor monoclonal antibody (BMA 031) despite isolated TNF release. Transplantation 1993;55:443-445.
32. Waid TH, Lucas BA, Thompson JS, et al. Treatment of acute cellular rejection with T10B9.1A-31 or OKT3 in renal allograft recipients. Transplantation 1992;53:80-86.
33. Chatenoud L, Baudrihaye MF, Chkoff N, Kreis H, Goldstein G, Bach JF. Restriction of the human in vivo immune response against the mouse monoclonal antibody OKT3. J Immunol 1986;137:830-838.
34. Baudrihaye MF, Chatenoud L, Kreis H, Goldstein G, Bach JF. Unusually restricted anti-isotype human immune response to OKT3 monoclonal antibody. Eur J Immunol 1984;14:686-691.
35. Chatenoud L, Jonker M, Villemain F, Goldstein G, Bach JF. The human immune response to the OKT3 monoclonal antibody is oligoclonal. Science 1986;232:1406-1408.
36. Abramowicz D, Crusiaux A, Goldman M. Anaphylactic shock after retreatment with OKT3 monoclonal antibody. N Engl J Med 1992;327:736.
37. Hricik DE, Mayes JT, Schulak JA. Inhibition of anti-OKT3 antibody generation by cyclosporine--results of a prospective randomized trial. Transplantation 1990;50:237-240.
38. Bolt S, Routledge E, Lloyd I, et al. The generation of a humanized, non-mitogenic CD3 monoclonal antibody which retains in vitro immunosuppressive properties. Eur J Immunol 1993;23:403-411.

39. Routledge EG, Falconer ME, Pope H, Lloyd IS, Waldmann H. The effect of aglycosylation on the immunogenicity of a humanized therapeutic CD3 monoclonal antibody. Tansplantation 1995;60:847-853.
40. Alegre ML, Peterson LJ, Xu D, et al. A non-activating "humanized" anti-CD3 monoclonal antibody retains immunosuppressive properties in vivo. Tansplantation 1994;57:1537-1543.
41. Hirsch R, Gress RE, Pluznik DH, Eckhaus M, Bluestone JA. Effects of in vivo administration of anti-CD3 monoclonal antibody on T cell function in mice. II. In vivo activation of T cells. J Immunol 1989;142:737-743.
42. Ferran C, Sheehan K, Dy M, et al. Cytokine-related syndrome following injection of anti-CD3 monoclonal antibody: further evidence for transient in vivo T cell activation. Eur J Immunol 1990;20:509-515.
43. Alegre M, Vandenabeele P, Flamand V, et al. Hypothermia and hypoglycemia induced by anti-CD3 monoclonal antibody in mice: role of tumor necrosis factor. Eur J Immunol 1990;20:707-710.
44. Durez P, Abramowicz D, Gerard C, et al. In vivo induction of interleukin 10 by anti-CD3 monoclonal antibody or bacterial lipopolysaccharide: differential modulation by cyclosporin A. J Exp Med 1993;177:551-555.
45. Yoshimoto T, Paul WE. CD4pos, NK1.1pos T cells promptly produce interleukin 4 in response to in vivo challenge with anti-CD3. J Exp Med 1994;179:1285-1295.
46. Flamand V, Abramowicz D, Goldman M, et al. Anti-CD3 antibodies induce T cells from unprimed animals to secrete IL-4 both in vitro and in vivo. J Immunol 1990;144:2875-2882.
47. Ferran C, Dy M, Sheehan K, et al. Cascade modulation by anti-tumor necrosis factor monoclonal antibody of interferon-gamma, interleukin 3 and interleukin 6 release after triggering of the CD3/T cell receptor activation pathway. Eur J Immunol 1991;21:2349-2353.
48. Charpentier B, Hiesse C, Lantz O, et al. Evidence that antihuman tumor necrosis factor monoclonal antibody prevents OKT3-induced acute syndrome. Transplantation 1992;54:997-1002.
49. Van Lier RA, Boot JH, de Groot ER, Aarden LA. Induction of T cell proliferation with anti-CD3 switch-variant monoclonal antibodies: effects of heavy chain isotype in monocyte-dependent systems. Eur J Immunol 1987;17:1599-1604.
50. Hirsch R, Bluestone JA, de Nenno L, Gress RE. Anti-CD3 F(ab')2 fragments are immunosuppressive in vivo without evoking either the strong humoral response or morbidity associated with whole mAb. Transplantation 1990;49:1117-1123.
51. Parlevliet KJ, Ten Berge IJ, Yong SL, Surachno J, Wilmink JM, Schellekens PT. In vivo effects of IgA and IgG2a anti-CD3 isotype switch variants. J Clin Invest 1994;93:2519-2525.
52. Chatenoud L, Thervet E, Primo J, Bach JF. Anti-CD3 antibody induces long-term remission of overt autoimmunity in nonobese diabetic mice. Proc Natl Acad Sci USA 1994;91:123-127.
53. Chatenoud L, Primo J, Bach JF. CD3 antibody-induced dominant self tolerance in overtly diabetic NOD mice. J Immunol 1997;158:2947-2954.
54. Woodle ES, Xu D, Zivin RA, et al. Phase I trial of a humanized, Fc receptor nonbinding OKT3 antibody, huOKT3gamma1(Ala-Ala) in the treatment of acute renal allograft rejection. Tansplantation 1999;68:608-616.
55. Friend PJ, Hale G, Chatenoud L, et al. Phase I study of an engineered aglycosylated humanized CD3 antibody in renal transplant rejection. Transplantation 1999;68:1632-1637.
56. Hirsch R, Archibald J, Gress RE. Differential T cell hyporesponsiveness induced by in vivo administration of intact or F(ab')2 fragments of anti-CD3 monoclonal antibody. F(ab')2 fragments induce a selective T helper dysfunction. J Immunol 1991;147:2088-2093.

57. Hughes C, Wolos JA, Giannini EH, Hirsch R. Induction of T helper cell hyporesponsiveness in an experimental model of autoimmunity by using nonmitogenic anti-CD3 monoclonal antibody. J Immunol 1994;153:3319-3325.

58. Herold KC, Bluestone JA, Montag AG, et al. Prevention of autoimmune diabetes with nonactivating anti-CD3 monoclonal antibody. Diabetes 1992;41:385-391.

59. Johnson BD, McCabe C, Hanke CA, Truitt RL. Use of anti-CD3 epsilon F(ab')2 fragments in vivo to modulate graft-versus-host disease without loss of graft-versus-leukemia reactivity after MHC-matched bone marrow transplantation. J Immunol 1995;154:5542-5554.

60. Swinnen LJ, Costanzo-Nordin MR, Fisher SG, et al. Increased incidence of lymphoproliferative disorder after immunosuppression with the monoclonal antibody OKT3 in cardiac-transplant recipients. N Engl J Med 1990;323:1723-1728.

61. Nicolls MR, Aversa GG, Pearce NW, et al. Induction of long-term specific tolerance to allografts in rats by therapy with an anti-CD3-like monoclonal antibody. Transplantation 1993;55:459-468.

62. Nooij FJ, Jonker M, Balner H. Differentiation antigens on rhesus monkey lymphocytes. II. Characterization of RhT3, a CD3-like antigen on T cells. Eur J Immunol 1986;16:981-984.

63. Neville Dm JR, Scharff J, Hu HZ, et al. A new reagent for the induction of T-cell depletion, anti-CD3-CRM9. Journal of Immunotherapy With Emphasis on Tumor Immunology 1996;19:85-92.

64. Hamawy MM, Knechtle SJ. trategies for tolerance induction in nonhuman primates. [Review] [26 refs. Curr Opin Immunol 1998;10:513-517.

65. Kirk AD, Burkly LC, Batty DS, et al. reatment with humanized monoclonal antibody against CD154 prevents acute renal allograft rejection in nonhuman primates [see comments. Nat Med 1999;5:686-693.

66. Contreras JL, Wang PX, Eckhoff DE, et al. Peritransplant tolerance induction with anti-CD3-immunotoxin: a matter of proinflammatory cytokine control. Tansplantation 1998;65:1159-1169.

67. Thomas FT, Ricordi C, Contreras JL, et al. Reversal of naturally occuring diabetes in primates by unmodified islet xenografts without chronic immunosuppression. Tansplantation 1999;67:846-854.

68. Castano L, Eisenbarth GS. Type-I diabetes: a chronic autoimmune disease of human, mouse, and rat. Annu Rev Immunol 1990;8:647-679.

69. Bach JF. Insulin-dependent diabetes mellitus as an autoimmune disease. Endocrine Rev 1994;15:516-542.

70. Leo O, Foo M, Sachs DH, Samelson LE, Bluestone JA. Identification of a monoclonal antibody specific for a murine T3 polypeptide. Proc Natl Acad Sci USA 1987;84:1374-1378.

71. Hirsch R, Eckhaus M, Auchincloss H JR, Sachs DH, Bluestone JA. Effects of in vivo administration of anti-T3 monoclonal antibody on T cell function in mice. I. Immunosuppression of transplantation responses. J Immunol 1988;140:3766-3772.

72. Chatenoud L, Bach JF. Antigenic modulation: a major mechanism of antibody action. Immunol Today 1984;5:20-25.

73. Chatenoud L, Baudrihaye MF, Kreis H, Goldstein G, Schindler J, Bach JF. Human in vivo antigenic modulation induced by the anti-T cell OKT3 monoclonal antibody. Eur J Immunol 1982;12:979-982.

74. Wong JT, Colvin RB. Selective reduction and proliferation of the CD4+ and CD8+ T cell subsets with bispecific monoclonal antibodies: evidence for inter-T cell-mediated cytolysis. Clin Immunol Immunopathol 1991;58:236-250.

75. Smith CA, Williams GT, Kingston R, Jenkinson EJ, Owen JJ. Antibodies to CD3/T cell receptor complex induce death by apoptosis in immature T cells in thymic cultures. Nature 1989;337:181-184.

76. Wesselborg S, Janssen O, Kabelitz D. Induction of activation-driven death (apoptosis) in activated but not resting peripheral blood T cells. J Immunol 1993;150:4338-4345.

77. Choy EH, Adjaye J, Forrest L, Kingsley GH, Panayi GS. Chimaeric anti-CD4 monoclonal antibody cross-linked by monocyte Fc gamma receptor mediates apoptosis of human CD4 lymphocytes. Eur J Immunol 1993;23:2676-2681.

78. Thomas JM, Neville DM, Contreras JL, et al. Preclinical studies of allograft tolerance in rhesus monkeys: a novel anti-CD3-immunotoxin given peritransplant with donor bone marrow induces operational tolerance to kidney allografts. Tansplantation 1997;64:124-135.

79. Smith JA, Tang Q, Bluestone JA. Partial TCR signals delivered by FcR-nonbinding anti-CD3 monoclonal antibodies differentially regulate individual Th subsets. J Immunol 1998;160:4841-4849.

80. Smith JA, Tso JY, Clark MR, Cole MS, Bluestone JA. Nonmitogenic anti-CD3 monoclonal antibodies deliver a partial T cell receptor signal and induce clonal anergy. J Exp Med 1997;185:1413-1422.

81. Plain KM, Chen J, Merten S, He XY, Hall BM. Induction of specific tolerance to allografts in rats by therapy with non-mitogenic, non-depleting anti-CD3 monoclonal antibody: association with TH2 cytokines not anergy. Tansplantation 1999;67:605-613.

82. Le Moine A, Flamand V, Demoor FX, et al. Critical roles for IL-4, IL-5, and eosinophils in chronic skin allograft rejection. J Clin Invest 1999;103:1659-1667.

83. Wissing KM, Desalle F, Abramowicz D, et al. Down-regulation of interleukin-2 and interferon-gamma and maintenance of interleukin-4 and interleukin-10 production after administration of an anti-CD3 monoclonal antibody in mice. Tansplantation 1999;68:677-684.

84. Boitard C, Yasunami R, Dardenne M, Bach JF. T cell-mediated inhibition of the transfer of autoimmune diabetes in NOD mice. J Exp Med 1989;169:1669-1680.

85. Hutchings PR, Cooke A. The transfer of autoimmune diabetes in NOD mice can be inhibited or accelerated by distinct cell populations present in normal splenocytes taken from young males. J Autoimmun 1990;3:175-185.

86. Yasunami R, Debray-Sachs M, Bach JF. Ontogeny of regulatory and effector T cells in autoimmune NOD mice. In: Shafrir E, editors. Frontiers in diabetes research. Lessons from animal diabetes III. London: Smith-Gordon, 1990:88-93.

87. Delovitch TL, Singh B. The nonobese diabetic mouse as a model of autoimmune diabetes: immune dysregulation gets the NOD. Immunity 1997;7:727-738.

88. Cobbold SP, Qin SX, Waldmann H. Reprogramming the immune system for tolerance with monoclonal antibodies. Semin Immunol 1990;2:377-387.

89. Strober S. Natural suppressor (NS) cells, neonatal tolerance, and total lymphoid irradiation: exploring obscure relationships. Annu Rev Immunol 1984;2:219-237.

MONOCLONAL ANTIBODY TARGETING OF THE IL-2R COMPLEX

Flavio G. Vincenti, M.D.

Introduction

Biologic agents have been used for induction therapy in renal transplantation since the 1970s. The primary objective of induction therapy has been to block T cell responses at the time of antigen presentation following allograft transplantation in an effort to reorient the host immune response toward accommodation rather than rejection. The first biologic agents that were used for induction were polyclonal antilymphocyte preparations obtained from horses or rabbits. The polyclonal antibodies result in T cell depletion thus depriving the host of immune reactive cells. However these polyclonal preparations are raised against antigens of whle cells and thus they target a variety of antigens including the costimulatory molecules, adhesion molecules and CD25. Cross-reactive antibodies also target neutrophils, red blood cells and platelets resulting in a number of hematologic abnormalities. OKT3, a murine anti-CD_3 monoclonal antibody, was introduced in 1986. The mechanism of action of OKT3 consists of T cell depletion and CD_3 modulation. While the polyclonal agents and OKT3 induce effective immunosuppression, they are also associated with opportunistic infections and post transplant lymphoproliferative disorders. In the latter part of the 1990s, humanized (fully humanized and chimeric) monoclonal antibodies targeting the interleukin 2 α receptor (IL-2R α) were introduced with the intent of inducing selective rather than broad immunosuppression. [1-4] The rationale for their use is shown in **Table 1**. The mechanism of action of the anti- IL-2R α monoclonal

Mohamed Sayegh and Giuseppe Remuzzi (editors), Current and Future Immunosuppressive Therapies Following Transplantation, 235-248.
© 2001 Kluwer Academic Publishers. Printed in the Netherlands.

Table 1. Rationale for Anti-IL2 α Therapy

- Cellular Selectivity
  IL-2R α chain expressed only on activated T cells
- IL-2R α forms part of the high affinity receptor complex for IL-2
- Interaction of IL-2 with its receptor is required for clonal expansion and continued viability of activated T cells. Blocking the interaction of IL-2 with IL-2R inhibits amplification of the of the immune response
- IL-2R α has no cytoplasmic tail and lacks transmembrane signaling functions
- No interference with stimulation of the IL-2R β γ used by NK and cytotoxic T cells (response to previous pathogens intact)

---

antibodies (mAbs) is probably complex but includes disrupting the high affinity IL-2R complex, down modulation of the α receptor and possible T cell depletion. Recent data suggests that these antibodies in addition to binding the α receptor may also block signaling from the β chain and thus may have broader interruption of the redundant cytokine-receptor complex. [5,6]

Clinical Experience of the Rodent Anti-IL-2R α Monoclonal Antibodies

In the late 1980s, several rodent anti-IL2-R α mAbs were introduced in clinical renal transplantation to test the hypothesis that blockade of the IL-2 activation pathway with monoclonal antibody therapy can provide effective yet safer immunosuppressive therapy. [7-10] The results from these trials, while promising, were not fully convincing (**Table 2**). In fact, the results of these early clinical trials as well as the increasing awareness of the redundancy of the cytokine receptor pathways led to widespread skepticism about the usefulness of blockade of the IL-2 pathway. This was further reinforced by the finding that IL-2 knockout mice were able to mount a vigorous rejection of allografts. However a close look at the rodent mAbs data showed that theses mAbs were effective while they were administered but the overall outcome of the patients treated with these antibodies was undermined by their immunogenicity. In these clinical trials, almost all patients developed a rapid immune response against the xenoantibodies (**Table 2**). Human anti-mouse or anti-rat antibodies accelerated the clearance of these mAbs and further reduced an already short half-life below the level necessary for clinical utility. Another potentially important factor limiting the efficacy of rodent monoclonal anti-bodies is that they are not effective at recruiting certain human immune effector functions such as antibody-dependent cell mediated

Table 2. Clinical Trials with Rodent Monoclonal Antibodies

Monoclonal Antibody	Study Design	Outcome	Percentage patients developing anti-isotypic antibodies
3383.1	Randomized trial comparing efficacy & safety	Similar efficacy as ATG but reduced toxicity	40%, anti-33B3.1 IgG &IgM by days 12-17
Anti-Tac	Randomized trial comparing efficacy & safety with cyclosporine triple therapy n=80	Significant reduction in early acute rejection, no difference in patient of graft survival or infectious episodes	70%, anti-mouse by day 30
L0-Tac-1	Randomized trial Comparing efficacy & safety with ALG n=40	Significant efficacy as ALG, reduced incidence of infectious episodes	89%,anti-L0-Tact-1 IgG, 67% anti-L0-Tact-1 IgM before day 14
BT563	Randomized double-blind trial,placebo controlled, n=56	Significant reduction in early acute rejection (p=0.011),no difference in patient or graft survival, acute rejection at one year, or infectious complications	60% by day 30

cytotoxicity (ADCC). Viewed from these prospectives it is clear that efficacy of IL-2R blockade could be dramatically improved by utilizing mAbs constructs that are more humanized. These expectations were fulfilled with the introduction of humanized anti-IL2-R α mAb daclizumab and chimeric mAb basiliximab. The differences between these two antibodies, daclizumab and basiliximab, are shown in **Table 3.**

Table 3. Difference Between Chimeric and Humanized IL2R α Monoclonal Antibodies

	Daclizumab	**Basiliximab**
Ig Framework	Humanized	Chimeric
Half-lifle	20 days	7 days
Conc. For Saturation	1	0.2
Affinity vs. murine Ab		
Regimen in Phase III	5 doses at 1 mg/kg	2 doses of 20 mg

Table 4. The Design of the Four Phase III Trials with Daclizumab and Basiliximab.

	Daclizumab	Basiliximab
Phase III Trials	1. U.S.-Canada-Sweden	1. U.S.
(participating centers)	2. Europe-Canada-Australia	2. Europe
Inclusion	1 & 2 only 1° cadaver recipients	1. 1° cadaver and living donor recipients
		2. only 1° cadaver recipients
Maintenance immunosuppression	1. Cyclosporine, azathioprine, prednisone	1 & 2: cyclosporine and prednisone
	2. Cyclosporine, prednisone	
No. of Patients	1 n = 260	1 n = 346
	2 n = 275	2 n = 376

Phase III Clinical Trials

Daclizumab and basiliximab were both initially tested in Phase I-II clinical tirals. [11, 12]   The regimen of daclizumab that was used in the Phase III trials, consisted of 1 mg/kg administered pre-operatively and at subsequent 4 bi-weekly intervals.   This regimen produced saturation of the IL-2R α on circulating lymphocytes for at least 90 days, a period of time when patients are most vulnerable for the occurrence of acute rejection.   The regimen of basiliximab that was used in the Phase III trials, was a fixed dose of 20 mg administered at day 0 and at day 4 post transplant which resulted in saturation of the IL-2R a on circulating lymphocytes for 25-35 days.   Each antibody was studied in two separate double-blind randomized clinical trials. [1-4] The details of the Phase III trials of daclizumad and basiliximab are shown in **Table 4**.   The one-year outcome of the pooled data of the Phase III trials of daclizumab and basiliximab are show in **Tables 5A** and **5B**.   In Summary, the addition of daclizumab or basiliximab to an immunosuppressive regimen consisting of cyclosporine and prednisone, or cyclosporine, azathioprine and prednisone decreased acute rejection rates by 30-40%, decreased the severity of acute rejection (as measured by the need for antilymphocyte therapy to reverse acute rejection) and delayed the onset of the episode of acute rejection.   The use of these antibodies were not associated with any cytokine mediated side effects, increase in infectious complications or opportunistic infections or post transplant lymphoproliferative

Table 5A. Daclizumab Phase III Pooled Data One Year Outcome

	Placebo % (n=268)		Daclizumab % (n=267)
Acute Rejection	43.3	.001	27.7
Median Time to Rejection (days)	40		18
Antilymphocyte Rx	15.3	.005	7.9
Cumulative steroid (6 mo.)	4562	.04	4137
Graft survival	86.6	.065	91.4
Patient survival	95.1	.022	98.5

diseases. That some degree of selective immunosuppression was achieved with these agents can be concluded from the enhanced immune prophylaxis to the allograft without consequences of over-immunosuppression.

The conclusion of the Phase III trials with daclizumab and basiliximab coincided with the introduction in clinical transplantation of mycophenolate mofetil as part of the triple therapy regimen in combination with cyclosporine and prednisone. In addition, tacrolimus began to be used in combination with mycophenolate mofetil and prednisone. These regimens were associated acute rejection rates below 20%. Thus it was not clear if the anti-IL-2R α mAbs could have an additive beneficial effect when added to the newer and more potent maintenance immunosuppressive regimens.

Table 5B. Basiliximab Phase III Pooled Data: One Year Outcome

	Placebo % (n=359)	*p value*	Basiliximab
Acute rejection	48%	<0.001	33%
Antilymphocyte Therapy	26%	<0.001	15%
Graft survival	87%	0.610	88%
Patient survival	97%	0.71	96%

Clinical Trials of Daclizumab and Basiliximab with Triple Therapy Maintenance Immunosuppression Regimens with the Newer Agents

In a Phase II blinded randomized trial, 75 patients treated with maintenance immunosuppression consisting of cyclosporine, mycophenolate mofetil and steroids were administered the same regimen of daclizumab or placebo as in the Phase III studies. [13] Patients receiving a first renal transplant from either a cadaver or a non-HLA identical living donor were enrolled in this double blind randomized study. The combination of daclizumab and mycophenolate mofetil was safe and well-tolerated. There were no pharmacokinetic interactions between daclizumab and mycophenolate mofetil and at 6 months biopsy-proven rejection was 12% versus 20% in the daclizumab and placebo groups, respectively. In a second trial reported by Lawen et al on behalf of the Simulect International Study Group, 123 patients were randomized before transplantation to either basiliximab (two doses, 20 mg at day 0 and day 4) or placebo. [14] Ninety-three patients were cadaveric recipients, 30 received kidneys from living donors. One hundred and nine patients were primary transplants and 14 re-transplants. The immunosuppression consisted of cyclosporine, mycophenolate mofetil and corticosteroids. The outcome at 6 months is shown in **Figure 1**. While these studies were not powered to show statistical difference it is clear that patients treated with daclizumab or basiliximab had an overall better outcome than placebo treated patients.

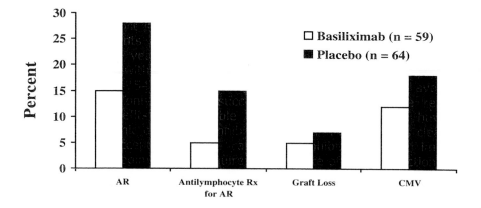

Figure 1. The six-month outcome of patients treated with basiliximab and placebo.

At the XVII International Congress of the Transplantation Society, Ciancio et al from the University of Miami presented data from a retrospective study utilizing daclizumab induction for primary kidney transplant recipients in addition to tacrolimus, mycophenolate mofetil and steroids as maintenance immunosuppression. [15] Two hundred nineteen primary kidney transplant recipients were treated with daclizumab induction (a regimen similar to the Phase III), mycophenolate mofetil and tacrolimus (started when the serum creatinine decreased to below 4 mg/dL) and corticosteroids. The mean follow-up was 11 months. The incidence of biopsy-proven acute rejection was 3.2%. Only 2 CMV infections occurred in this group and no malignancies were noted.

More recently daclizumab has been used in a limited dosing regimen, usually 2 doses administered pre-operatively and at 1-2 weeks after transplantation. This regimen provides saturation of the IL-2R α on circulating lymphocytes for a minimum of 70 days following renal transplantation (Vincenti et al, unpublished data). A large experience of this regimen was recently reported by Dr. Deierhoi and associates from the University of Alabama at Birmingham. [16] One hundred and sixty-nine primary and secondary cadaver recipients transplanted between May 1998 and September 1999 were treated with a two-dose regimen of daclizumab and maintenance immunosuppression consisting of cyclosporine, mycophenolate mofetil and prednisone. These patients were compared with 124 patients who were transplanted from May 1997 to April 1998 with the same maintenance immunosuppression regimen but who had induction therapy with OKT3 for 10 to 14 days. The one-year outcome is shown in **Table 6**. Although this is a retrospective analysis, it clearly demonstrates that induction with daclizumab was superior to OKT3 both in terms of efficacy and safety. This study also demonstrates the effectiveness of the two-dose regimen of daclizumab.

Table 6. Clinical Experience: Two-Dose Regimen of Daclizumab in Cadaveric Renal Transplantation

	Historical Controls OKT3 (n = 124)	Daclizumab (n = 169)	*P value*
Time period	5/97 to 4/98	5/98 to 9/99	
Graft survival, 1y	89%	93%	P = 0.049
Acute rejection, 1y	32%	18%	P = 0.004
Infections, 1y	39%	27%	P = 0.03
Readmissions, 6 mos	50%	32%	P = 0.003

The Anti-IL2-R Monoclonal Antibodies Are as Effective as the Depleting Agents

Are the humanized and chimeric anti-IL-2R α as effective as the depleting antilymphocyte agents in prophylaxis for acute rejection. As described above in the study by Deierhoi et al, [16] induction with two doses of daclizumab was shown to be superior to induction with OKT3. However, this study was a retrospective analysis and therefore it cannot fully validate the superiority of one agent over the other. More relevant data is available from two basiliximab studies comparing basiliximab to thymoglobulin or ATGAM. In a multicenter prospective randomized trial, 103 primary cadaver transplants were randomized to basiliximab (Group I) or to thymoglobulin 1-1.5 mg/kg administered fcor 6-14 days (Group II). [17] In Group I cyclosporine was started at day 0 and in Group II cyclosporine was delayed until 6-10 when the serum creatinine was less than 250 μmol/L. The outcome at 6 months is shown in **Table 7**. While the overall outcome in patients treated with basiliximab and theymoglobulin was comparable, there were less CMV infections in the basiliximab-treated group. The second study randomized patients at 6 centers from November 1997 to April 1998 in an open label trial to either basiliximab (20 mg on Day 0 and Day 4) and early cyclosporine or to ATGAM and cyclosporine which was delayed until the serum creatinine was less than 3 mg/DL. [18] Patients in both arms received mycophenolate mofetil and steroids. Seventy patients were randomized to basiliximab, 65 to ATGAM. The incidence of biopsy-proven rejection at 12 months was 19% for basiliximab and 20% for ATGAM. Thus censored graft survival was 97% and 98% respectively. There were no significant differences found in renal function or patterns of adverse events. The authors concluded that, based on its convenient 2-dose regimen and comparable effectiveness to ATGAM, basiliximab may be the preferred therapy. While additional data is still needed, the retrospective

Table 7. Six Months Outcome of the Basiliximab (Group I) and Thymoglobulin (Group II) Trial

	Group I 36	Group II 37
Patient Survival	97%	100%
Graft Survival	94%	100%
DGF	14%	24%
Acute rejection	8%	5%
CMV infection	N = 2	N = 9
CMV syndrome	N = 1	N = 9

daclizumab study from the University of Alabama and the prospective basiliximab trials suggest that at the very least the anti-IL-2R α are comparable in effectiveness to the depleting antilymphocyte agents but may be associated with less complications, are clearly easier to administer and are more cost-effective.   Two clinical indications that require additional studies are immunologic high-risk patients (high PRA, second transplants) and delayed graft function.   In a pilot study reported by Hong and Kahan, an initial calcineurin-free strategy for induction immunosuppression was used for delayed graft function in cadaver kidney transplants. [19] In 24 patients deemed to be at high risk for delayed graft function, immunosuppression therapy was initiated with basiliximab, corticostyeroids and sirolimus, (initial dose 15 mg and therafter 5-10 mg a day to achieve trough concentration between 5-20 ng/mL). Cyclosporine therapy was withheld until the serum creatinine dropped below 2.5 mg/dL.   The cyclosporine-free interval ranged from 4-159 days. Only three acute rejection episodes occurred during the cyclosporine-free period: two in retransplanted patients and one occurred in an African-American patient with systemic lupus erythematosus.   The authors conclude that this calcineurin inhibitors-free regimen could be useful and effective in patients with delayed graft function. At the University of California, San Francisco we are currently using a combination of an anti IL-2R α mAb, sirolimus, mycophenolate mofetil and steroids for patients with delayed graft function.

Future Indications

The long half-life and the prolonged biologic effects of the anti-IL-2R α mAbs can provide the opportunity to utilize an immunosuppression regimen that minimize the sue of drugs that are toxic and in particular nephrotoxic. The role of the new anti-IL-2R mAbs in regimen-sparing steroids and calcineurin inhibitors is undergoing careful clinical experimentation.

Steroids Sparing Elimination Studies

The use of the anti-IL2R mAbs antibodies may allow complete avoidance or very early withdrawal of corticosteroids from immuno-suppression regimens.   While the majority of steroid sparing studies withdraw steroids late after transplantation (3-12 months), there maybe several advantages for complete avoidance or very early with-drawal of corticosteroids.   Complete avoidance or very early with-drawal of corticosteroids may be safer than late withdrawal of cortico-steroids because acute rejection may occur early on and be more readily diagnosed as patients are more intensively followed-up early in the course after transplantation.   In addition, corticosteroids may interfere with some toleregenic pathways and therefore steroids avoidance may in fact enhance long term clinical tolerance. Finally prevention of corticosteroids side effects is more effective if steroids are complete eliminated or withdrawn very early after transplantation. Two separation studies, one with basiliximab and the second with daclizumab have attempted to eliminate corticosteroids from the immunosuppression regimen. [20,21]

An open label pilot study conducted at 6 Canadian centers was performed to determine whether substituting daclizumab for cortico-steroids would result in acceptable freedom from rejection while reducing morbidity associated with steroid use. [20]   Fifty-seven primary renal allografts were enrolled in the study and received an immunosuppression regimen that consisted of daclizumab 1 mg/kg in 5 doses (similar to the Phase III tiral), 2 gm of mycophenolate mofetil and cyclosporine without corticosteroids. Twenty-eight patients received cadaver organs, 29 received organs from living donors. Twenty-six percent of patients had delayed graft function and required dialysis after transplantation. At one year patient survival was 95% and graft survival was 89% (3 deaths, 2 technical, 1 poor donor). Fourteen patients (25%) had a single rejection episode: 11 in the first three months, 2 between months 4-6, and 2 after six months of transplantation. Thirteen of the 14 rejection episodes were reversed with steroids and one required OKT3. In another multicenter study of primary renal transplants, patients were treated with basiliximab in 2 doses (similar to the Phase II trial), mycophenolate mofetil and cyclosporine for the prevention of acute rejection. [21] Patients were then randomized to either standard steroid therapy with slow taper versus rapid withdrawal of steroids with complete discontinuation at day 5 post-transplant.   The patients received the same dose of corticosteroids the first three days after transplantation with the rapid withdrawal arm receiving steroids for an additional 2 days followed by complete discontinuation. Forty-three patients were randomized to the conventional steroid arm and 40 patients were randomized to the rapid withdrawal arm. At one year the acute rejection rates were similar in the two groups 18% versus 20% (standard steroid therapy versus rapid withdrawal, respectively). The majority of rejections in the steroid withdrawal group were mild and were reversible with steroid therapy. The only graft loss that occurred was due to a patient death in the standard steroid therapy group.   In summary, these studies demonstrate that steroid avoidance or rapid withdrawal after transplantation can be achieved with induction therapy with the anti-IL-2R α mAbs and should be seriously considered for patients at low immunologic risk (primary transplants, non-blacks, low PRA). However longer term follow-up will be required to determine the safety of these regimens.

Calcineurin Inhibitors-Free Regimens

The adoption of calcineurin inhibitors as the mainstay of immuno-suppression since the early 1980s has resulted in a significant decreased incidence of acute rejection and improvement of short-term graft survival. However because of the irreversible nephrotoxicity associated with the chronic use of the calcineurin inhibityors, attempts are being made to decrease reliance on calcineurin inhibitors in immunosuppression regimens. [22,23] Since the calcineurin inhibitors block interleukin 2 production, it is theoretically possible that the sue of anti-IL-2R a mAbs that block IL-2 binding to its receptor could be substituted for the calcineurin inhibitors, particularly early in the post-transplant period, when the risk of acute rejection is relatively high. A multicenter trial explored calcineurin inhibitors avoidance in renal transplantation utilizing a regimen of daclizukmab, mycophenolate mofetil, and corticosteroids in an attempt to provide effective im-munosuppression without the use of calcineurin inhibitors. [22] Ninety-eight patients of primary cadaver or living donor kidneys at low immunologic risks were enrolled in a calcineurin inhibitor avoidance study. The immunosuppression regimen consisted of daclizumab ad-ministered for a total of 5 doses at bi-weekly intervals, mycophenolate mofetil 3 gm/day for the first 6 months and 2 gm thereafter in conventional corticosteroid therapy. Patients who underwent rejection episodes could be started on calcineurin inhibitors. The primary efficacy endpoint of the study was biopsy-proven rejection during the first 6 months after transplantation. The majority of rejection episodes were Banff grade 1 and 2A and were fully reversed with corticosteoids. The median time to the first biopsy-proven rejection among patients who experienced this event during the first 6 months was 39 days. At one year, patient survival was 97% and graft survival was 96%. Only two grafts were lost secondary to rejection. At one year post-transplant, 62% of patients had received calcineurin inhibitors for more than 7 days. At one year post-transplant, the mean serum creatinine in the non-rejectors with no calcineurin inhibitors used was 113 μmol/L, and in the rejectors 154 μmol/L. Thus this calcineurin inhibitors avoidance study, while only partially successful in preventing acute rejection provided benefits to a sizable minority of patients who have not required chronic calcineurin inhibitor therapy. However it is clear that the wider acceptance of a calcineurin inhibitor sparing immuno-suppression regimens will require a lower rate of acute rejection. One approach would be to add to this regimen a very low dose of calcineurin inhibitors that may not result in overt nephrotoxicity. There is some experimental evidence that low dose cyclosporine is synergistic with the sue of the anti-IL-2R α mAbs. [24] In fact a multicenter study is currently underway to explore the combination of daclizumab, myco-phenolate mofetil and low dose cyclosporine (with one arm continuing low dose cyclosporine while in the second arm cyclosporine would be discontinued altogether at 6 months).

A possibly more intriguing approach is to utilize sirolimus in a calcineurin-free regimen consisting of an anti-IL-2R mAb, mycophenolate mofetil and corticosteroids. The immunologic advantages of this combination may be the blockade of interleukin 2 binding to its receptor as well as interrupting signaling from the β γ chains (thus interrupting multiple cytokins signaling). [25]   The combination of high dose sirolimus, mycophenolate mofetil and corticosteroids was compared to cyclosporine, mycophenolate mofetil and corticosteroids in a multicenter randomized trial. [23] The incidence of biopsy-proven acute rejection was 27% versus 18% in the sirolimus and cyclosporine-treated patients, respectively.   Thus the combination of sirolimus and mycophenolate mofetil without calcineurin inhibitors can provide effective immunosuppression.   However, the acute rejection episodes occurring with this combination tended to be more severe (10 of the 11 were grade II) and over 40% of patients had to discontinue this regimen in part because of side effects. The addition of an anti-IL-2R mAb may allow lower dosage of sirolimus, better acceptance and tolerability of this regimen and possibly decrease the severity of the acute rejections. [26] At the University of California, San Fransisco, we have initiated a prospective study utilizing daclizumab, sirolimus (initial dose 15 mg followed by 10 mg per day) and 2 gm of mycophenolate mofetil with low dose steroids to assess the feasibility, tolerability and initial effectiveness of this calcineurin inhibitors-free regimen.   This immunosuppression strategy is particularly beneficial for patients with delayed graft function where the use of depleting antilymphocyte biologics and calcineurin inhibitors can be completely eliminated.

At the present time several new monoclonal antibodies are being tested in early Phase I trials including humanized anti-LFA1, humanized anti-B7.1 and B7.2 and second generation CRL4Ig. These antibodies should be optimally used in calcineurin inhibitors-free regimens but may require the concomitant use of the ani-IL-2R mAbs. The anti-IL-2R mAbs have been shown to be effective, safe and flexible agents in immunoprophylaxis in renal transplaintation. It is likely that they will play an important role in immunoprophylaxis in renal transplantation for many years.

References

1. Nashan B, Moor R, AmlotP, et al. Randomised trial of bsiliximab versus placebo for control of acute cellular rejection in renal allograft recipients. Lancet 1997;350:1193-1198.
2. Vincenti F, Kirkman R, Light S, et al. Interleukin-2-receptor blockade with daclizumab to prevent acure rejection in renal transplantation. N Engl J Med 1998;338:161-165.
3. Nashan B, Light S, Hardie IR, et al. Reduction of acute renal allograft rejection by daclizumab. Transplantation 1999;67:110-115.
4. Kahan BD, Rajagopalan PR, Hall M. Reduction of the occurrence of acute cellular rejection among renal allograft recipients treated with basiliximab, a chimeric anti-interleukin-2-receptor monoclonal antibody. Transplantation 1999;67:276-284.
5. Boelaars-van Haperen MJAM, BaanCC, van Riemsdijk IC, et al : Treatment with the chimeric anti-IL2Rα antibody basiliximab prevents the development of renal rejection by affecting the IL-2 and IL-15 pathway. XVIII International Congress of the Transplantation Society (Abstract OAP17) pg. 28, Aurg. 27-Sept. 1, 2000.
6. Goebel J, Stevens E, Forrest K, et al: Daclizumab (dac) blocks early interleukin (IL)-2 receptor ® signaling. XVII International Congress of the Transplantation Society (Abstract #P0528), pg. 316, Aug. 27-Sept. 1, 2000.
7. Souillou JP, Cantarovich D, LeMauff B, et al. Randomized controlled trial of monoclonal antibody against rejection of renal allografts. N Eng J Med 1990;322:1175.
8. Krikman RL, Shapiro ME, Carpenter DB, et al. A randomized prospective trial of anti-Tac monoclonal antibody in human renal transplantation. Transplantation 1991; 51:107-113.
9. Kriaa F, Hiesse C, Alard P, et al. Prophylactic use of the anti-IL-2-receptor monoclonal antibody LO-Tact-I in cadaveric renal transplantation: results of a randomized study. Transplant Proc 1993;25:817-819.
10. van Gelder T, Zietse R, Mulder AH, et al. A double-blind, placebo-controlled study of monoclonal anti-interleukin-2 receptor antibody (BT563) administration to prevent acute rejection after kidney transplantation. Transplantation 1995;60:248-252.
11. Vincenti F, Lantz M, Birnbaum J, et al. A phase I tirla of humanized anti-interleukin 2 receptor antibody in renal transplantation. Transplantation 1997;63:33-38.
12. Amlot PL, Rawlings E, Fernando ON, et al. Prolonged action of chiameric IL-2 receptor (CD25) monoclonal antibody used in cadaveric renal transplantation. Transplantation, 1995;60:748-56.
13. Kirkman RL, Bumgardner G, Gaston RS, et al. Addition of daclizumab to mycophenolate mofetil, cyclosporine, and steroids in renal transplantation: pharmacokinetics, safety and efficacy. (Submitted for publication, Clinical Transplantation).
14. Davies E, Lawen J, Mourad G, et al. Basiliximab (Simulect®) is safe and effective in combination with Neoral®, steroids, and CellCept® for the prevention of acute rejection episodes in renal transplantation. Interim results of a double-blind, randomized clinical trial. (Abstract #A3672) Amer. Soc Nephrology 32nd annual meeting, Nov. 1-8, 1999.
15. Ciancio G, Miller A, Cespedes M, et al: Daclizumab induction for primary kidney transplant recipients using tacrolimus, mycophenolate mofetil and steroids as maintenance immunosuppression. XVIII International Congress of the Transplantation Society. (Abstract OAP27), pg. 46, Aug. 27-Sept. 1, 2000.
16. Deierhoi MH, Hudson SL, Gaston RS: Clinical experience with a two dose regimen of daclizumab in cadaveric renal transplantation. (Abstract #574) pg. S75, AST

Transplant 2000.

17. Lebranchu Y, Hurault de Ligny B, Toupance O, et al. A multicenter randomized trial of Simulect® versus Thymoglobuline® in renal transplantation, (Abstract #567) pg. S74, AST Transplant 2000.

18. Sollinger H, Kaplan B, Pewscovitz M, et al: A multicenter, randomized trial of Simulect® with early Neoral® vs. ATGAM® with delayed Neoral in renal transplantation,. XVIII International Congress of the Transplantation Soceity (Abstract #0113) pg. 29, Aug. 27-Sept 1, 2000.

19. Hong JC, Kahan BD. Interleukin-2 receptor monoclonal antibodies and sirolimus: a novel induction immunosuppression strategy. Transplantation & Immunology Letter XVI:7-9, 2000.

20. Landsberg DN, Cole EH, Russell D, et al. Renal transplantation without steroids – one year results of a multicentre Canadian pilot study. (Abstract #86), pg. S49, AST Transplant 2000.

21. Vincenti F, Monaco A, Grinyo J, et al. Rapid steroid withdrawal versus standard steroid treatment in patients treated with Simulect®, Neoral®, and Cellcept® for the prevention of acute rejection in renal transplantation: a multicenter, randomized trial. (Abstract #83) pg. S49, AST Transplant 2000.

22. Vincenti F, Ramos E, Brattstrom C, Cho S, Ekberg H, Grinyo J, Johnson R, Kuypers D, Stuart F, Khanna A, Navarro M, Nashan B. Multicenter trial exploring calcineurin inhibitors avoidance in renal transplantation. In Press, Transplantation, 2000.

23. Kreis H, Cisterne J-M, Land @, et al. Sirolimus inassociation with mycophenolate mofetil induction for the prevention of acute graft rejection in renal allograft recipients. Transplantation 69:1252-1260.

24. Tellides G, Dallman MJ, Morris PJ. Synergistic interaction of cyclosporine A with interleukin 2 receptor monoclonal antibody therapy. Transplantation Proc 1988;20 (Suppl 2):202-206.

25. Baan CC, Knoop CJ, van Gelder T, et al. Anti-CD25 therapy reveals the redundancy of the intragraft cytokine network after clinical heart transplantation. Transplantation 1999;67:870-876.

26. Chang, GJ, Harish H, Mahanty, Vincenti F, et al. A calcineurin inhibitor-sparing regimen with sirolimus, mycophenolate mofetil, and anti-CD25 mAb provides effective immunosuppression in kidney transplant recipients with delayed or impaired graft function. Clinical Transplantation 2000; 14:545-549.

MONOCLONAL ANTIBODY TARGETING OF ADHESION MOLECULES

Markus H. Frank and David M. Briscoe

Introduction

The process of adhesion has been described in the medical literature for more than 100 years as a characteristic component of all forms of inflammation. Over the past few decades, multiple investigators have defined series of families of adhesion molecules that provide for intimate cell-cell contact and facilitate interactions among another series of activation molecules. To this end, the process of adhesion is intimately associated with activation and there has been some debate as to whether certain molecules provide for selective adhesion or for selective activation [1-7]. For instance, the adhesive interactions between MHC molecules and the T cell receptor, discussed in detail in Chapter X are critical for the activation of lymphocytes. But these interactions are of very low affinity and thus require the function of families of high affinity adhesion molecules to enable close approxima-tion of these molecules and activation events. Furthermore, biological processes have evolved to facilitate these processes in as much as the interaction between cognate antigen and the T cell receptor is a process that facilitates the expression of high affinity adhesion molecules; and disruption of adhesion (such as ICAM-1-mediated adhesion, discussed below) may dysregulate activation. To this end it must be emphasized that adhesion events interrelate with activation responses and it is important to consider the entire adhesion process as fundamental to any bidirectional cell-cell activation response.

Mohamed Sayegh and Giuseppe Remuzzi (editors), Current and Future Immunosuppressive Therapies Following Transplantation, 249-263.
© *2001 Kluwer Academic Publishers. Printed in the Netherlands.*

In this chapter we will focus our discussion on leukocyte-endothelial adhesion events. Activation of endothelial cells and the expression of endothelial cell adhesion molecules are critical for the effective recruitment of leukocytes into inflammatory sites. The anatomic location of the vascular endothelial cell provides it with the unique ability to interact with all leukocytes in the course of an immune response. Indeed, the endothelial cell is functional in all aspects of the immune response, from the initial recruitment of cells into a site of inflammation, to the reciprocal activation of leukocytes and endothelial cells, to the angiogenesis of the chronic healing inflammatory reaction [6]. Critical to this function are leukocyte-endothelial cell adhesion and multiple regulated families of adhesion molecules. For this reason, vascular endothelial cell adhesion molecules have been proposed to be a highly attractive target for the therapeutic manipulation of immune responses, including therapeutic intervention in organ transplantation [7-10]. In transplanted vascularized grafts, adhesion molecules are expressed by endothelial cells lining post capillary venules and bind counterreceptors on recipient leukocytes to function in the extravasation of leukocytes into the allograft and their subsequent migration through the extracellular matrix. In addition, adhesion molecules support signaling functions in antigen presentation and T cell costimulation that are essential for the bi-directional activation of endothelial cells and leukocytes. Monoclonal antibodies that specifically target several of these critically important molecules have been studied in clinical trials. In this chapter, we summarize the current understanding of the role of endothelial cell adhesion molecules in immune inflammation and allograft rejection, and we review the rationale for experimental strategies that target these molecules in allotransplantation.

The Role of Adhesion Molecules in Inflammation and Allograft Rejection

It is now generally accepted that leukocyte emigration from the bloodstream to extravascular sites of inflammation or immune reactivity is a multistep process, in which the initial contact of circulating immune cells with activated microvascular endothelium results in low-affinity rolling interactions followed by firm cellular adhesion and subsequent transendothelial diapedesis and subendothelial migration [11]; several distinct classes of adhesion molecules that participate at various stages in this adhesion cascade have been identified: Initial leukocyte rolling under laminar flow conditions within the blood vessel has been shown to be mediated mainly by low affinity interactions between the selectin family (P-, E-, and L-selectin) and its ligands [11-16], although interactions between $\beta 1$ integrins on lymphocytes and vascular cell adhesion molecule (VCAM)-1 have also been described to support rolling [17]. P-and E-selectin are predominantly expressed by cytokine

(IL-1, TNF-α)- or inflammatory mediator (Thrombin, Histamine, LTC$_4$, LPS)-activated endothelium, and serve as adhesion receptors for P-selectin glycoprotein ligand (PSGL)-1, L-selectin and the carbohydrate ligand Sialyl Lewis X , and possibly additional molecules expressed on circulating leukocytes [7, 18-21]. All three selectins have been shown to facilitate leukocyte rolling *in vitro*, and L- and P-selectin have also been shown to mediate leukocyte rolling and recruitment *in vivo* [22]. While P-selectin expression is rapidly induced on activated endothelial cells and platelets by mobilization from intracellular stores, E-selectin expression by activated endothelium is transcriptionally regulated and occurs only several hours upon activation, suggesting a role for this molecule in the later recruitment of leukocytes [5]. Firm leukocyte adherence and arrest on activated endothelium follows initial rolling interactions, and this process is mediated by integrin receptors and their ligands. The CD11/CD18 β2 integrins (lymphocyte function associated antigen-1 (LFA-1, CD11aCD18); macrophage antigen complex-1 (Mac-1, CD11bCD18) and very late antigen-4 (VLA-4) (β1 integrin) are expressed by leukocytes upon cytokine- and/or antigen-dependent stimulation, and respectively bind ICAM-1 and VCAM-1 induced on activated endothelium in part by signaling from selectin engagement, and by soluble cytokine and chemokine mediators released locally at sites of leukocyte-endothelial cell interactions [23-28]. While adherence to endothelium is obligate for subsequent diapedesis and transmigration to occur, it is not a sufficient prerequisite. Additional changes in and interactions with cell-cell junctional adhesion molecules are thought to be necessary. Transmigration is a complex process that involves another series of molecular interactions including interactions among platelet-endothelial cell adhesion molecule (PECAM)-1 [29], and a series of molecular zipper molecules including the vascular endothelial cell cadherin complex (VE-cadherin), alpha-, beta-, and gamma-catenin, and p120/p100 [30]. PECAM-1 is constitutively expressed on endothelial cells and on a subset of leukocytes at high levels, forming homotypic interactions at endothelial cell junctions, and has been shown to facilitate endothelial cell junction rearrangement [31,32]. VE-cadherin localizes to adherens junctions surrounding vascular endothelial cells; and recent studies have demonstrated transient and focal dissociation and reassociation of the VE-cadherin complex during leukocyte transmigration [30]. In addition, other cell surface and soluble mediators including families of chemokines facilitate leukocyte migration through the extracellular matrix and retention at the site of inflammation .

It is now widely appreciated that the multistep cascade of leukocyte-endothelial adhesion interactions in inflammation applies to the extravasation of T lymphocytes as well, and it is likely that the same mechanisms underlie the peripheral recruitment of alloreactive T cells to the allograft [6,33]. In addition, adhesion molecule-mediated lymphocyte/microvascular graft endothelial cell interactions may initiate or sustain allograft rejection by mechanisms other than mere recruitment, including graft endothelial cell/lymphocyte interactions necessary for recipient T cell alloactivation and costimulation [4,9]. Thus, adhesion molecule-facilitated interactions, from the initial lymphocyte interaction with microvasculature graft endothelial cells to the reciprocal activation of lymphocytes by endothelial cells, are critical in several pathways leading to acute and chronic allograft rejection.

The expression of adhesion molecules and their association with the recruitment of leukocytes to allografts undergoing rejection has been studied in both animal and humans following transplantation. When naive T cells are activated by alloantigen in lymphoid tissues, they differentiate into effector T cells or memory T cells. Unlike naive T cells, which home to lymph nodes, differentiated T cells are preferentially recruited to peripheral sites of inflammation [4]. The preferential interaction of previously activated T cells with the endothelium at inflammatory sites may be explained, in part, by the restricted expression of functional ligands for endothelial cell E- and P-selectin only on memory or effector T cells [34]. It has been demonstrated that functional selectin ligands are expressed by Th1 cells but not Th2 cells; furthermore, *in vivo* studies in mice suggest that Th1 cells are recruited to peripheral delayed-type-hypersensitivity sites in a selectin-dependent manner while Th2 cells are not, pointing to a critical role of selectin-mediated interactions in determining the balance of intragraft Th1 or Th2 responses, which may be important for shaping the outcome of the rejection response [35-37]. Although endothelial E-selectin expression is rarely observed in biopsies in association with acute rejection, it is known to occur early following transplantation, usually preceding acute rejection episodes [38,39]. This observation is consistent with the role of the selectin interactions in early lymphocyte recruitment. In contrast, expression of ICAM-1 and VCAM-1 on endothelial cells is observed in close association with acute rejection [39-45]. However, while ICAM-1, constitutively expressed at low levels on endothelium, is augmented throughout the graft microvasculature bed both before and during acute rejection episodes, the de novo VCAM-1 expression found predominantly on post-capillary venules exhibits close temporal and topologic association with T cell infiltrates and the rejection process itself [46,47]. In the case of renal transplantation, during both allograft rejection and reperfusion injury, ICAM-1 and VCAM-1, in addition to being overexpressed in renal microvascular endothelial cells, are also upregulated in renal tubular cells [46]. Indeed, several studies have demonstrated a direct pathophysiologic role for the CD11/CD18 and ICAM-1 pathways in renal ischemia/reperfusion injury [48-53], implicating an important role of these pathways for delayed graft function of this etiology, in addition to rejection as an underlying factor. Expression of E-selectin, ICAM-1 and VCAM-1 is usually downregulated following acute rejection episodes; however, prolonged persistence of

ICAM-1 and VCAM-1 expression following human cardiac transplantation has been correlated with the development of chronic rejection, thus suggesting a link between endothelial cell activation and ongoing intragraft immune events [6].

In addition to facilitating leukocyte recruitment to the allograft, endothelial cell/leukocyte adhesion and transmigration events support the ability of endothelial cells to facilitate T cell activation via the direct and the indirect pathway of allorecognition. The ability of endothelial cells to activate T cells via the direct pathway of allo-recognition is well documented [6]. Endothelial cells act as effective antigen presenting cells by providing both antigen-dependent signals (signal 1) and costimulatory signals (signal 2), mediated by distinct molecules. Expression of MHC class II molecules by allogeneic endothelial cells supports their antigen presenting capacity [54-56], while cell surface expression of accessory adhesion molecules promotes costimulatory signals. The best characterized costimulatory signal in the direct pathway of T cell activation is provided the interaction of endothelial LFA-3 with T cell CD2 [57-59] , but endothelial ICAM-1 and VCAM-1 also contribute in this process by interacting with T cellular LFA-1 and VLA-4, respectively [60-64]. Since endothelial cells, however, do not express the B7 family of molecules, which potently costimulate T cell activation through interaction with T cellular CD28, they are limited in their ability to fully costimulate CD4+ T cell activation "in cis". The recent demonstration that leukocyte/endothelial cell interactions can promote B-7 expression on T cells and monocytes suggests that an important function of the endothelium may be to induce local expression of B7-family molecules and provide for costimulation locally at the site of inflammation [65]. Furthermore, recent evidence suggests that specific endothelial cell/monocyte interactions may facilitate monocyte differentiation into myeloid-derived dendritic cells expressing B7 and ICAM-1 costimulatory molecules and MHC class II [66]. Myeloid-derived dendritic cells use another series of molecules to reverse transmigrate out of the graft across lymphatic endothelial cells, and upon migration from graft tissue to lymphatic tissue present allo-antigen to recipient T cells [67]. Taken together, these findings indicate that critical components of subsequent activation responses are dependent on initial and specific endothelial cell/monocyte inter-actions that facilitate recruitment, transendothelial trafficking into and out of sites of inflammation [1].

Targeting Adhesion Molecules in Allotransplantation - Animal Studies

The role of leukocyte adhesion molecules in lymphocyte recruitment and activation as well as the observed overexpression during rejection responses have provided a rationale for assessing the potential therapeutic effects of specific adhesion molecule blockade *in vivo* in animal models of organ transplantation. *In vivo* studies, using specific monoclonal antibodies (mAb) directed against ICAM-1 and its ligand CD11CD18, VCAM-1 and its ligand VLA-4, either as monotherapy or in combination, have been performed in various animal models (mouse, rat, rabbit, non-human primates) of renal and cardiac allograft transplantation, and to a lesser extent of other organs such as skin, pancreatic islets and cornea.

In a rat cardiac allograft model, targeting of ICAM-1 by post-transplant 10 day mAb monotherapy has been shown to reduce the degree of graft T cell infiltration by both CD4+ and CD8+ subsets, to reduce myocardial necrosis, vascular injury and intravenous thrombi, and to induce a modest prolongation of allograft survival to 18 d from 10 d in treatment versus control groups [68]. Other investigators, in a rat model of small bowel transplantation, reported that a post-transplant 5 day course of anti-ICAM-1 mAb attenuated rejection in the early post-transplant period, although no changes were observed between treatment and control groups at day 15 post transplantation [69]. In addition, in nonhuman primates with renal allografts, anti-ICAM-1 mAb monotherapy for a 12 d duration significantly prolonged allograft survival from 9 to 24 days, attenuated graft T cell infiltration, although not blocking it completely, and reduced arterial endothelial inflammation [42]. In addition, ICAM-1 inhibition in this study successfully reversed preexisting rejection in a subset of treated animals. Anti-ICAM-1 mAb was found on circulating recipient T cells as well, pointing to a potential additional role of the antibody in interfering with antigen presentation and/or T cell interactions. No additional benefit was derived from pretransplant graft perfusion with anti-ICAM-1 mAb in this study. In contrast, other investigators found that pretransplant perfusion of the donor organ alone with anti-ICAM-1 mAb, in the absence of systemic recipient administration, had no prolonging effect on allograft survival in a rat renal transplant model [70]; indeed, in a particular rat strain combination this treatment adversely affected the graft by causing vascular damage by both Fc-mediated and Fc-independent mechanisms.

Another approach in targeting the ICAM-1/CD11CD18 pathway in allotransplantation has been to block the ICAM-1 ligand CD11CD18 by mAbs directed against CD18 or LFA-1 (CD11aCD18). In a rabbit heterotopic cardiac allograft model, Sadahiro et al. compared the relative efficacy of anti-ICAM-1 and anti-CD18, and found that T cellular rejection grade and vascular rejection were significantly lower in animals treated with anti-CD18 than with anti-ICAM-1 [71]. This study pointed to the possibility of a functional redundancy of ICAM-1 in the immune response, raising the possibility that the observed relative greater efficacy of LFA-1 inhibition resulted from the fact that LFA-1 is the ligand not only for ICAM-1, but also ICAM-2 and ICAM-3, and possibly others. In a rat heterotopic heart allograft model, anti-CD18 mAb monotherapy was shown to exhibit immmunesuppressive effects

[72]. Two other studies [73,74] found significant prolongation of mouse cardiac allograft survival by LFA-1 mAb monotherapy. In a mouse islet allograft transplantation model, anti-LFA-1 mAb significantly prolonged allograft survival, and in a subset of animals induced indefinite graft survival with donor-specific tolerance [75]. Dissection of the tolerogenic effect of anti-LFA-1 mAb in this subset of animals indicated prevention of T cell activation mediated by a T cell receptor engagement in treated animals that led to antigen-specific unresponsiveness maintained by transferable suppressor cells.

The observed beneficial, yet incomplete, therapeutic effects of either anti-ICAM-1 or anti-LFA mAb monotheray in certain animal models of allotransplantation have prompted investigation of potential synergistic effects of these treatment modalities. While both agents target the ICAM-1/LFA-1 pathway, the differential tissue expression of ICAM-1 and LFA-1, the differential targeting by anti-ICAM-1 or LFA-1 mAbs of predominantly donor or recipient tissue-expressed antigens, and the redundancy of LFA-1 ligands have provided a rationale for combination treatment. Several studies have been performed in vivo in various animal models of allotransplantation, with varying efficacy depending on the model used. In a mouse cardiac allograft model, a 6 d posttranplant course of combined anti-LFA-1 and anti-ICAM-1 mAb therapy induced donor-specific tolerance and indefinite graft survival, whereas administration of either antibody alone prolonged graft sur-vival but was insufficient for tolerance induction [76]. In a follow-up study directed at elucidating the mechanisms of tolerance induction, tolerance could not be abrogated by injection of either naive recipient lymphocytes or sensitized lymphocytes taken from untreated recipient strain mice that rejected donor strain hearts [77]. In addition, mixed lymphocyte culture showed that splenocytes from treated allograft recipient mice showed normal allogeneic response without donor alloantigen specificity, raising the possibility that the mechanism of tolerance in this model depended on both absent donor-specific sen-sitization and also inhibition of T cell recruitment in the immune res-ponse effector arm. In contrast, in a fully mismatched mouse skin allograft model, no significant prolongation of graft survival was observed using this combination treatment regimen [78]. Prolongation of skin graft survival in the treatment groups was observed, however, in subsets of animals when either MHC class I or class II-mismatched strains were used. In another study, treatment with anti-ICAM-1 and anti-LFA-1 mAbs alone or in combination had no effect on allograft survival after heart transplantation between fully incompatible rat strains [79], indicating the existence of specific species-dependent differences in the role of these adhesion molecules in transplant rejection.

Endothelial VCAM-1 as discussed above has been found to be both temporally and spatially associated with T cells in allografts. Furthermore, it has been shown that the induction of VCAM-1 is most intense and is persistent in allografts in comparison to isografts where its expression is early and transient. This suggests that a factor produced by activated T cells may induce local VCAM-1 to facilitate ongoing mononuclear cell recruitment. Blockade of the VCAM-1/VLA-4 cell adhesion pathway has been studied in animal models. In a murine cardiac allograft model, treatment with anti-VCAM-1 mAb induced long-term graft acceptance associated with inactivity of graft-infil-trating T cells, with absent IL-2 receptor expression and lack of IL-2, IL-4 and IFN- production [80]. In another study, both anti-VCAM-1 or anti-VLA-4 mAb monotherapy resulted in moderate prolongation of mouse cardiac allograft survival, and combination therapy was synergistic, resulting in further prolongation of allograft survival [81].

Targeting both the ICAM-1/CD11CD18 and VCAM-1/VLA-4 adhesion pathways concurrently has been assessed as well. In a rat cardiac allograft model, anti-LFA-1 and anti-VLA-4 combination therapy resulted in a modest prolongation of graft survival [82]. No additional benefit was detected in a follow-up study when a mAb to Mac-1 (CD11bCD18), a monocyte adhesion receptor and mediator of monocyte migration, was added to the regimen [83]. In a rabbit cardiac allograft model, anti-LFA-1 and anti-VLA-4 combination therapy reduced vascular and cellular rejection responses assessed at 1 week post transplantation; allograft survival, however, was not reported in this study [71].

Adhesion Molecule Blockade in Renal Transplantation in Human Clinical Trials

There is general interest in the use of adhesion molecule antagonists in immune inflammation, especially chronic inflammatory conditions and allograft rejection. The rationale for its use is based first on the functional preclinical animal studies as outlined above, and second on the findings of adhesion molecule expression in rejecting human allografts. Third, its use has been designed on the basis of immunologic deficiencies observed in patients with Leukocyte Adhesion Deficiencies (LAD). One such deficiency called LAD-1 results from a mutated CD18 gene and is characterized by a deficiency in $\beta2$ integrin-mediated adhesion [84,85]. These patients have recurrent infections, abscesses and cell-mediated immune deficiencies that ultimately lead to chronic illness and death. Another such deficiency called LAD-2 results from a mutation in glycosylation of sialyl x moieties and results in recurrent infections [86,87]. Also, inhibition of $\beta2$ integrin-mediated adhesion inhibits the human MLR. Thus, it was anticipated that these agents would be immunosuppressive and studies to assess the efficacy of anti-ICAM-1 mAb and anti-LFA-1 mAb therapy were commenced in patients following human renal transplantation.

In a phase I dose-finding study of 18 kidney transplant recipients, murine anti-ICAM-1 mAb (BIRR1, Enlimomab) was given prophylactically as add-on therapy to high-risk patients who were highly immunized, were retransplant recipients, received renal allografts from unstable donors, or received grafts with cold ischemia times longer than 36 h [88]. The use of 360 mg or 560 mg enlimomab, including a loading dose of 160 mg before the operation and 40 mg or 80 mg for the following 5 days, was associated with adequate serum levels of the anti-ICAM-1 antibody, and graft outcome was better than in the groups who received lower loading doses. These results established a dosing schedule and the clinical safety of enlimomab, and suggested that anti-ICAM-1 mAb therapy may be useful in controlling allograft rejection and possibly in limiting reperfusion injury in a selected high-risk population. A multicenter randomized, double-blind trial assessing the efficacy of the anti-ICAM-1 mAb (enlimomab) for the prevention of acute rejection and delayed onset graft function in human cadaveric renal transplantation in an unselected population of patients was subsequently performed [89]. In an initial report it appeared that similar to observations in animals the predominant effect of the treatment was to prevent ischemia reperfusion injury and to attenuate the development of delayed graft function. However, a larger study involving a total of 262 recipients of cadaveric kidneys that received either enlimomab or a placebo for six days and triple immuno-suppressive therapy of cyclosporine, azathioprine and prednisolone showed no significant difference in the incidences of first acute rejection at three months between the two groups, and enlimomab did not reduce the risk of delayed onset of graft function. In addition, no differences in patient survival or graft survival were observed at one year. Thus, in the interpretation of these data the general consensus was that anti-adhesion molecule therapy with this combination may be of benefit exclusively in selected patients at high risk for rejection or delayed graft function, rather than the general renal transplant population.

The therapeutic potential of CD11aCD18 blockade has been examined in human transplant recipients as well. A dose-searching trial of an anti-LFA1 mAb (odulimomab) in first kidney transplant recipients indicated a good tolerability and safety of this mAb [90]. Clinical trials have assessed the effect of anti-LFA-1 mAb blockade in the treatment of acute rejection in kidney transplantation, and the efficacy of the antibody as part of an induction treatment protocol in first kidney transplants for the prophylaxis of acute allograft rejection. While anti-LFA-1 was unable to reverse ongoing acute rejection episodes in one study [91], a phase I, multicenter trial using anti-LFA-1 as induction therapy in renal transplants demonstrated similar efficacy of anti-LFA-1 mAb compared with antithymocyte globulin and a tendency of improved prevention of delayed graft function [92]. Thus, again it appears that there is some redundancy in the function of adhesion molecules and that it is likely that combination therapy will be necessary for the best results. These studies are currently being planned.

Summary and Future Directions

Pathophysiological considerations based on available *in vitro* evidence concerning the role of cellular adhesion molecules in leukocyte recruitment and T cell activation provide a strong rationale for the potential therapeutic usefulness of specific adhesion molecule inhibition strategies in clinical organ transplantation. While the use of some of the available monoclonal antibody agents has been very promising in some animal models of allotransplantation, including the induction of long-term allograft survival and donor-specific tolerance, initial human clinical trials involving the most promising of currently available agents have revealed only limited efficacy in a subset of the general renal transplant population. Current evidence points to a potential usefulness of adhesion molecule blockade in controlling allograft rejection and possibly in limiting reperfusion injury in a selected high-risk population, and also as a potential alternative agent in transplant induction therapy. No human clinical trial has as of yet assessed the preventive or therapeutic potential of combination therapy using adhesion molecule-directed antibodies with established safety profiles in humans. A barrier to greater clinical utility of cell adhesion molecule-targeted approaches is the demonstrated existence of functional redundancy of some of the molecules and the possible functional redundancy of others, thus limiting the possibilities of specific efficient blockade of some of the critical pathways involved. Future identification of novel related proteins and further elucidation of the multiple complex functions that adhesion molecules serve in alloimmunity will help in the development of more targeted and efficient strategies.

References

1. Briscoe, D.M., Recent Insights into the Roles of the Endothelium in Allorecognition. Graft, 1999. 2(6): p. 261-262.
2. Pober, J.S., Immunobiology of human vascular endothelium. Immunol Res, 1999. 19(2-3): p. 225-32.
3. Rabb, H. and J.V. Bonventre, Leukocyte adhesion molecules in transplantation. Am J Med, 1999. 107(2): p. 157-65.
4. Briscoe, D.M., S.I. Alexander, and A.H. Lichtman, Interactions between T lymphocytes and endothelial cells in allograft rejection. Curr Opin Immunol, 1998. 10(5): p. 525-31.
5. Fuggle, S.V. and D.D. Koo, Cell adhesion molecules in clinical renal transplantation. Transplantation, 1998. 65(6): p. 763-9.
6. Briscoe, D.M., et al., The problem of chronic rejection: influence of leukocyte-endothelial interactions. Kidney Int Suppl, 1997. 58:p.S22-7.
7. Carlos, T.M. and J.M. Harlan, Leukocyte-endothelial adhesion molecules. Blood, 1994. 84(7): p. 2068-101.
8. Pober, J.S. and R.S. Cotran, The role of endothelial cells in inflammation. Transplantation, 1990. 50(4): p. 537-44.
9. Pober, J.S., et al., Can graft endothelial cells initiate a host anti-graft immune response? Transplantation, 1996. 61(3): p. 343-9.
10. Imhof, B.A. and D. Dunon, Leukocyte migration and adhesion. Adv Immunol, 1995. 58: p. 345-416.
11. Springer, T.A., Traffic signals for lymphocyte recirculation and leukocyte emigration: the multistep paradigm. Cell, 1994. 76(2): p. 301-14.
12. Yamada, S., et al., Rolling in P-selectin-deficient mice is reduced but not eliminated in the dorsal skin. Blood, 1995. 86(9): p. 3487-92.
13. Ley, K. and T.F. Tedder, Leukocyte interactions with vascular endothelium. New insights into selectin-mediated attachment and rolling. J Immunol, 1995. 155(2): p. 525-8.
14. Arbones, M.L., et al., Lymphocyte homing and leukocyte rolling and migration are impaired in L- selectin-deficient mice. Immunity, 1994. 1(4): p. 247-60.
15. Mayadas, T.N., et al., Leukocyte rolling and extravasation are severely compromised in P selectin-deficient mice. Cell, 1993. 74(3): p. 541-54.
16. Labow, M.A., et al., Characterization of E-selectin-deficient mice: demonstration of overlapping function of the endothelial selectins. Immunity, 1994. 1(8): p. 709-20.
17. Luscinskas, F.W., H. Ding, and A.H. Lichtman, P-selectin and vascular cell adhesion molecule 1 mediate rolling and arrest, respectively, of CD4+ T lymphocytes on tumor necrosis factor alpha-activated vascular endothelium under flow. J Exp Med, 1995. 181(3): p. 1179-86.
18. Pober, J.S., et al., Overlapping patterns of activation of human endothelial cells by interleukin 1, tumor necrosis factor, and immune interferon. J Immunol, 1986. 137(6): p. 1893-6.
19. Thornhill, M.H., et al., Tumor necrosis factor combines with IL-4 or IFN-gamma to selectively enhance endothelial cell adhesiveness for T cells. The contribution of vascular cell adhesion molecule-1-dependent and -independent binding mechanisms. J Immunol, 1991. 146(2): p. 592-8.
20. Thornhill, M.H. and D.O. Haskard, IL-4 regulates endothelial cell activation by IL-1, tumor necrosis factor, or IFN-gamma. J Immunol, 1990. 145(3): p. 865-72.
21. Briscoe, D.M., R.S. Cotran, and J.S. Pober, Effects of tumor necrosis factor, lipopolysaccharide, and IL-4 on the expression of vascular cell adhesion molecule-1 in vivo. Correlation with CD3+ T cell infiltration. J Immunol, 1992. 149(9): p. 2954-60.

22. Ley, K., et al., Sequential contribution of L- and P-selectin to leukocyte rolling *in vivo*. J Exp Med, 1995. 181(2): p. 669-75.
23. Springer, T.A., Adhesion receptors of the immune system. Nature, 1990. 346(6283): p. 425-34.
24. Hemler, M.E., VLA proteins in the integrin family: structures, functions, and their role on leukocytes. Annu Rev Immunol, 1990. 8: p. 365-400.
25. Hynes, R.O., Integrins: versatility, modulation, and signaling in cell adhesion. Cell, 1992. 69(1): p. 11-25.
26. Marlin, S.D. and T.A. Springer, Purified intercellular adhesion molecule-1 (ICAM-1) is a ligand for lymphocyte function-associated antigen 1 (LFA-1). Cell, 1987. 51(5): p. 813-9.
27. Diamond, M.S., et al., ICAM-1 (CD54): a counter-receptor for Mac-1 (CD11b/CD18). J Cell Biol, 1990. 111(6 Pt 2): p. 3129-39.
28. de Fougerolles, A.R., et al., Characterization of ICAM-2 and evidence for a third counter-receptor for LFA-1. J Exp Med, 1991. 174(1): p. 253-67.
29. Muller, W.A., The role of PECAM-1 (CD31) in leukocyte emigration: studies *in vitro* and *in vivo*. J Leukoc Biol, 1995. 57(4): p. 523-8.
30. Allport, J.R., W.A. Muller, and F.W. Luscinskas, Monocytes induce reversible focal changes in vascular endothelial cadherin complex during transendothelial migration under flow. J Cell Biol, 2000. 148(1): p. 203-16.
31. Del Maschio, A., et al., Polymorphonuclear leukocyte adhesion triggers the disorganization of endothelial cell-to-cell adherens junctions. J Cell Biol, 1996. 135(2): p. 497-510.
32. Bianchi, E., et al., Through and beyond the wall: late steps in leukocyte transendothelial migration. Immunol Today, 1997. 18(12): p. 586-91.
33. Bradley, L.M. and S.R. Watson, Lymphocyte migration into tissue: the paradigm derived from CD4 subsets. Curr Opin Immunol, 1996. 8(3): p. 312-20.
34. Lichtman, A.H., et al., CD45RA-RO+ (memory) but not CD45RA+RO- (naive) T cells roll efficiently on E- and P-selectin and vascular cell adhesion molecule-1 under flow. J Immunol, 1997. 158(8): p. 3640-50.
35. Lichtman, A.H. and A.K. Abbas, T cell subsets: recruiting the right kind of help. Curr Biol, 1997. 7(4): p. R242-4.
36. Borges, E., et al., P-selectin glycoprotein ligand-1 (PSGL-1) on T helper 1 but not on T helper 2 cells binds to P-selectin and supports migration into inflamed skin. J Exp Med, 1997. 185(3): p. 573-8.
37. Austrup, F., et al., P- and E-selectin mediate recruitment of T-helper-1 but not T-helper-2 cells into inflammed tissues. Nature, 1997. 385(6611): p. 81-3.
38. Brockmeyer, C., et al., Distribution of cell adhesion molecules (ICAM-1, VCAM-1, ELAM-1) in renal tissue during allograft rejection. Transplantation, 1993. 55(3): p. 610-5.
39. Taylor, P.M., et al., Induction of vascular adhesion molecules during rejection of human cardiac allografts. Transplantation, 1992. 54(3): p. 451-7.
40. Briscoe, D.M., et al., Predictive value of inducible endothelial cell adhesion molecule expression for acute rejection of human cardiac allografts [published erratum appears in Transplantation 1995 Mar 27;59(6):928]. Transplantation, 1995. 59(2): p. 204-11.
41. Alpers, C.E., et al., Expression of vascular cell adhesion molecule-1 in kidney allograft rejection. Kidney Int, 1993. 44(4): p. 805-16.
42. Cosimi, A.B., et al., *In vivo* effects of monoclonal antibody to ICAM-1 (CD54) in nonhuman primates with renal allografts. J Immunol, 1990. 144(12): p. 4604-12.
43. Kanagawa, K., et al., Identification of ICAM-1-positive cells in the nongrafted and transplanted rat kidney--an immunohistochemical and ultrastructural study. Transplantation, 1991. 52(6): p. 1057-62.

44. Wuthrich, R.P., Intercellular adhesion molecules and vascular cell adhesion molecule-1 and the kidney [editorial]. J Am Soc Nephrol, 1992. 3(6): p. 1201-11.
45. Pelletier, R.P., et al., Importance of endothelial VCAM-1 for inflammatory leukocytic infiltration *in vivo*. J Immunol, 1992. 149(7): p. 2473-81.
46. Briscoe, D.M., et al., Expression of vascular cell adhesion molecule-1 in human renal allografts. J Am Soc Nephrol, 1992. 3(5): p. 1180-5.
47. Briscoe, D.M. and R.S. Cotran, Role of leukocyte-endothelial cell adhesion molecules in renal inflammation: *in vitro* and *in vivo* studies [published erratum appears in Kidney Int 1993 Sep;44(3):658]. Kidney Int Suppl, 1993. 42: p. S27-34.
48. Kelly, K.J., et al., Antibody to intercellular adhesion molecule 1 protects the kidney against ischemic injury. Proc Natl Acad Sci U S A, 1994. 91(2): p. 812-6.
49. Rabb, H., et al., Antibodies to ICAM-1 protect kidneys in severe ischemic reperfusion injury. Biochem Biophys Res Commun, 1995. 211(1): p. 67-73.
50. Linas, S.L., et al., Ischemia increases neutrophil retention and worsens acute renal failure: role of oxygen metabolites and ICAM 1. Kidney Int, 1995. 48(5): p. 1584-91.
51. Haller, H., et al., Antisense oligonucleotides for ICAM-1 attenuate reperfusion injury and renal failure in the rat. Kidney Int, 1996. 50(2): p. 473-80.
52. Rabb, H., et al., Role of CD11a and CD11b in ischemic acute renal failure in rats. Am J Physiol, 1994. 267(6 Pt 2): p. F1052-8.
53. Kelly, K.J., et al., Intercellular adhesion molecule-1-deficient mice are protected against ischemic renal injury. J Clin Invest, 1996. 97(4): p. 1056-63.
54. Pober, J.S., et al., Ia expression by vascular endothelium is inducible by activated T cells and by human gamma interferon. J Exp Med, 1983. 157(4): p. 1339-53.
55. Pardi, R., J.R. Bender, and E.G. Engleman, Lymphocyte subsets differentially induce class II human leukocyte antigens on allogeneic microvascular endothelial cells. J Immunol, 1987. 139(8): p. 2585-92.
56. Collins, T., et al., Immune interferon activates multiple class II major histocompatibility complex genes and the associated invariant chain gene in human endothelial cells and dermal fibroblasts. Proc Natl Acad Sci U S A, 1984. 81(15): p. 4917-21.
57. Hughes, C.C., C.O. Savage, and J.S. Pober, Endothelial cells augment T cell interleukin 2 production by a contact- dependent mechanism involving CD2/LFA-3 interaction. J Exp Med, 1990. 171(5): p. 1453-67.
58. Hughes, C.C., C.O. Savage, and J.S. Pober, The endothelial cell as a regulator of T cell function. Immunol Rev, 1990. 117: p. 85-102.
59. Hughes, C.C. and J.S. Pober, Costimulation of peripheral blood T cell activation by human endothelial cells. Enhanced IL-2 transcription correlates with increased c-fos synthesis and increased Fos content of AP-1. J Immunol, 1993. 150(8 Pt 1): p. 3148-60.
60. van Seventer, G.A., et al., Analysis of T cell stimulation by superantigen plus major histocompatibility complex class II molecules or by CD3 monoclonal antibody: costimulation by purified adhesion ligands VCAM-1, ICAM-1, but not ELAM-1. J Exp Med, 1991. 174(4): p. 901-13.
61. Van Seventer, G.A., et al., The LFA-1 ligand ICAM-1 provides an important costimulatory signal for T cell receptor-mediated activation of resting T cells. J Immunol, 1990. 144(12): p. 4579-86.
62. Damle, N.K., et al., Differential costimulatory effects of adhesion molecules B7, ICAM-1, LFA-3, and VCAM-1 on resting and antigen-primed CD4+ T lymphocytes. J Immunol, 1992. 148(7): p. 1985-92.
63. Damle, N.K., et al., Costimulation via vascular cell adhesion molecule-1 induces in T cells increased responsiveness to the CD28 counter-receptor B7. Cell Immunol, 1993. 148(1): p. 144-56.

64. Damle, N.K., et al., Costimulation with integrin ligands intercellular adhesion molecule-1 or vascular cell adhesion molecule-1 augments activation-induced death of antigen-specific CD4+ T lymphocytes. J Immunol, 1993. 151(5): p. 2368-79.
65. Denton, M.D., et al., Endothelial cells modify the costimulatory capacity of transmigrating leukocytes and promote CD28-mediated CD4(+) T cell alloactivation. J Exp Med, 1999. 190(4): p. 555-66.
66. Ferrero, E., et al., CD14+ CD34+ peripheral blood mononuclear cells migrate across endothelium and give rise to immunostimulatory dendritic cells. J Immunol, 1998. 160(6): p. 2675-83.
67. Randolph, G.J., et al., Differentiation of monocytes into dendritic cells in a model of transendothelial trafficking [see comments]. Science, 1998. 282(5388): p. 480-3.
68. Kobayashi, H., et al., Prolongation of rat cardiac allograft survival by a monoclonal antibody: anti-rat intercellular adhesion molecule-1. Cardiovasc Surg, 1993. 1(5): p. 577-82.
69. Yamataka, T., et al., The effect of anti-ICAM-1 monoclonal antibody treatment on the transplantation of the small bowel in rats. J Pediatr Surg, 1993. 28(11): p. 1451-7.
70. Kanagawa, K., et al., Strain combination-dependent genesis of necrotizing arteritis in anti- ICAM-1 antibody-perfused renal allografts in the rat. Pathol Int, 1995. 45(3): p. 196-201.
71. Sadahiro, M., T.O. McDonald, and M.D. Allen, Reduction in cellular and vascular rejection by blocking leukocyte adhesion molecule receptors. Am J Pathol, 1993. 142(3): p. 675-83.
72. Kameoka, H., et al., The immunosuppressive action of anti-CD18 monoclonal antibody in rat heterotopic heart allotransplantation. Transplantation, 1993. 55(3): p. 665-7.
73. Nakakura, E.K., et al., Potent and effective prolongation by anti-LFA-1 monoclonal antibody monotherapy of non-primarily vascularized heart allograft survival in mice without T cell depletion. Transplantation, 1993. 55(2): p. 412-7.
74. Nakakura, E.K., et al., Long-term survival of solid organ allografts by brief anti-lymphocyte function-associated antigen-1 monoclonal antibody monotherapy. Transplantation, 1996. 62(5): p. 547-52.
75. Nishihara, M., et al., Awareness of donor alloantigens in antiadhesion therapy induces antigen- specific unresponsiveness to islet allografts. Transplantation, 1997. 64(7): p. 965-70.
76. Isobe, M., et al., Specific acceptance of cardiac allograft after treatment with antibodies to ICAM-1 and LFA-1. Science, 1992. 255(5048): p. 1125-7.
77. Isobe, M., et al., Assessment of tolerance induction to cardiac allograft by anti-ICAM-1 and anti-LFA-1 monoclonal antibodies. J Heart Lung Transplant, 1997. 16(11): p. 1149-56.
78. Isobe, M., et al., Acceptance of primary skin graft after treatment with anti-intercellular adhesion molecule-1 and anti-leukocyte function- associated antigen-1 monoclonal antibodies in mice. Transplantation, 1996. 62(3): p. 411-3.
79. Brandt, M., et al., Treatment with monoclonal antibodies to ICAM-1 and LFA-1 in rat heart allograft rejection. Transpl Int, 1997. 10(2): p. 141-4.
80. Orosz, C.G., et al., Treatment with anti-vascular cell adhesion molecule 1 monoclonal antibody induces long-term murine cardiac allograft acceptance. Transplantation, 1993. 56(2): p. 453-60.
81. Isobe, M., et al., Immunosuppression to cardiac allografts and soluble antigens by anti- vascular cellular adhesion molecule-1 and anti-very late antigen-4 monoclonal antibodies. J Immunol, 1994. 153(12): p. 5810-8.
82. Paul, L.C., et al., The efficacy of LFA-1 and VLA-4 antibody treatment in rat vascularized cardiac allograft rejection. Transplantation, 1993. 55(5): p. 1196-9.

83. Paul, L.C., et al., Anti-integrin (LFA-1, VLA-4, and Mac-1) antibody treatment and acute cardiac graft rejection in the rat. Transpl Int, 1996. 9(4): p. 420-5.

84. Anderson, D.C., et al., The severe and moderate phenotypes of heritable Mac-1, LFA-1 deficiency: their quantitative definition and relation to leukocyte dysfunction and clinical features. J Infect Dis, 1985. 152(4): p. 668-89.

85. Anderson, D.C. and T.A. Springer, Leukocyte adhesion deficiency: an inherited defect in the Mac-1, LFA-1, and p150,95 glycoproteins. Annu Rev Med, 1987. 38: p. 175-94.

86. Etzioni, A., Adhesion molecule deficiencies and their clinical significance. Cell Adhes Commun, 1994. 2(3): p. 257-60.

87. Price, T.H., et al., *In vivo* neutrophil and lymphocyte function studies in a patient with leukocyte adhesion deficiency type II. Blood, 1994. 84(5): p. 1635-9.

88. Haug, C.E., et al., A phase I trial of immunosuppression with anti-ICAM-1 (CD54) mAb in renal allograft recipients. Transplantation, 1993. 55(4): p. 766-72; discussion 772-3.

89. Salmela, K., et al., A randomized multicenter trial of the anti-ICAM-1 monoclonal antibody (enlimomab) for the prevention of acute rejection and delayed onset of graft function in cadaveric renal transplantation: a report of the European Anti-ICAM-1 Renal Transplant Study Group. Transplantation, 1999. 67(5): p. 729-36.

90. Le Mauff, B., et al., A dose-searching trial of an anti-LFA1 monoclonal antibody in first kidney transplant recipients. Kidney Int Suppl, 1996. 53: p. S44-50.

91. Le Mauff, B., et al., Effect of anti-LFA1 (CD11a) monoclonal antibodies in acute rejection in human kidney transplantation. Transplantation, 1991. 52(2): p.291-6.

92. Hourmant, M., et al., A randomized multicenter trial comparing leukocyte function-associated antigen-1 monoclonal antibody with rabbit antithymocyte globulin as induction treatment in first kidney transplantations. Transplantation, 1996. 62(11): p. 1565-70.

COSTIMULATION BLOCKADE

Roy D. Bloom and Laurence A. Turka

New Paradigms in Immunosuppression

Five decades of clinical transplantation have seen a dramatic improvement in many aspects of patient outcome, largely attributable to better
quality immunosuppressive agents and their more judicious use. The
success of contemporary immunosuppression is underscored by a
reduction in the incidence of acute rejection rates between 1988 and
1998 from 60 to 20 percent and an improvement in one-year renal
allograft survival rates to around 90 percent over the past 2 decades
[1,2]. Over the same period, despite substantial evidence implicating
acute rejection as a major risk factor for chronic allograft nephropathy,
the early benefits of our current immunosuppressive agents have not
been maintained in the long-term. Historically, the immunosuppressive
arsenal has encompassed predominantly steroid-based therapy initially
and subsequently, the introduction of antimetabolites, calcineurin phosphatase inhibition, as well as antilymphocyte antibodies. Most of these
agents are broadly acting and non-specific in their immunosuppressive
effect. Consequently, these drugs have been associated with the spectrum of risks of global over-immunosuppression, including the development of life-threatening infectious complications and the increased risk
of certain malignancies. Besides risk related to excessive immunosuppression, these medications have all been implicated in the plethora of
serious non-immune related adverse effects, including perturbations in
metabolic pathways (diabetes mellitus, osteopenia, hyperlipidemia),
renal function (renal failure, hypertension), as well as several

*Mohamed Sayegh and Giuseppe Remuzzi (editors), Current and Future
Immunosuppressive Therapies Following Transplantation, 265-277.*
© *2001 Kluwer Academic Publishers. Printed in the Netherlands.*

cosmetically disfiguring manifestations (weight gain, skin friability and bruising, hirsutism and alopecia).

The introduction of costimulation blockade obviously represents a novel and dramatic paradigm shift in the application of immunosuppression in the clinical arena. Antigen-specific immunosuppression offers the potential to avert complications related to global over-immunosuppression, in addition to being associated with a marked reduction in the protean non-specific side effects of our contemporary agents. The exciting results observed thus far with costimulatory blockade in rodent models bode well for success in primates, both non-human and human. To date a handful of studies (see **Table 1**) have been performed in this population with molecules that inhibit T cell costimulation, and the early indications continue to be encouraging for their future use. This article will outline the immunobiology of T cell activation with a focus on the role of costimulatory signals in this process, review the small animal and primate experience to date using agents which block costimulatory signals, and discuss what we believe is the promise and the potential problems of applying this approach to clinical transplantation medicine.

Table 1. Summary of clinical studies with costimulation blockade in Primates.

Study	Species	# subjects	Costimulation Blockade*	Disease State	Outcome
Kirk et al	Monkey	9	Anti-CD154 (6 mos)	KTX	All experienced LT rejection-free survival
Kenyon et al	Baboon	3	Anti-CD154 (10 d)	Islet Txp	Delayed, though did not prevent, AR in al
Kenyon et al	Monkey	6	Anti-CD154 (6 mos)	Islet Txp	All engrafted; 50% LT, rejection-free survival
Levisetti et al	Monkey	5	CTLA-4Ig (2 wks)	Islet Txp	No LT engraftment
Guinan et al	Human	12	CTLA-4Ig (ex vivo)ª	BMT	All engrafted; decreased GVHD, 45% LT survival
Abrams et al	Human	43	CTLA-4Ig (5 wks)	Psoriasis	46% patients > 50% disease activity reduction

KTX=kidney transplant; txp=transplantation, BMT=bone marrow transplantation; AR=acute rejection; LT=long term; GVHD=Graft-versus-host-disease. * time period in parentheses refers to total duration of treatment with costimulation blockade. ªex vivo incubation of donor cells with CTLA-4Ig.

Role of Costimulatory Signals in T cell Activation

T cells require two signals for optimal antigen-specific activation. The first signal is antigen itself, and this signal is delivered when the T cell receptor (TCR) is engaged by a peptide fragment located in the antigen-binding groove of a major histocompatibility complex (MHC)-encoded molecule [3]. TCR ligation transduces a signal to the T cell interior through a series of associated proteins such as the CD3 molecules, ZAP-70, and lck [4]. They in turn activate several signal transduction pathways including phospholipase C, and the ras and MAP kinase pathways. Collectively, these events are sufficient to induce a resting T cell to enter G1 phase of the cell cycle, and to express early activation genes such as CD69 and CD25 (the IL-2R alpha chain). However, these signals by themselves are unable to support full and sustained T cell responses. Unless antigen-density is high, thereby binding a large number of TCRs, cytokine gene induction is only minimal, and may be insufficient to support T cell proliferation [5,6]. Even at an antigen-density sufficient to induce cytokine gene expression and T cell proliferation, the T cell response is transient as the expanded population of T cells becomes anergic and/or undergoes apoptosis [7]. Full and complete T cell responses require both TCR engagement, as well as the delivery of costimulatory signals.

The best-characterized costimulatory pathway is mediated by the CD28 receptor on the surface of T cells [8,9,10]. CD28, a member of the immunoglobulin supergene family, is expressed on all rodent T cells, and 80% of human T cells (virtually all CD4+ T cells and half of CD8+ T cells). It has two ligands, CD80 (B7-1) and CD86 (B7-2), both of which are primarily expressed on activated antigen presenting cells (APCs), but which have been variably reported on other cell types including endothelial cells, renal tubular cells, thymic epithelial cells and myocytes. CD86 is expressed earlier during APC activation than CD80, however they appear to deliver similar signals to the T cell. Upon activation, T cells express another relevant molecule on their surface, CTLA-4 (CD152) [9,11,12]. CTLA-4 exhibits a high degree of sequence and structural homology to CD28, and indeed shares the same ligands, binding CD80 and CD86 with an even higher affinity than does CD28. CTLA-4 is preformed in resting T cells, but is restricted to a largely cytoplasmic location. Following T cell activation is it translocated to the cell surface. Unlike the activating properties of CD28, CTLA-4 transduces a negative signal to the cell interior [13]. This signal turns off IL-2 and IL-2R gene expression, and is dominant over both TCR and CD28 signals [14]. This leads to a model in which T cells initially become activated by TCR ligation and CD28 costimulation, but in which T cell responses subsequently are terminated through CTLA-4.

The production of mice with targeted deletions of each of these genes helps reveal their relative roles. Both CD80 and CD86 single knockout mice have generally intact immune responses, reflecting no double the relative redundancy of these two pathways [15-17]. However, CD80/CD86 double knockout mice are profoundly immune deficient, with respect to T cell dependent responses, including allograft rejection, confirming the requirement of this pathway for intact cellular immunity [18]. Mice with targeted deletions of CD28 and CTLA-4 have been produced as well [19]. Curiously, the CD28 knockout mouse is not as globally immunodeficient and CD80/CD86 double knockout mice. For example, these mice are able to reject allografts and fight viral infections [18,20]. This surprising finding has several possible explanations. First, it raises the question as to whether the CTLA-4 molecule might, under certain circumstances, be able to transduce an activating signal to T cells, an hypothesis which is supported by a small number of studies [21]. A second possibility is that there are CD80/CD86 ligands other than CD28 or CTLA-4, and that these provide stimulatory signals. However, the failure of many efforts to identify other ligands in this system argues strongly against this hypothesis. Finally, some investigators suggest that T cells from CD28 knockout mice might be immunologically "abnormal" as a result of maturation without receipt of CD28 signals. These cells may not be dependent on CD28 costimulation, perhaps making use of other costimulatory pathways which, in normal mice, cannot substitute for CD28.

Indeed, it appears that a number of other costimulatory pathways exist for T cells, although their relative roles in normal T cell responses are not completely defined. The most prominent such pathway is mediated by interaction of CD154 on T cells, with its ligand CD40, expressed on antigen-presenting cells, and selected other cell types such as endothelial cells and keratinocytes. CD154 is a member of the tumor-necrosis factor (TNF) family, and CD40 belongs to the TNF-receptor family [22]. Interaction of these two molecules leads to a number of critical events during an immune response. CD40 stimulation induces CD80 and CD86 expression on APCs, is required for immunoglobulin isotype switching in B cells, promotes B cell proliferation and survival, induces adhesion molecule expression on macrophages, dendritic cells, and endothelial cells, and induces macrophage IL-12 production. All of these events promote and augment the development of inflammatory responses. Thus, while upregulation of CD28 ligands (i.e., CD80 and CD86) on APCs is certainly an important component of the role of the CD154:CD40 pathway in T cell mediated responses, it is by no means the only component. Consistent with this, simultaneous blockade of both the CD28 and the CD154 pathways has additive effects in a variety of circumstances, including a number of models of transplantation tolerance (see below) [23]. Finally, it should be noted that the effects of CD154 engagement on the T cell itself are not well understood. All the events described above occurring conesquent to CD154:CD40 binding focus on the effects of this pathway on the APC (or other CD40-expressing cell). At the present time, it is not known what if any signals are transduced by CD154 to the T cell.

In addition to the CD28:B7 and CD154:CD40 systems, a number of other pathways have been shown to transduce activating signals to T cells. These include receptor:ligand pairs which, like CD154:CD40 are members of the TNF:TNFR family, such as FasL:Fas, 4-1BB:4-1BBL; and CD30:CD30L, as well as other systems such as HSA:CD44H [24,25]. As presently understood, these interactions are not as important as the CD28 or CD154 pathways for T cell responses, particularly in previously unprimed animals. However, important roles for each of these other pathways have been suggested in either of two circumstances: augmenting the expansion and function of memory T cells, and supporting T cell responses in the absence of CD28 costimulation. Given the somewhat artificial nature of these experiments, particularly using CD28-deficient mice, the physiological role of these other pathways during *in vivo* immune responses remains to be clarified.

Costimulation Blockade in Small Animals

The first studies of costimulation blockade to inhibit *in vivo* immune responses in the transplant setting were performed in rodent models [26,27]. These studies tested the effects of blocking the CD28:B7 pathway, and used either monoclonal antibodies to the B7 molecules, or CTLA4Ig, a fusion protein consisting of the binding region of human CTLA-4 linked to a human IgG1 constant region tail [28]. CTLA4Ig binds both B7 molecules with a higher affinity than does CD28, serving as a soluble competitive inhibitor of CD28 costimulation. Furthermore, by virtue of its immunoglobulin tail, CTLA4Ig, like monoclonal antibodies, has a long circulating half-life, making it suitable for *in vivo* studies. These initial studies demonstrated that blocking CD28 costimulation prevented the rejection of human islet xenografts in mice, and fully MHC-mismatched vascularized cardiac allografts in rats [26,27]. Subsequent studies have extended these findings, utilizing either CTLA4Ig, anti-CD80 and/or CD86 monoclonal antibodies, or anti-CD154 monoclonal antibody in models of heart, islet, liver, kidney, lung, skin, and intestinal transplantation [29]. Collectively, a number of general conclusions can be drawn from this work. First, costimulatory blockade prevents rejection in virtually all models of organ and tissue transplantation in rodents. However, use of a single agent alone rarely induces transplantation tolerance (defined as indefinite graft survival without evidence of chronic rejection, and spontaneous acceptance of addition transplants from the same donor type). The most effective strategies to induce tolerance with costimulatory blockade have been either to combine CD28 and CD154 blockade (using CTLA4Ig plus anti-CD154 monoclonal antibody), or to use a single agent and concomitantly administer donor cells (in the form of splenocytes or bone marrow) at the time of transplantation [30,31]. Either of these approaches is able to induce long-term graft survival/tolerance in most situations, the most notable exception being skin transplantation in which ultimate graft loss cannot be forestalled.

An interesting approach to transplantation tolerance using costimulatory blockade has been to use these agents to facilitate the creation of hematopoietic chimerism, by permitting the engraftment of donor marrow without the need for myeloablative preconditioning [32]. This type of approach may be extremely useful in clinical practice, as the use of donor bone-marrow is amongst the most effective strategies to induce tolerance in primates, however the toxicity of the cytoreductive preconditioning regimens has precluded their introduction into widespread clinical trials.

Costimulation Blockade in Primates – The Initial Experience

The first published clinically relevant study of costimulation blockade in non-human primates involved renal transplantation between HLA disparate Rhesus monkeys [33]. In this pilot observation where monkeys treated with no immunosuppression experienced rapid rejection, renal allografts were transplanted into nephrectomized animals under cover of varying combinations and dosages of CTLA4Ig and anti-CD154, with no additional contemporary immunosuppression. Initially, animals received either CTLA4Ig or anti-CD154 alone administered in an induction style approach, at the time of surgery and then, intermittently for varying time intervals thereafter, ranging from 5-14 days. Each treatment strategy prolonged graft survival although the limited monotherapy approach ultimately resulted in allografts rejection in all cases. However, anti-CD154 monotherapy, which resulted in rejection-free survival of 95-100 days, appeared to be more effective than CTLA4Ig. Moreover, treatment of the acute rejection episodes in the former group with a further 14 day course of anti-CD154 effected normalization of graft function and long term survival.

These investigators next examined the effect of simultaneous administration of anti-CD154 and CTLA4Ig in a similar induction approach to that described above [33]. The two animals rejected at day 35 and 100 respectively, although once again, a repeat course of combined antibody therapy effectively restored serum creatinine to its baseline. A second pair of animals received an extended regimen of combination antibody therapy, with further administration of each reagent at later time points within the first post-transplant month. Both animals experienced extended rejection-free survival though, intriguingly, maintained *in vitro* responsiveness throughout the study period to both donor as well as third party. Whether this observation reflects differences in activation between donor parenchymal cell *in vivo* and donor lymphoid cells *in vitro* remains unknown. The renal allograft histology from all the long-term survivors demonstrated preserved renal architecture, although grafts had isolated nests of lymphocytes in the interstitium. Significantly, there were no changes of chronic allograft nephropathy. The exciting potential of this pilot study obviously had to be tempered by the very small sample sizes, markedly limiting meaningful data interpretation. On the other hand however, costimulation-blockade appeared to be safe, with minimal toxicity, little effect on either T or B cell subsets and effective in both preventing and treating acute rejection.

Blockade of the CD40-CD154 Pathway

Armed with this preliminary information, this same group of investigators has subsequently broadened their observation in a larger scale study using the same transplant system described above [34]. In this second study treated animals were given an 'extended' course of anti-CD154 monotherapy, administered both immediately before and after transplantation, on four occasions during the first post-transplant month, then monthly for 5 months. All nine monkeys treated with this regimen remained rejection-free. Aside from an anesthetic death in one animal, all experienced prolonged survival, stable and normal renal function and were unhindered by infection, malignancy or wound-healing related problems. Of the surviving monkeys, five that had completed their treatment protocol had been off anti-CD154 for as long as one year without any problems or the need for additional immuno-suppression. Unlike a briefer course of combination anti-CD154 and CTLA4Ig given in the previous study, more prolonged administration of anti-CD154 alone resulted in a diminution in donor-specific MLRs *in vitro*. However, all animals developed donor-specific antibodies in relatively low titers although there was no IgG deposition detectable within the renal allograft on serial protocol biopsies. In fact, the only histological changes were seen on light microscopy, characterized by focal mononuclear cell infiltration in all cases, with diminution over time. The infiltrate comprised MHC class II expressing CD4+ or CD8+ T cells as well as B cells. This leukocyte activity did not appear to cause significant tissue injury, with preservation of normal architecture and the absence of chronic allograft nephropathy on the sequential biopsies.

In contrast to the anti-CD154 monotherapy treated animals, 3 additional groups received conventional immunosuppression (short course MMF-steroids, chronic MMF-steroids or tacrolimus) in conjunction with costimulation-blockade. The monkeys in the combination therapy groups generally had inferior outcomes, with complications typical of those observed in our current clinical settings. The most notable adverse effect was acute rejection, while life-threatening infections, as well as tacrolimus-related nephrotoxicity occurred as well. Overall, this set of studies corroborated the earlier findings suggesting that administration of anti-CD154 alone appeared to be safe, with a conspicuous absence of commonly observed clinical complications. Long-term treatment did not appear to be necessary as rejection did not occur even several months following withdrawal of the drug and its clearance from the circulation. However, small study group sizes precluded definitive conclusions regarding use of anti-CD154 with conventional therapy.

More recently, 2 further pilot studies have examined the effect of anti-CD154 on intrahepatic islet allograft transplantation in a baboon and rhesus monkey model respectively [35,36]. In the former study, anti-CD154 was given as an induction regimen for the first 10 post-transplant days [35]. All animals transplanted with this regimen experienced engraftment and insulin independence. However, all ultimately experienced delayed acute rejection (compared to either the untreated or tacrolimus treated controls) although as described above, a further short course of anti-CD154 effectively reversed the rejection in 85% of the animals. The baboons continued to have recurrent intermittent episodes of anti-CD154-responsive acute rejection, which was generally accompanied by a reduction in functional islet mass and ultimately, the need for reinstitution of long term insulin for maintenance of chronic euglycemia. Hepatic tissue obtained early in the post-transplant course demonstrated viable engrafted islets variably surrounded by non-infiltrating CD4+ and CD8+ T cells. It is worth noting that the last two islet allograft recipients received donor bone marrow and were given an extended monthly maintenance antibody dose for the first 6 post-transplant month. In contrast to the data in murine models, infusion of donor-derived bone marrow did not prolong or promote graft acceptance. Moreover, all animals experienced a marked reduction in circulating CD4+ lymphocytes.

The second set of intrahepatic islet experiments, in rhesus monkeys, was conducted by the same investigators [36]. In this study, however, all animals received the extended induction course of anti-CD154. Unlike with the baboon study, all monkeys experienced prolonged rejection-free engraftment and insulin independence. Three of the animals remained insulin independent and rejection-free despite discontinuation of anti-CD154 at the end of the first post-transplant year. A feature common to both of these non-human primate islet studies is the lack of any systemic or infectious complications. Anti-CD154 was not associated with any islet toxicity or diabetogenicity and no antibodies against this costimulation blocker were detected. Over time, periodic MLC screening in all animals revealed decreasing reactivity to donor cells. Third party reactivity was maintained in the rhesus monkeys, suggesting some degree of donor specificity in the maintenance of the islet grafts in these animals.

Blockade of the CD28-B7 Pathway

In addition to successful interruption of the above CD40/CD154 costimulatory pathway, there are a few primate studies that have examined blockade of the CD28-B7 interaction. Levisetti and colleagues used CTLA4Ig in a cynomologous monkey islet allograft model, with administration of this antibody at the time of transplantation and then for 2 additional weeks [37]. Islet allograft survival was prolonged in only 40% of recipients, with no evidence of long term engraftment at all. Very recently, two clinical studies utilizing CTLA4Ig have been published [38,39]. One of these studies was performed in a histoincompatible allogeneic bone marrow transplantation setting in 12 recipients, all of whom were high risk candidates for graft-versus-host disease (GVHD) [38]. Prior to transplantation, harvested donor bone marrow was incubated *ex vivo* with irradiated recipient cells in the presence of CTLA4Ig. Tolerance specific to recipient alloantigens was induced in donor marrow, as defined by a reduction of the frequency of donor T cells recognizing recipient alloantigens, while *in vitro* responsiveness to third-party alloantigens was unaffected. From a clinical outcomes standpoint in this non-randomized, uncontrolled study, both the incidence and severity of GVHD was remarkably diminished compared to the expected frequency. Infection developed in only 3 of 11 patients, all of whom successfully recovered following treatment. Engraftment occurred in all patients although overall long term patient survival was 45% with complete remission in all these survivors.

The second study, a phase I clinical trial in patients with psoriasis vulgaris, was unique in that it was the first report describing the effects of blocking T cell costimulation in human subjects [39]. In this dose-escalating study, forty six percent of patients overall achieved a more than 50% reduction in disease activity clinically, although at the 2 highest dosages, a benefit was seen in over 80% of patients. CTLA4Ig was well tolerated, with no evidence of malignancy, infection or the development of anti-CTLA4Ig antibodies. CTLA4Ig appeared to be ineffective in suppressing fully primed T cell-dependent humoral immune responses. Once again, a potentially long term benefit from this therapy was seen even after CTLA4Ig serum levels were undetectable, suggestive of the induction of chronic hyporesponsiveness.

Costimulation Blockade in Perspective at the Turn of the Century

The early primate data with costimulation blockade holds tremendous promise for both clinical transplantation, as well as the diverse spectrum of immunologically mediated diseases. The benefits thus far demonstrated appear to be substantial, while relatively few risks have been uncovered at this early juncture. With relevance to clinical transplantation, the published studies to date all demonstrate a high level of safety with at least equivalent, if not superior, outcomes compared to the currently accepted treatment standards for each clinical situation. The primate transplant studies indicate that anti-CD154 is effective both for the prevention of, as well as the reversal of, biopsy-proven acute rejection. The immunomodulatory effect appeared to be antigen-specific and in the majority of the studies long-term sequential biopsies revealed no evidence of chronic allograft injury. Notably, since the enhanced clinical outcomes occurred in a conventional immunosuppression-free milieu, avoidance of commonly observed clinical side effects would represent a potentially significant advancement in patient care.

On the other hand, it is important to put these new biologic agents into an appropriate perspective. The above observations represent the earliest and most preliminary experience with primates and certainly do not constitute definitive studies. In addition, numerous barriers and hurdles have to be cleared prior to the more widespread application of these humanized antibodies in clinical transplantation. While anti-CD154 has been associated with successful outcomes thus far, there remain several issues of concern regarding its mechanism of action. These include the presence in the recipient circulation of apparently inert donor-specific antibodies whose functional significance is not apparent. Second, co-administration of traditional, non-specific immunosuppressive agents commonly used in current clinical practice appeared to compromise the beneficial effect of anti-CD154 although, once again, the underlying mechanism remains uncertain. At a fundamental level, whether costimulation blockade truly induces tolerance and can avoid the use of chronic conventional immunotherapy is unknown. Certainly, antigen-specific tolerance, a major goal of costimulation blockade, has not been unequivocally established in the primate studies conducted thus far. Moreover, even if it were achieved, tolerance to antigens present at time of transplantation could have catastrophic consequences in the event that there happened to be undesirable viral (e.g. CMV) or tumor antigens in the circulation at that time. Such potential complications highlight the importance of a clear comprehension of mechanisms underlying the effectiveness of costimulation blockade prior to its introduction into the wider community at large.

Additional basic questions that require addressing pertain to optimal dosing strategies. In particular, the need for combined versus monotherapy with CTLA4Ig and/or anti-CD154, the timing and duration of administration, as well as the requirement for adjunctive immunosuppression. On one hand, while an induction therapy approach carries the disadvantage of serial intravenous injections over several months' duration (at least), a potential benefit of such a protocol is that patient compliance can be easily tracked. Even then, once these above obstacles have been satisfactorily resolved, selection of patients for trials of costimulation blockade will become an issue.   Will this therapy be appropriate for low risk, primary renal allograft recipients in whom the likelihood of excellent long term graft survival is already excellent? Will it be worth attempting this strategy in high risk, poorly matched, highly sensitized individuals undergoing re-transplantation? Finally, in concert with a continually declining incidence of acute rejection, one-year renal allograft survival rates are now above 90% in many centers in the United States and long term outcomes are likewise improving.   Effectively, the bar has been raised against which future immunomodulatory agents will be compared.   Therefore, demonstrating a significant outcomes benefit of costimulation blockade will provide a challenge going forward, unless i) good markers of chronic allograft loss can be identified and tracked as surrogates and/or ii) avoidance of our conventional agents and their adverse effects can be cleanly and unequivocally demonstrated.

References

1. Cecka, J.M., The UNOS Scientific Renal Transplant Registry. Clinical Transplantation, 1997: p. 1-14.
2. United States Renal Data System, 1998 USRDS Annual Data Report, . 1998, National Institutes of Health, National Institute of Diabetes and Digestive and Kidney Diseases: Bethesda, MD.
3. Janeway, C.H. and K. Bottomly, Signals and Signs for Lymphocyte Responses. Cell, 1994. 76: p. 275-285.
4. van Leeuwen, J.E. and L.E. Samelson, T cell antigen-receptor signal transduction. Curr Opin Immunol, 1999. 11(3): p. 242-8.
5. DeSilva, D.R., K.B. Urdahl, and M.K. Jenkins, Clonal anergy is induced *in vitro* by T cell receptor occupancy in the absence of proliferation. J. Immunol., 1991. 147: p. 3261-7.
6. Jenkins, M.K., et al., T cell unresponsiveness *in vivo* and *in vitro*: fine specificity of induction and molecular characterization of the unresponsive state. Immunol. Rev., 1987. 95: p. 113.
7. Noel, P.J., et al., CD28 costimulation prevents cell death during primary T cell activation. Journal of Immunology, 1996. 157: p. 636-642.
8. Bluestone, J.A., New perspectives of CD28-B7-mediated T cell costimultion. Immunity, 1995. 2(6): p. 555-559.
9. June, C.H., et al., The B7 and CD28 receptor families. Immunology Today, 1994. 15(7): p. 321-31.
10. Viola, A. and A. Lanzavecchia, T cell activation determined by T cell receptor number and tunable thresholds. Science, 1996. 273: p. 104-106.
11. Lee, K.M., et al., Molecular basis of T cell inactivation by CTLA-4. Science, 1998. 282(5397): p. 2263-6.
12. Bluestone, J.A., Is CTLA-4 a master switch for peripheral T cell tolerance?. J. Immunol., 1997. 158(5): p. 1989-93.
13. Krummel, M.F. and J.P. Allison, CTLA-4 Engagement Inhibits IL-2 Accumulation and Cell Cycle Progression upon Activation of Resting T Cells. J. Exp. Med., 1996. 183: p. 2533-2540.
14. Lin, H., et al., Cytotoxic T lymphocyte antigen 4 (CTLA4) blockade accelerates the acute rejection of cardiac allografts in CD28-deficient mice: CTLA4 can function independently of CD28. J Exp Med, 1998. 188: p. 199-204.
15. Freeman, G.J., et al., Uncovering of functional alternative CTLA-4 counter-receptor in B7-deficient mice. Science, 1993. 262: p. 907-909.
16. Sharpe, A.H., Analysis of lymphocyte costimulation *in vivo* using transgenic and 'knockout' mice. Curr Opin Immunol, 1995. 7(3): p. 389-95.
17. Schweitzer, A.N., et al., Role of costimulators in T cell differentiation: studies using antigen- presenting cells lacking expression of CD80 or CD86. J Immunol, 1997. 158(6): p. 2713-22.
18. Mandelbrot, D.A., et al., Expression of B7 molecules in recipient, not donor, mice determines the survival of cardiac allografts [In Process Citation]. J Immunol, 1999. 163(7): p. 3753-7.
19. Shahinian, A., et al., Differential T cell costimulatory requirements in CD28-deficient mice. Science, 1993. 261: p. 609-612.
20. Kawai, K., et al., Skin allograft rejection in CD28-deficient mice. Transplantation, 1996. 61: p. 352-355.
21. Wu, Y., et al., CTLA-4-B7 interaction is sufficient to costimulate T cell clonal expansion. J Exp Med, 1997. 185: p. 1327-35.
22. Durie, F.H., et al., The role of CD40 in the regulation of humoral and cell-mediated immunity. Immunology Today, 1994. 15(9): p. 406-411.

23. Sayegh, M.H. and L.A. Turka, The role of T cell co-stimulatory activation pathways in transplant rejection. N Engl J Med, 1998. 338: p. 1813-1821.
24. Watts, T.H. and M.A. DeBenedette, T cell co-stimulatory molecules other than CD28. Curr Opin Immunol, 1999. 11(3): p. 286-93.
25. Liu, Y., et al., Distinct costimulatory molecules are required for the induction of effector and memory cytotoxic T lymphocytes. J Exp Med, 1997. 185: p. 251-262.
26. Lenschow, D., et al., Long-Term Survival of Xenogeniec Pancreatic Islet Grafts Induced by CTLA4Ig. Science, 1992. 257: p. 789-792.
27. Turka, L.A., et al., T cell activation by the CD28 ligand B7 is required for cardiac allograft rejection *in vivo*. Proc Natl Acad Sci USA, 1992. 89: p. 11102-11105.
28. Linsley, P.S., et al., CTLA-4 is a second receptor for the B cell activation antigen B7. J Exp Med, 1991. 174: p. 561-569.
29. Sayegh, M.H. and L.A. Turka, T cell costimulatory pathways: Promising novel targets for immunosuppression and tolerance induction. J Am Soc Nephrol, 1995. 6: p. 1143-1150.
30. Sayegh, M., et al., Donor antigen is necessary for the prevention of chronic rejection in CTLA4Ig-treated murine cardiac allografts. Transplantation, 1998. 64: p. 1646-1650.
31. Larsen, C.P., et al., Long-term acceptance of skin and cardiac allografts after blocking CD40 and CD28 pathways. Nature, 1996. 381: p. 434-438.
32. Wekerle, T., et al., Extrathymic T cell deletion and allogeneic stem cell engraftment induced with costimulatory blockade is followed by central T cell tolerance. J Exp Med, 1998. 187(12): p. 2037-44.
33. Kirk, A., et al., CTLA4-Ig and anti-CD40 ligand prevent renal allograft rejection in primates. Proc. Natl. Acad. Sci. (USA), 1997. 94: p. 8789-8794.
34. Kirk, A.D., et al., Treatment with humanized monoclonal antibody against CD154 prevents acute renal allograft rejection in nonhuman primates [In Process Citation]. Nat Med, 1999. 5(6): p. 686-93.
35. Kenyon, N.S., et al., Long-term survival and function of intrahepatic islet allografts in baboons treated with humanized anti-CD154. Diabetes, 1999. 48(7): p. 1473-81.
36. Kenyon, N.S., et al., Long-term survival and function of intrahepatic islet allografts in rhesus monkeys treated with humanized anti-CD154. Proc Natl Acad Sci U S A, 1999. 96(14): p. 8132-7.
37. Levisetti, M., et al., Immunosuppressive effects of hCTLA4Ig in a non-human primate model of allogeneic pancreatic islet transplantation. J Immunol, 1997. 159: p. 5187-5191.
38. Guinan, E.C., et al., Transplantation of anergic histoincompatible bone marrow allografts. New England Journal of Medicine, 1999. 340(22): p. 1704-1714.
39. Abrams, J.R., et al., CTLA4Ig-mediated blockade of T cell costimulation in patients with psoriasis vulgaris. The Journal of Clinical Investigation, 1999. 103(9): p. 1243-1252.

IMMUNOMODULATORY FUNCTION OF MHC PEPTIDES

Barbara Murphy and Alan Krensky

Abstract

Our continuing dependence on long-term broad spectrum immunosuppression, coupled with a growing understanding of the mechanisms mediating the alloimmune response, has led to an increasing focus on the development of alternative, more specific forms of immunotherapy in the hope of inducing transplant tolerance. In recent years it has become apparent that the peptide bound by the MHC molecule plays a major influential role in the initial T cell receptor interaction with the MHC/peptide complex, and also in the subsequent T cell response. There is now extensive experimental evidence in vitro and in vivo, that varying the nature of the bound peptide provides an effective means of manipulating the immune response. It would appear, however, that the role of peptides as immunosuppressants is not limited to the disruption of antigen recognition alone, but rather they may exert their effects through many diverse mechanisms including inhibition of cell cycle progresssion, altered signal transduction and the induction of apoptosis. The potential, therefore, exists that peptides, or compounds derived from them, may represent an exciting new form of immunotherapy.

Introduction

The development of newer forms of immunosuppression in the last decade has resulted in substantial improvements in graft and patient survival, and made transplantation more accessible to patients

Mohamed Sayegh and Giuseppe Remuzzi (editors), Current and Future
Immunosuppressive Therapies Following Transplantation, 279-292.
© 2001 Kluwer Academic Publishers. Printed in the Netherlands.

previously considered unsuitable. With this success has come the all too great awareness of the debilitating, and often life threatening, side effects arising from the administration of broad spectrum immunosuppression. We are now faced with the challenge of using the information which we have gained in our understanding of the processes leading to allograft rejection, so that we may develop more specific forms of immunosuppression and ultimately attain the goal transplant tolerance. Through the use of X-ray cyrstallography the structure of both class I and II Major Histocompatibility Complex (MHC) molecules, and the manner in which they interact with the T-cell receptor (TCR) have been elucidated [1-4]. Peptides bind in a groove in the MHC molecule created by a pair of alpha helices located above a β pleated sheet. This binding groove contains pockets which confer constraints on the peptides which may bind to a particular MHC allele [5]. Peptides in turn influence the interaction of the TCR with the MHC / peptide complex through residues which orient themselves outward from the binding groove, known as TCR contact residues. In addition, it has been demonstrated that very subtle structural changes in the peptide side chains may influence the surface conformation of the MHC molecule [6]. The response of the T cell following recognition of MHC/peptide complex varies depending on

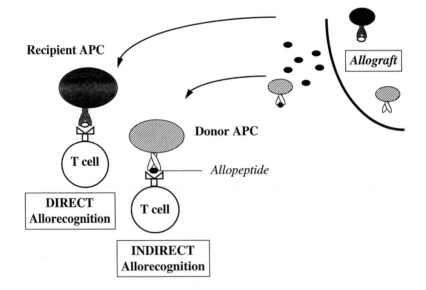

Figure 1. Direct and Indirect Allorecognition. The direct pathway involves recognition of the intact foreign MHC molecule by the recipient T cell with any variety of natural peptides in the antigen presenting groove of the MHC molecule. In contrast, in indirect recognition foreign MHC sequences are presented as peptides in the context of self MHC

nature and concentration of the presented peptide [7,8]. This knowledge has highlighted the possibility of manipulating the immune response through the use of peptides. Simultaneous to these developments the processes by which we recognise foreign MHC have been determined. Allorecognition provides an exception to the rule of "self restricted" T cell recognition, since in the "direct" pathway of allorecognition recipient T cells recognise intact donor MHC with its associated peptide on the surface of donor antigen presenting cells. The second pathway, the "indirect pathway", is in keeping with the traditional mechanism whereby we recognise nominal antigen. In this pathway donor antigen is shed from the graft, taken up, processed and presented in the context of recipient MHC (**Figure 1**) [9,10]. In both pathways of allorecognition the peptide plays an integral role in the response of recipient T cells. Much experimental evidence has been accumulated demonstrating that both the allo- and autoimmune responses may be inhibited in vivo and in vitro though the administration of MHC derived peptide. Despite the initial premise that peptides would exert their effect through binding to the MHC molecule disrupting subsequent T cell recognition, it has now become apparent that their effects are more far reaching, including: inhibition of antigen processing, disruption of cell surface molecular interactions, altered T cell signalling, prevention of cell cycle progression and induction of apoptosis. Immunomodulatory MHC derived peptides can be divided into two broad groups (1) polymorphic peptides which exert their effect through binding to the MHC molecule, and (2) non-polymorphic peptides with diverse mechanisms of action (**Figure 2**). The use of these two groups of peptides as immunosuppressants will be reviewed in this chapter.

Polymorphic MHC Class I Derived Peptides.

Induction of antigen specific unresponsiveness by intrathymic injection was first reported by Posselt et al [11]. They and other groups have now shown that intrathymic injection of various donor cell preparations can induce systemic and antigen-specific unresponsiveness to cardiac [12, 13], liver (14), renal [15, 16] and skin [17] allografts. Although it is clear that intrathymic injection of live donor cells is not necessary since intrathymic injection of synthetic MHC class I or II peptides is now an effective source of donor antigen. Shirwan et al reported long-term cardiac allograft survival after intrathymic injection of a mixture of three MHC class I allopeptides, which had been previously shown to be immunodominant in the same rodent transplant model [18]. Analysis of intragraft cytokine expression was characterised by the predominance of Th2 type cytokines in long-term surviving allografts, while control animals expressed Th1 cytokines, thus implying the effect of intrathymic class I MHC peptides is mediated through immune deviation

[19]. Chowdhury et al. demonstrated that intrathymic administration of three non-immunogenic WAG peptides in a WF to ACI cardiac transplant model resulted in a modest prolongation of graft survival, with long-term graft survival following co-administration of a single dose of ALS [20]. More recently they have used three immunogenic peptides, also derived from the WAG rat, to induce permanent cardiac allograft survival and WF-specific tolerance following intrathymic injection. Furthermore, a single immunogenic peptide was capable of producing similar results. Thus, both immunogenic and non-immunogenic components of the hypervariable WAG RT1-A molecule can induce transplant tolerance when administered intrathymically. Ohajekwe et al. demonstrated that thymic tolerance could still be achieved with administration of alloantigens post-transplant when given in combination with low doses of anti-lymphocyte serum (ALS) [21]. This observation is particularly important since it makes application of this treatment more clinically feasible.

Zavazava and colleagues provide data which highlights the differential effects of peptides derived from different regions of the MHC class I (RT1.A^a) molecule [22, 23]. Subcutaneous immunisation of a peptide derived from a conserved region of the α1-domain of the α-helical region (residues 56-80) induced a concentration-dependent downregulation of proliferation in an MLR. Immunisation with a second peptide, however, which corresponded to residues 96-120 from the beta pleated sheet of the α 2-domain resulted in strong sensitisation. Administration of these two peptides together with a single dose of ALS resulted in permanent graft survival when a combination of these peptides in a DA to LEW rat cardiac transplant model. What is interesting is the route of administration that was effective. Peptide 1 which was immunosuppressant following immunisation, and is derived from a relatively conserved region similar to the ALLOTRAP^{TM} peptides, was injected intrathymically, while the second peptide, which was immunogenic, was injected intraperitoneally. Reversal of the routes did not alter graft survival [24]. This is contrary to other class I MHC peptide data.

Ghobrial et al. have developed a novel method of inducing tolerance to allografts using transfecting hepatoma cells which produce soluble "allochimeric" MHC proteins. These allochimeric proteins incorporate a polymorphic region of donor class I MHC into a backbone of the recipient class I MHC. Subcutaneous administration caused significant prolongation of allograft survival, however, a more striking effect was seen following a single intraportal injection in conjunction with subtherapeutic cyclosporine [25]. Subsequently, a baculovirus expression system was used to produce chimeric proteins with varying degrees of amino acid substitutions [26]. A single intraportal injection of one peptide at the time of transplantation in conjunction with low dose cyclosporine produced long term survival in four of six animals. Thus, peptides derived from MHC class I sequences incorporating specific donor amino acid substitutions can be processed and presented by recipient antigen presenting cells (APC's). These "neoantigens" can induce long term engraftment.

MacDonald et al recently described another method of manipulating indirect allorecognition by administering peptides derived from mismatched donor class I MHC antigen in the form of immunogenic allopeptides conjugated to an anti-IgD monoclonal antibody pretransplant, thereby delivering the peptides to resting B cells which lacked the necessary costimulatory molecules [27]. Although this resulted in a reduction in the anti-MHC class I alloantibody response no effect on graft survival was seen. Targeting CD4+ T cell help for antibody production may prove useful in transplant and autoimmune models.

Polymorphic MHC Class II Derived Peptides

Self-MHC restricted recognition of MHC class II derived allopeptides has been demonstrated following priming by either vascularized cardiac [28] or renal [29] allografts. Intrathymic administration of immunogenic polymorphic MHC class II allopeptides in the rat renal allograft model was shown to induce antigen specific unresponsiveness [30]. In addition, intrathymic injection of a single immunogenic class II peptide results in specific inhibition of primed T cell proliferative responses to the peptide *in vitro* [30], as well inhibition of DTH responses *in vivo* [31]. The induction phase of this acquired thymic tolerance required an intact thymus, implying that it was mediated by peripheral T cell

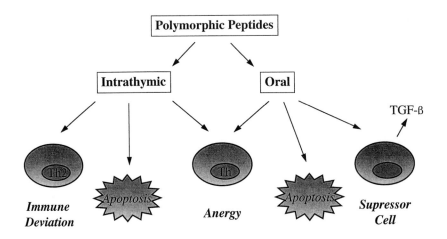

Figure 2. Proposed mechanisms of action for tolerance induction following either intrathymic or oral administration of polymorphic peptides

anergy. The maintenance phase, however, was thymus-independent, suggesting deletion of specific alloreactive T cell clones [32,33]. The tolerogenicity of orally delivered synthetic polymorphic class II MHC allopeptides has also been investigated [34,35]. Oral administration of a mixture of the peptides representing two MHC class II alleles significantly inhibited the DTH response to the allopeptides as well as to allogeneic cells [35]. The tolerogenic effect was antigen-specific and, as with intrathymic administration, was induced by the immunogenic polymorphic MHC class II peptides. Immunohistology of DTH skin lesions showed that, in contrast to the intrathymic model, oral tolerance is associated with a state of 'immune deviation' with a predominance of Th2 cytokine production [31].

Evidence indicating that indirect recognition early post-transplantation is limited to a small number of dominant peptides would suggest that it is possible to induce tolerance through the manipulation of the indirect pathway [36]. A small number of relevant allopeptides may be provided either by oral or intrathymic administration. Since peptides binding to the same class II MHC molecule can compete with each other for presentation to T cells, priming of T cells may be inhibited *in vivo* by co-administration of antigen and an excess of a competitor peptide, so-called "MHC blockade". [37]. This method has been successful *in vivo* in several autoimmune models, including experimental allergic encephalomyelitis (EAE) [38,39] and autoimmune diabetes [40]. In "high zone" tolerance high concentrations of antigen stimulate T cell activation followed by apoptotic cell death [41]. This method has been successfully used in an EAE model in which administration of high concentrations of myelin basic protein are associated with activation-induced apoptosis of reactive T cells and concomitant decrease in incidence and severity of disease [42]. Alternatively, inhibition of the T cell response with antigen analogs in which the major T cell contact residues have been modified can produce powerful antagonists. In this case, the peptide does not interfere with the TCR/APC interaction; rather, early events in T cell activation are inhibited [43]. This method had been shown to inhibit direct alloreactivity by cytotoxic T lymphocytes *in vitro* [44].

Dunsavage et al. have used a peptide derived from a polymorphic region of a class II MHC allele associated with diabetes mellitus in a NOD mouse model. Immunisation with the peptide induced peptide-specific antibodies and memory T cells which were associated with protection from development of diabetes [45]. Clinical evaluation of this peptide vaccine approach is currently in progress. Rheumatoid arthritis patients who received multiple doses of a 20 amino acid peptide derived from the third hypervariable region of the disease-associated MHC class II molecule showed encouraging results in a recent placebo-controlled phase II clinical trial [46]. The mechanism mediating the effect is not fully understood but is a promising new strategy for modulating self-antigen presentation to autoreactive T cells in autoimmune disease.

Non-Polymorphic MHC Class-I Derived Peptides.

Initial studies by Clayberger et al. showed that synthetic peptides corresponding to certain polymorphic regions of the α_1 or α_2 domain of HLA-A2 inhibited lysis by cytotoxic T lymphocytes (CTL) apparently by competing with the specific allele for binding to the TCR [Clayberger, 1987 #102; Parham, 1987 #101. The use of these peptides was limited by the allele-specific nature of their inhibition. Although subsequent studies demonstrated that synthetic peptides corresponding to residues 222-235 of the HLA class I sequence, the CD8 binding loop, were able to inhibit CTL differentiation they did not affect cytolysis by mature CTL [47]. More recently, *in vitro* and *in vivo*, there have been extensive studies focused on peptides corresponding to residues 75-84 of the α_1 helix of HLA class I molecules which have been shown to inhibit class I restricted immune responses in a allele non-specific manner. Both HLA-B7.75-84 and HLA-B2702.75-84 peptides (ALLOTRAP™ peptides, Sangstat Medical Corporation, Menlo Park, CA) prevented the differentiation of precursors into effector cytotoxic T lymphocytes (CTL) *in vitro*, while HLA-B2702.75-84 inhibited lysis by established CTL, and inhibited natural killer cell-mediated cytotoxicity [48]. These peptides have immunomodulatory effects in several rodent transplant models when given alone or in combination with low dose cyclosporine [49-51]. They induced specific tolerance in several of these models, with acceptance of a second allograft from the same donor, while third party

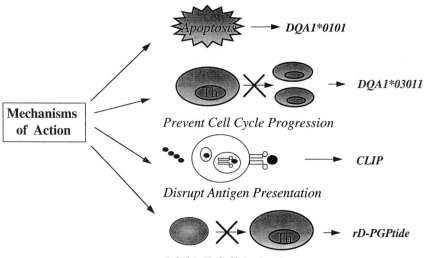

Figure 3. Mechanisms of action of selected MHC-derived immunomodulatory peptides.

grafts were rejected. More recent data showed that the D-isomer, which is more resistant to proteolytic breakdown, is more potent than the original L-isomer peptide [52]. These data provided the impetus to conduct a randomised, double-blind, placebo controlled study of the safety and the pharmacokinetics of HLA-B2702.75-84 in human recipients of a first renal allograft [53]. Patients received a dose of 7mg/kg administered immediately after transplantation and at 24 hour intervals thereafter varying from 2 doses to 10 depending on the treatment group. There were no toxic effects during the three month follow up. No phenotypic differences were found in the lymphocyte population following administration of HLA-B2702.75-84 as compared to placebo. However, in those patients that received a 10 day treatment, there was a significant reduction in NK cytotoxicity noted from day 15 through two months after the end of treatment, a finding which is consistent with *in vitro* data in humans [48] and *in vivo* findings in animals [54]. In fact, there was a tendency toward more acute rejection episodes and viral infections in the treatment groups. Interestingly, those patients in whom a rejection episode did occur showed no significant difference in NK cytotoxicity when compared to patients with no rejection episodes. The clinical significance of these results is uncertain. Nevertheless, they provide encouraging results for the potential clinical application of peptide based therapies in humans.

Investigations into the mechanism mediating the effect of these peptides demonstrated binding of HLA-B2702.75-84 to two proteins of molecular weight 70 and 74 KD from T cell lysates [55]. These proteins were shown to be members of the heat shock protein (HSP) 70 family. Peptide binding was sequence specific with strict correlation between peptide binding and immunomodulatory effect. Based on these results, it was postulated that the class I HLA-derived peptides act intracellularly by binding to HSP's in a similar manner to the binding of cyclosporine and FK506 to cyclophilin and FKBP, respectively. More recent studies in which the effects of a panel of peptides on CTL cytotoxicity, graft survival, and binding to HSP70 were studied, indicate that their immunomodulatory activity correlated poorly with binding to HSP70. D-isomers of the original inhibitory peptides proved more effective at inhibiting CTL cytotoxicity while showing no binding to HSP70 [56]. Other proposed mechanisms of action include the inter- action with the NK inhibitory receptor or modulation of the heme oxygenase-1 (HO-1) an inducible HSP [57]. It has been suggested that HO-1 exerts its effects through the intermediate metabolites in the conversion of heme to biliveredin. They are known to inhibit complement, IL-2 production, antibody dependent and independent cell-mediated cytoxicity, and proliferative responses [57]. Computer- assisted rational design of analogs of the lead compound, HLA- B2702.75-84, have been shown to prolong cardiac allograft survival in a mouse model, with the dose required and the efficacy varying with the individual compounds [58].

Non-Polymorphic Class II MHC-Derived Peptides

Murphy et al. investigated the possible immunoregulatory role of pep-tides derived from conserved regions of class II MHC molecules [59]. They demonstrated that three peptides derived from a highly conserved region of the class II MHC alpha chain inhibited the rat MLR in a dose dependent manner, with the human HLA-DQA1*0101 peptide also inhibiting the human and mouse MLR. No effect was seen on mitogen induced T cell proliferation, while that produced by stimulation with superantigen was inhibited, implying that the peptide interferes with the MHC-TCR interaction. HLA-DQA1*0101 inhibited CTL generation in a dose response fashion, with no reduction in preformed cytotoxic T lymphocyte killing, suggesting the inhibitory effect is targeted at CD4+ T cell help for CD8+ T cells. Although the inhibition of the MLR by HLA-DQA1*0101 was not reversed by IL-2, a stimulatory anti-CD28 monoclonal antibody (mAb) completely abrogated the inhibitory effect. The provision of excess costimulation can overcome some defects in T cell activation by weak agonists [60]. It is possible therefore that HLA-DQA1*0101 peptide interferes with the TCR - MHC interaction, thus altering the pattern T cell activation, this effect is then overcome or compensated for by stimulation with anti-CD28 mAb. An alternative explanation is that anti-CD28 mAb rescues the cells from apoptosis through the induction of Bcl-x$_L$. The induction of apoptosis, as assessed by cell cycle analysis following propidium iodide uptake, showed that stimulation of primed T cells in the presence of HLA-DQA1*0101 resulted in marked apoptosis at 24 hours with some evidence as early as 1 hour. On the other hand incubation of naive cells with the peptide showed no evidence of apoptosis. No difference in the level of expression of several pro- and anti-apoptotic molecules was found at the RNA level. Interestingly, stimulation of primed T cell in the presence of HLA-DQA1*0101 resulted in a dramatic increase in the production of IL-1β suggesting a possible role for IL-1β in the induction of apoptosis by DQA1*0101 through a Fas/FasL dependent pathway. These data demonstrate that synthetic peptides derived from highly conserved regions of the class II MHC alpha chain can alter CD4+ T lymphocyte alloimmune responses *in vitro*, and this effect is mediated by the induction of apoptosis in activated T cells. Further studies are required to determine the binding site and the exact mechanism of action of this peptide.

Using a synthetic class II MHC peptide from the same region of another allele, DQA1*3011(DQ 65-79), Boytim et al. demonstrated that anti-CD3 mAb, mitogen, and alloantigen induced T cell proliferation could be inhibited in an allele independent manner [61]. Delayed addition of the peptide up to 24 hours after stimulation with anti-CD3 has a minimal effect on inhibition. In addition, inhibition of anti-CD3 mAb induced proliferation is not reversed by anti-CD28 mAb or IL-2.

These results are in contrast to those shown by Murphy et al with by DQA1*0101, not only from the aspect of the effect of IL-2 and CD28, but also since delayed addition of the peptide to the MLR by as little a 5 minutes reduced the inhibitory effect seen [59]. Cells which were initially stimulated in the presence of DQA1*3011(DQ 65-79) are unresponsive to restimulation. Cell cycle analysis showed that the peptide prevented DNA replication by blocking the G1 to S transition, suggesting that the peptide may work in manner similar to rapamycin. This was confirmed by the finding that DQA1*3011(DQ 65-79) inhibited cyclin-dependent kinase 2 via a block in the degradation of the inhibitory protein p27. The effects, however, unlike rapamycin, are not mediated through binding to FKBP since the peptide did not compete for binding with FK506. Recently, using a yeast two-hybrid system proliferating cell nuclear antigen (PCNA) was identified as a DQA1*3011(DQ 65-79) binding protein, suggesting that the peptide interferes with the normal interaction of cyclins, cyclin-dependent kinases, and PCNA [62].

Peptide Inhibitors of Coreceptor Interactions.

MHC derived peptides may also exert their effects on the immune response through disruption of critical protein-protein interactions. Clayberger et al. have shown that generation of CTL could be inhibited by a synthetic peptide corresponding to the CD8 binding loop of HLA class I, but killing by established CTL was not affected. Furthermore they showed that peptides corresponding to a CD4 binding region of class II MHC (residues 134-152 of HLA-DRβ) inhibited differentiation of CTL precursors, lymphocyte proliferation and proliferation by an antigen-specific CD4+ T cell clone [47]. Korngold and colleagues have used computer based technology to design a peptide analog mimicking the CDR3-D1 region of the murine CD4 molecule [63]. This peptide, referred to as rD-mPGPtide, corresponded to residues 86-94 of the mouse CD4 molecule and consists of D-amino acids to increase resistance to proteolytic breakdown. In addition a proline-glycine-proline-cysteine sequence was added to allow tertiary structural constraints and cyclization. rD-mPGPtide blocks *in vitro* the activation of CD4+ T cells after TCR engagement and inhibits the MLR. Administration of rD-mPGPtide *in vivo* to murine recipients limited the development of graft-versus-host disease (GVHD) and enhanced engraftment [64,65]. A single dose markedly inhibited the development of CD4+ lymphocyte mediated experimental allergic encephalomyelitis (EAE) and was effective whether administered prior or subsequent to disease development [63,66]. The effect was specific and responses to other antigens remained intact. In addition, it has also been shown to significantly prolong skin allograft survival in a mouse model. Unlike anti-CD4 mAb, rD-mPGptide is nonimmunogenic and inhibits only the activated antigen-specific T cells rather than all CD4+ T cells, it does not cause CD4 depletion [66]. Although the exact mechanism of action mediating the inhibitory effect of rD-mPGptide has not been elucidated it has been proposed that it may function by uncoupling CD4-CD4 dimerization and therefore preventing a stable APC-T-cell interaction. This group has also used nuclear magnetic resonance data to develop other peptides mimicking the CD4 interaction site with similarly good results in three CD4+ T cell dependent mouse models, EAE, skin allograft rejection across a class II antigen mismatch, and GVHD across a haplomismatched MHC difference [67]. In fact non-peptidic CD4 inhibitors are now being developed using computer screening mechanisms [68].

This same group has used these techniques to design similar peptide analogues which mimic the putative interaction sites of CD8 and the class I MHC molecule [69]. This group of peptides effectively inhibited both preformed CTLs and CTL generation. A single dose of one of these peptides significantly prolonged skin allografts in a class I MHC mismatched mouse model. These experiments emphasise the exciting opportunities which are possible in the development of new immuno-therapies through the use of computer modelling technologies, in conjunction with our expanding understanding of structure-function relationships in the immune response. In addition, they may be modified by incorporating organic molecules, so that the resulting peptidomimetic would be orally active, thus offering considerable advantage over other existing approaches such as monoclonal anti-bodies. An example of such is demonstrated by Falcioni et al., who developed a group of peptidomimetic compounds which compete for presentation by the group of DR alleles associated with rheumatoid arthritis [70]. These compounds were modified so as to be cathepsin resistant, thus preventing degradation in the endosomal compartment of APC's. They were effective inhibitors of proliferation to a number of antigens presented by the alleles in question.

Other Peptides

A further example of how our knowledge of the processes involved in the processing, presentation, recognition and subsequent responses to antigen can help in the development of agents which disrupt these events is the use of Class II-associated invariant chain peptide (CLIP) to interrupt binding of antigen to MHC class II. CLIP plays an important in MHC class II expression and antigen presentation within APCs. Zechel et al showed that a synthetic peptide with a sequence derived from the CLIP inhibited antigen-specific T cell response *in vitro* and *in vivo* following immunisation [71]. The peptide presumably exerted it effect by inhibiting the loading of antigenic peptides onto MHC class II molecules and the subsequent expression of the MHC molecule-peptide complexes on the cell surface. These studies have not yet been extended to an *in vivo* transplant model.

Conclusions

There is extensive evidence that MHC-derived peptides may regulate the immune response to both allo- and autoantigen. These effects are mediated through targeting a wide range of sites involved in the recognition of antigen, and the subsequent T cell response. Although these peptides offer many advantages as immunomodulatory agents, including specificity, tolerance induction and lack of toxicity, there are several hurdles to be overcome. A potential problem is bioavailability. Specifically, will oral administration be feasible, and how do we maintain a therapeutic plasma level in view of the likely degradation by proteases? In addition, potential problems with the production of large quantities of highly purified peptide must be dealt with. The use of computer based rational designs and modifications offer the opportunity to overcome some of these problems, and enhance the function of peptides which have already been tested. The likelihood is that MHC-derived peptides will provide the initial inspiration for the development of more effective agents, or serve to highlight target sites. Since we have shown that peptides inhibit the immune response at several key sites, consideration must also be given to combining peptide therapies. For example two non-polymorphic MHC class II peptides, DQA1*0101 and DQA1*3011 could be combined. In this manner T cells which are activated would undergo apoptosis induced by DQA1*0101, while T cells that escape this effect would be prevented from proliferating by the second peptide DQA1*3011. Many aspects of the immunomodulatory effects of MHC-derived peptides have yet to be discovered. The exact mechanisms of action, the binding sites, the interactions with conventional immunosuppression and their effectiveness *in vivo* in humans are beginning to be elucidated. Nevertheless, peptides offer us the possibility of a new, diverse and exciting group of immunosuppressants.

References

1. Nashan B, Moor R, AmlotP, et al. Randomised trial of bsiliximab versus placebo for control of acute cellular rejection in renal allograft recipients. Lancet 1997;350:1193-1198.
2. Vincenti F, Kirkman R, Light S, et al. Interleukin-2-receptor blockade with daclizumab to prevent acure rejection in renal transplantation. N Engl J Med 1998;338:161-165.
3. Nashan B, Light S, Hardie IR, et al. Reduction of acute renal allograft rejection by daclizumab. Transplantation 1999;67:110-115.
4. Kahan BD, Rajagopalan PR, Hall M. Reduction of the occurrence of acute cellular rejection among renal allograft recipients treated with basiliximab, a chimeric anti-interleukin-2-receptor monoclonal antibody. Transplantation 1999;67:276-284.
5. Boelaars-van Haperen MJAM, BaanCC, van Riemsdijk IC, et al : Treatment with the chimeric anti-IL2Rα antibody basiliximab prevents the development of renal rejection by affecting the IL-2 and IL-15 pathway. XVIII International Congress of the Transplantation Society (Abstract OAP17) pg. 28, Aurg. 27-Sept. 1, 2000.
6. Goebel J, Stevens E, Forrest K, et al: Daclizumab (dac) blocks early interleukin (IL)-2 receptor ® signaling. XVII International Congress of the Transplantation Society (Abstract #P0528), pg. 316, Aug. 27-Sept. 1, 2000.
7. Souillou JP, Cantarovich D, LeMauff B, et al. Randomized controlled trial of monoclonal antibody against rejection of renal allografts. N Eng J Med 1990;322:1175.
8. Krikman RL, Shapiro ME, Carpenter DB, et al. A randomized prospective trial of anti-Tac monoclonal antibody in human renal transplantation. Transplantation 1991; 51:107-113.
9. Kriaa F, Hiesse C, Alard P, et al. Prophylactic use of the anti-IL-2-receptor monoclonal antibody LO-Tact-I in cadaveric renal transplantation: results of a randomized study. Transplant Proc 1993;25:817-819.
10. van Gelder T, Zietse R, Mulder AH, et al. A double-blind, placebo-controlled study of monoclonal anti-interleukin-2 receptor antibody (BT563) administration to prevent acute rejection after kidney transplantation. Transplantation 1995;60:248-252.
11. Vincenti F, Lantz M, Birnbaum J, et al. A phase I tirla of humanized anti-interleukin 2 receptor antibody in renal transplantation. Transplantation 1997;63:33-38.
12. Amlot PL, Rawlings E, Fernando ON, et al. Prolonged action of chiameric IL-2 receptor (CD25) monoclonal antibody used in cadaveric renal transplantation. Transplantation, 1995;60:748-56.
13. Kirkman RL, Bumgardner G, Gaston RS, et al. Addition of daclizumab to mycophenolate mofetil, cyclosporine, and steroids in renal transplantation: pharmacokinetics, safety and efficacy. (Submitted for publication, Clinical Transplantation).
14. Davies E, Lawen J, Mourad G, et al. Basiliximab (Simulect®) is safe and effective in combination with Neoral®, steroids, and CellCept® for the prevention of acute rejection episodes in renal transplantation. Interim results of a double-blind, randomized clinical trial. (Abstract #A3672) Amer. Soc Nephrology 32nd annual meeting, Nov. 1-8, 1999.
15. Ciancio G, Miller A, Cespedes M, et al: Daclizumab induction for primary kidney transplant recipients using tacrolimus, mycophenolate mofetil and steroids as maintenance immunosuppression. XVIII International Congress of the Transplantation Society. (Abstract OAP27), pg. 46, Aug. 27-Sept. 1, 2000.
16. Deierhoi MH, Hudson SL, Gaston RS: Clinical experience with a two dose regimen of daclizumab in cadaveric renal transplantation. (Abstract #574) pg. S75, AST

Transplant 2000.

17. Lebranchu Y, Hurault de Ligny B, Toupance O, et al. A multicenter randomized trial of Simulect® versus Thymoglobuline® in renal transplantation, (Abstract #567) pg. S74, AST Transplant 2000.

18. Sollinger H, Kaplan B, Pewscovitz M, et al: A multicenter, randomized trial of Simulect® with early Neoral® vs. ATGAM® with delayed Neoral in renal transplantation,. XVIII International Congress of the Transplantation Soceity (Abstract #0113) pg. 29, Aug. 27-Sept 1, 2000.

19. Hong JC, Kahan BD. Interleukin-2 receptor monoclonal antibodies and sirolimus: a novel induction immunosuppression strategy. Transplantation & Immunology Letter XVI:7-9, 2000.

20. Landsberg DN, Cole EH, Russell D, et al. Renal transplantation without steroids – one year results of a multicentre Canadian pilot study. (Abstract #86), pg. S49, AST Transplant 2000.

21. Vincenti F, Monaco A, Grinyo J, et al. Rapid steroid withdrawal versus standard steroid treatment in patients treated with Simulect®, Neoral®, and Cellcept® for the prevention of acute rejection in renal transplantation: a multicenter, randomized trial. (Abstract #83) pg. S49, AST Transplant 2000.

22. Vincenti F, Ramos E, Brattstrom C, Cho S, Ekberg H, Grinyo J, Johnson R, Kuypers D, Stuart F, Khanna A, Navarro M, Nashan B. Multicenter trial exploring calcineurin inhibitors avoidance in renal transplantation. In Press, Transplantation, 2000.

23. Kreis H, Cisterne J-M, Land @, et al. Sirolimus inassociation with mycophenolate mofetil induction for the prevention of acute graft rejection in renal allograft recipients. Transplantation 69:1252-1260.

24. Tellides G, Dallman MJ, Morris PJ. Synergistic interaction of cyclosporine A with interleukin 2 receptor monoclonal antibody therapy. Transplantation Proc 1988;20 (Suppl 2):202-206.

25. Baan CC, Knoop CJ, van Gelder T, et al. Anti-CD25 therapy reveals the redundancy of the intragraft cytokine network after clinical heart transplantation. Transplantation 1999;67:870-876.

26. Chang, GJ, Harish H, Mahanty, Vincenti F, et al. A calcineurin inhibitor-sparing regimen with sirolimus, mycophenolate mofetil, and anti-CD25 mAb provides effective immunosuppression in kidney transplant recipients with delayed or impaired graft function. Clinical Transplantation 2000; 14:545-549.

TOLERANCE: IS IT TIME TO MOVE TO THE CLINIC?

Markus H. Frank and Mohamed H. Sayegh

Introduction

Tolerogenic manipulation of the immune response remains the major barrier to successful organ transplantation. The introduction of cyclosporine into clinical use in the early 1980s [1] and the development of newer immunosuppressive drugs [2] has led to a significant reduction in acute rejection rates and improvement in short-term allograft survival. However, achieving long-term graft survival and overcoming chronic rejection remain difficult tasks [3,4]. Lifelong non-specific immunosuppressive therapy following organ transplantation is associated with an increased risk of infection, malignancy and cardiovascular disease, and hence considerable morbidity and mortality. The development of strategies to induce donor-specific tolerance has therefore become the major goal of transplantation research.

Billingham, Brent, and Medawar in 1953 were the first to describe a state of actively acquired "immunological tolerance" in mice that had been injected in utero or during the neonatal period with bone marrow derived donor cells [5]. Such animals would later accept an allograft taken from the same inbred strain from which the original cells were harvested, while maintaining the ability to reject third party strain grafts. Since these observations, extensive research has focused on developing strategies to understand the mechanisms of tolerance and to induce tolerance in adult animals. Immunologically, tolerance can be regarded as a state of specific unresponsiveness to the antigens of the graft in the absence of maintenance immunosuppression [6].

*Mohamed Sayegh and Giuseppe Remuzzi (editors), Current and Future
Immunosuppressive Therapies Following Transplantation, 293-313.*
© 2001 Kluwer Academic Publishers. Printed in the Netherlands.

However, since tolerance can be mediated by an active regulatory immune response, perhaps a better definition suggested by Suthanthiran is: the absence of a destructive immune response against the graft in an immunocompetent host (7). In experimental animals, criteria for donor-specific tolerance are the absence of acute rejection with prolongation of graft survival and acceptance of second test grafts from the original donor, while maintaining the ability to reject third party grafts [8]. Donor-specific tolerance holds the promise to not only prevent acute allograft rejection, but also the alloantigen-dependent component of chronic allograft dysfunction, the major cause of late graft dysfunction and loss in solid organ transplantation [9].

Immunologic donor-specific tolerance may be mediated by thymic deletional mechanisms (central tolerance) or be induced/maintained by various mechanisms in the peripheral blood and extrathymic lymphoid tissue [8], including anergy, deletion and regulation. Hence, strategies directed at inducing experimental tolerance are primarily aimed at effecting the deletion or inactivation of existing peripheral donor-reactive T cells, and/or at modulating the developing T cell repertoire such as to effect the central or peripheral deletion and/or inactivation of newly emerging donor-reactive T cells. Although several distinct strategies have been successful in inducing tolerance in rodents, it has proven to be much more difficult to translate such strategies into primates and humans. Nevertheless, recent advances in our understanding of the cellular and molecular mechanisms of alloimmunity and tolerance have resulted in the refinement of existing strategies and spurred the development of novel approaches, that may in the future be successfully translated into humans. Here, we will briefly summarize our current understanding of the mechanisms that underlie immunological tolerance and provide an overview of clinically relevant strategies aimed at transplantation tolerance induction that hold the promise of applicability in human allograft recipients.

Self Tolerance

In self-tolerance, the physical elimination of certain T cells that interact with self-major histocompatibility complex (MHC) molecules within the thymus plays an important role in the development of tolerance to self-antigens in the fetal/neonatal period [10]. Phenotypic expression of T cells is determined by the sum of random T cell receptors (TCR) gene rearrangements [11]. T cell precursors originate in the bone marrow and migrate to the thymus where they initially fail to express the CD4 and CD8 T cell markers that are associated with maturity. These double negative T cells then undergo proliferation and maturation and acquire both CD4 and CD8 T cell markers to become so-called double-positive cells. Through random TCR gene rearrangements, these thymocytes express TCRs with varying affinity for self-MHC+peptide. Central to the mechanisms of self-tolerance is the avidity with which the TCR interacts with the self-MHC+peptide. This is determined by both the structure of the TCR for the antigen as well as the density of TCRs present on the T cell [12,13]. Thymocytes that either lack affinity or have very high affinity for the complex are negatively selected and undergo deletion by programmed cell death (apoptosis). Those thymocytes with low avidity for the complex are positively selected and become a set of T cells that function with self-MHC but lack sufficient autoreactivity to result in autoimmune disease. Some lower avidity TCRs may escape at this stage only to be deleted later with the increase in TCR expression that occurs with the transition from double positivity (CD4+/CD8+) to single positivity (CD4+/CD8- or CD4-/CD8+) as thymocytes migrate from the cortex to the medulla of the thymus. Positively selected medullary thymocytes acquire MHC class II restricted helper (CD4$^+$) or MHC class I restricted cytotoxic (CD8$^+$) functions and migrate to the periphery as immunocompetent T cells. Between 95-99% of thymocytes are deleted in the thymus, with only the small remainder becoming mature T cells that migrate to the periphery. It is thought that autoimmunity arises when some autoreactive T cells escape thymic negative selection.

There are two types of thymic antigen presenting cells (APCs): bone marrow derived macrophages/dendritic cells and epithelial cells [14]. There is evidence that each type has a different function in the induction of self-tolerance and in T cell repertoire selection. Positive selection is thought to be mediated by thymic epithelial cells, whereas negative selection is thought to be mediated by bone marrow-derived cells. Since the thymus involutes after puberty, clonal deletion may play only a minor role in the development of tolerance in the adult. However, cells that are important in the induction of thymic (central) deletional tolerance may still be functional.

In addition to central mechanisms, self tolerance may be mediated by peripheral mechanisms, including T cell anergy, deletion and regulation (**Figure 1**). T cells which recognize antigen presented by costimulator signal-deficient APCs do not proliferate and differentiate and are rendered incapable of responding to the antigen (anergic), even during subsequent antigen presentation by competent APCs. Peripheral deletion of antigen-specific T cells can result from activation-induced cell death (AICD) upon high affinity binding and repeated stimulation by Fas-FasL interactions or by passive cell death. In addition, antigen-specific regulatory cells, possibly Th2 suppressor T cells, can inhibit the induction or function of peripheral antigen-specific effector T cells [15]. These peripheral mechanisms likely contribute to the maintenance of self-tolerance and prevention of autoimmunity and are likely of importance in acquired transplantation tolerance as well.

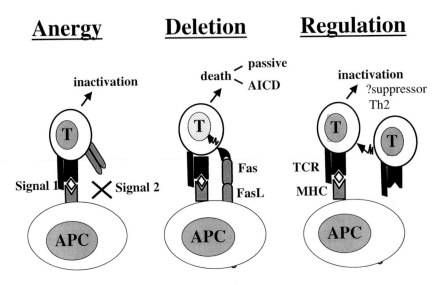

Figure 1: Peripheral mechanisms of Tolerance: T cells which recognize antigen presented by costimulator signal (signal 2)-deficient APCs do not proliferate and differentiate and are rendered incapable of responding to the antigen (anergic), even during subsequent antigen presentation by competent APCs (left panel). Peripheral deletion of antigen-specific T cells can result from activation-induced cell death (AICD) upon high affinity binding and repeated stimulation with Fas-FasL interactions, or by passive cell death (middle panel). Antigen-specific regulatory cells, possibly Th2 suppressor T cells, can inhibit the induction or function of peripheral antigen-specific effector T cells (right panel). Abbreviations: APC – antigen presenting cell, T – T cell, FasL – Fas Ligand, AICD – activation induced cell death, TCR – T cell receptor, MHC – major histocompatibility complex.

Transplantation Tolerance – Mechanisms and Experimental Strategies

Therapeutically induced transplantation tolerance, in analogy to self tolerance, may be mediated by thymic deletional mechanisms (central tolerance) or be induced/maintained throughout the peripheral blood and extrathymic lymphoid tissue (peripheral tolerance) by a complex interplay of several distinct mechanisms, including deletion, anergy, and regulation/suppression of alloreactive immune cells. Various experimental strategies have been developed which are directed at one or more of these mechanisms; here, we will review those that hold the greatest promise for potential clinical applicability in the near future.

Bone marrow chimerism: The creation of bone marrow chimeras in experimental animals can induce central allograft tolerance involving thymic deletional mechanisms analogous to self-tolerance [16]. Bone marrow chimeras can be achieved by donor marrow infusion into a recipient animal treated with a myeloablative regimen such as total body irradiation. Donor APCs from this inoculum migrate to the thymus of the reconstituted animal where they will be seen as self. Thereafter, the resultant animal will be specifically tolerant to donor alloantigen, presumably by deletion of alloreactive T cells in the thymus (negative selection). Besides the potential complication of graft versus host disease, which can be prevented by T cell depletion of the bone marrow preparation, chimeric animals may have deficient T cell responses to nominal antigens. Since T cells are positively selected during normal maturation to recognize foreign antigens in association with the self-MHC molecules expressed on thymic epithelium, and since bone marrow derived APCs in chimeras are of donor origin whereas the thymic epithelial APCs remain of recipient origin, mature T cells will be positively selected to respond only to antigens presented by the recipient MHC molecule, but not to antigen presented in association with donor-MHC on APCs derived from the donor bone marrow. As a result, the T cell immune response is suppressed [16]. To overcome this problem, another approach has been the creation of mixed allogeneic chimeras by reconstituting myeloablated animals with a mixture of both syngeneic plus allogeneic bone marrow [17]. The reconstituted animals have a mixture of APCs derived from both recipient and donor and therefore have normal T cell function. This strategy has been successful in both rodents and non-human primates, in allo- as well as xeno- transplant models [16], but the clinical applicability of myeloablative strategies has been uncertain because of the potential for serious side effects and the temporal requirements of the conditioning regimen. Non-myeloablative conditioning regimen involving irradiation have been successful in non-human primates as well, and the applicability of such approaches has been extended from solid organ transplantation to cellular grafts, with successful induction of tolerance to a pancreatic islet allograft in a non-human primate using hematopoetic mixed multilineage chimerism and a non-myeloablative conditioning regimen [18]. However, because of the potential side effects of the use of radiation in humans, a focus of recent research has been the induction of stable mixed hematopoietic chimerism tolerance using allogeneic bone marrow transplantation in conjunction with various non-myeloablative biologic and pharmacologic synergistic therapies [19], described in the next section. These approaches allow for host bone marrow suppression and stable mixed chimerism with minimal side effects and have shown promise in non-human primates as a pre-clinical strategy [20, 21].

Costimulatory Blockade: Although there are several experimental strategies that may hold promise for the achievement of tolerance induction in transplantation, T cell costimulatory blockade of the CD80/CD86 – CD28/CTLA4 and CD40 – CD40L pathways is perhaps the most promising and will likely be tested clinically in the near future

[22]. T cells require two distinct signals for full activation. The first signal is provided by the engagement of the TCR with the MHC+peptide complex on APCs, and a costimulatory signal is provided by engagement of one or more T cell surface receptors with their specific ligands on APCs [23]. TCR ligation in the absence of additional signals provided by the MHC-expressing APC results in antigen-specific unresponsiveness or anergy [24]. While several receptor:ligand interactions have been suggested to provide costimulatory signals to T cells (CD2:LFA-3, LFA-1:ICAM-1), the best characterized costimulatory signal involves binding of the T cell surface molecule CD28 to either of its ligands, B7-1 or B7-2, expressed on the surface of professional bone marrow derived APCs [23]. The uniqueness of this costimulatory pathway has been clearly demonstrated in studies indicating that signaling through CD28 prevents T cell anergy and death induced by TCR signaling alone [25,26]. CD28 has a high degree of homology (32% identity at the amino acid level) to another gene called CTLA4 [27]. Unlike CD28, which is expressed on resting T cells, CTLA4 appears to be expressed on the cell surface only after initial T cell activation. CTLA4 appears to down-regulate immune responses by binding with high affinity to its B7 counter-receptors [28,29]. CTLA4 gene knockout mice show a variety of lymphoproliferative disorders and early death [30], while administration of blocking anti-CTLA4 monoclonal antibodies (to block negative T cell signaling) worsens autoimmune disease [31] and prevents induction of peripheral tolerance [32], implying a critical physiologic role for CTLA4 in terminating T cell responses [33]. Ligation of CD28 by B7-1 or B7-2 is blocked by CTLA4Ig, a recombinant fusion protein that contains the extracellular domain of soluble CTLA4 used to an Ig heavy chain [34]. CTLA4Ig binds to both B7-1 and B7-2 and acts as a competitive inhibitor of CD28 binding to B7-1 and B7-2, resulting in T cell anergy in vitro [35,36]. T cell costimulatory blockade by systemic administration of CTLA4Ig has been very effective in preventing experimental acute rejection, prolonging graft survival and inducing specific tolerance in some transplantation models [37]. Studies from our laboratory have demonstrated that CD28-B7 T cell costimulatory blockade by CTLA4Ig prevents development of chronic rejection in rat models of cardiac as well as renal transplantation [38,39]. More interestingly, CD28-B7 blockade late after acute injury interrupts progression of chronic rejec-tion in an experimental chronic renal allograft rejection model [40].

A second costimulatory pathway, provided by the interaction of CD40 with its ligand, CD40L, is of significance in the process of allograft rejec-tion and tolerance [23]. CD40, a member of the tumor necrosis factor (TNF) receptor family, is expressed on B cells and other APCs, including dendritic cells and endothelial cells [41]. CD40L (a member of the TNF family, also known as gp39), is expressed early on activated T cells [41]. Binding of CD40L to CD40 is critical in providing T cell help for B cell Ig production and class switching [42]; a defect in CD40L is responsible for the hyper-IgM syndrome in humans [43]. The role of CD40L in T cell activation has been uncertain. Studies using CD40L knockout mice have demonstrated an inability of CD40L deficient T cells to undergo effective clonal expansion [44,45]. It has been questioned, however, whether CD40L acts directly to transduce a costimulatory signal to the T cell or indirectly, since ligation of CD40 on APCs is a strong inducer of B7 expression [46,47]. Therefore, CD40L on the T cell might merely serve to induce CD28-ligands or other costimulatory molecules on APCs. Several studies in experimental transplantation models indicate that CD40L blockade can prevent acute rejection and prolong allograft survival [48-50].

While the exact mechanisms mediating induction of tolerance by CD28-B7 T cell costimulatory blockade in vivo remain unclear, recent findings have significantly furthered our understanding. It has been suggested that CTLA4Ig induces T cell anergy and prevents expansion of antigen-specific T cells in vivo [51]. In the mouse heart transplant model, the induction of unresponsiveness requires an intact CTLA4 negative signaling pathway [52]. In addition, two important recent studies have suggested that apoptosis of alloreactive T cells is required for induction of peripheral transplantation tolerance. Wells et al. found that mice with defective passive or active T cell apoptotic pathways were resistant to induction of transplantation tolerance by costimulatory pathway blockade [53-55]. Li et al demonstrated in a mouse skin allograft model that costimulatory blockade was ineffective at tolerance induction in the absence of peripheral activation-induced cell death (AICD) prevented by concurrent cyclosporine administration. Importantly, concurrent sirolimus administration, which did not prevent AICD, facilitated tolerance induction [54-56]. Studies from our laboratory in the rat acute renal allograft rejection model indicate that systemic tolerance induced by the administration of CTLA4Ig is associated with selective inhibition of Th1 and sparing of Th2 cytokines in the target organ [57]. Similar data have been reported in a cardiac transplant model with CD40L blockade [48,58]. However, a causal relationship of a Th2 switch and transplantation tolerance has not been established. Nevertheless, recent studies have begun to elicit the roles of the CD28-B7 and CD40L-CD40 pathways in regulating Th1 versus Th2 alloimmune responses, since studies in cytokine gene knockout animals have highlighted the complex roles of cytokines in allograft rejection and tolerance. In a murine cardiac allograft model, using recipient STAT 4 and STAT6 knockout (KO) mice, deficient in producing Th1 or Th2 cytokines, respectively, a lesser tolerogenic effect of CD28-B7 blockade in Th2- but not Th1-deficient mice versus wildtype has been observed [59]. In addition, studies from our laboratory have indicated a diminished tolerogenic effect of CD40L-CD40 blockade in Th2-deficient mice [60]. Taken together, these data suggest a lesser effectiveness of costimulatory blockade in a predominant Th1 cytokine environment in vivo. However, complete absence of IL-2 has been observed to enhance the generation or maintanance of allospecific T cell memory, suggesting that IL-2 targeting immunosuppressive strategies may impair the potential for tolerance induction [61]. Larsen et al. [62] have addressed the potential for synergy between B7 and CD40L blockade by demonstrating that inhibition of these two pathways leads to prolonged allogeneic mouse skin and cardiac allograft survival. An interesting finding in this study was that only combination therapy with both anti-CD40L and CTLA4Ig was able to prevent graft arteriosclerosis and fibrosis (chronic rejection). One of the interesting observations in several of the experimental studies with T cell costimulatory blockade is the fact that administration of donor antigen appears to synergize with CTLA4Ig or anti-CD40L in promoting long term graft survival [48,50,63]. In some models, the administration of donor cells was necessary to prevent the development of chronic rejection [64,65]. In other models, a novel critical role of CD8+ dependent allograft rejection resistant to conventional costimulation blockade is emerging. In certain mouse strain combinations in a cardiac allograft transplantation model the failure of CD40-CD40L blockade to inhibit alloantigen-specific CD8+ T cell responses has been described, and there appears to be no requirement for CD40-CD40L-mediated activation of donor passenger leukocytes for induction of CD8+ T cell responses to donor antigen following transplant-ation [66]. In a murine allograft model, CD8+ T cells have been reported to mediate acute allograft rejection when normal CD4+ function is impaired by either CD40L costimulatory blockade, CD28 deficiency or CD4+ depletion [67]. Others have recently reported that conventional CD80/CD86 – CD28/CTLA4 and CD40 – CD40L pathway-directed costimulatory blockade was ineffective in prolonging allograft survival in a murine islet allograft transplantation model using CD8+ TCR transgenic mice, capable only of CD8+-mediated rejection, as recipients, whereas full efficacy was observed in wild-type recipients, identifyng a potential for costimulation blockade escape by alloreactive T cells [68]. Interestingly, the costimulatory molecule ICOS, a recently identified proposed third member of T cell specific cell surface receptors CD28 and CTLA4 [69], appears functional in CD8+ responses [68] and has been proposed as a potential additional target for more enhanced costimulatory blockade protocols. Taken together, these observations suggest a potential benefit of adding reagents directed at CD8+ T cell function to costimulatory blockade-based tolerogenic regimen.

Immunomodulatory Peptides: Observations that some peptides bound to MHC molecules are derived from MHC sequences themselves has prompted the study of the immunoregulatory properties of MHC derived peptides. In transplantation, two pathways of allorecognition are recognized [23,70,71]. The direct pathway involves recipient T cells recognizing intact allo-MHC molecules complexed with peptide on the surface of donor cells. The indirect pathway involves recipient APCs processing and presenting alloantigens (mainly allo-MHC peptides) to recipient CD4+ cells. In the latter situation, T cell responses to an alloantigen may be limited to one or only a few dominant peptide determinants. Therefore, tolerizing to these peptide determinants alone may then successfully inhibit at least indirect T cell alloresponses [72] Strategies designed to induce allogeneic unresponsiveness using peptides derived from both polymorphic and non-polymorphic portions of Class I and II MHC have been studied [73]. Boytim et al. were able to block allo-nonspecific induced T cell proliferation with a synthetic peptide corresponding to the alpha helical region of HLA-DQ by interrupting cell-cycle progression [74]. Similarly, Murphy et al. were able to alter T cell alloimmune responses in vitro with synthetic peptides derived from a highly conserved region of the class II MHC alpha chain through the induction of apoptosis [75]. In vivo studies have demonstrated reduced delayed type hypersensitivity responses to a mixture of polymorphic class II MHC allopeptides in peptide immunized rats with oral administration of the peptide mixture prior to immunization [76]. Since indirect allorecognition may play a role in chronic rejection, synthetic MHC peptides may also be used in the future to develop predictive assays that link T cell activity to the subsequent risk of developing chronic rejection posttransplant [77,78]. Whether tolerizing to MHC peptides, by oral administration for example, will have an impact on delaying progression of chronic rejection remains to be seen. Immunomodulatory and tolerogenic properties of MHC class I protein and derived peptides have been studied as well. Perez et. al have reported prolonged allograft survival and in vitro donor-specific hyporesponsiveness in response to i.v. and oral administration of allochimeric MHC class I proteins with transient cyclosporine A treatment [79]. Increased graft survival by i.p administered donor-derived MHC class I molecules with transient cyclosporine A therapy has also been reported in a rat heterotopic cardiac allograft model, but donor-specific graft tolerance was not achieved in this model with delayed rejection of a syngeneic skin graft [80]. In a novel and promising approach, Garrovillo et al. have demonstrated in a rat cardiac allograft model that intrathymic injection of class I MHC allopeptide-pulsed self dendritic cells can induce acquired thymic tolerance via indirect allorecognition of foreign antigen in the thymus [81]. The same group, building on these findings, has most recently reported that the interaction of thymic dendritic cells with allopeptide-primed peripheral self T cells may contribute to the induction of antigen-specific T cell tolerance by central (thymic) inactivation or deletion of alloreactive peripheral T cells. However, for donor-specific graft tolerance to be achieved in all animals in this model, concomitant ALS immunosuppression was required [82].

Shirwan et al. have demonstrated by adoptive transfer experiments the presence of an immunoregulatory suppressor cell generated in a host by intrathymic immunization with MHC class I derived allopeptide, capable of transferring donor-specific tolerance to secondary/tertiary allograft recipients, thus pointing to the thymic generation of specific cellular suppressor mechanisms in this model [83]. Together, these findings identify an important function of the thymus in the central generation of suppressor T cells via the indirect pathway, in addition to its role in central deletional mechanisms in tolerance induction. In MHC class II-mediated tolerance, apoptosis has recently been described to play a major role, and novel findings by Qingsheng et al. indicate the importance of caspase-independent pathways in this process [84]. Future studies will delineate further the various mechanisms involved in MHC derived peptide-induced transplantation tolerance, and help in guiding the rational design of concomitant immunosuppressive strategies for potential clinical applicability of these promising approaches.

Transplantation Tolerance – Moving Closer To the Clinic

Despite the fact that it has been relatively easy to induce true tolerance in small experimental animals, translating these studies into larger animals and non-human primates prior to potential application in humans has been much more difficult to achieve, although groundbreaking advances have recently been made as will be outlined below. In addition, due to the lack of reliable clinical predictive assays for rejection or tolerance in human transplant recipients where rechallenging with a second test graft to prove tolerance is not feasible, the introduction of tolerogenic strategies into the clinical arena will need to rely on concurrent conventional immunosuppressive therapy. This challenge is heightened by the fact that some common immunosuppressive agents may actually abrogate the induction of tolerance [62,64,85]. Thus, current research focuses on developing non-myeloablative tolerogenic strategies that are effective in large animal models even when combined with conventional immuno-suppressive therapy of proven clinical efficacy. Several promising strategies are evolving which involve single or synergistic tolerogenic strategies in conjunction with pharmacologic immunosuppression.

The induction of stable mixed hematopoietic chimerism tolerance using allogeneic bone marrow transplantation in conjunction with non-myeloablative biologic and pharmacologic synergistic therapies is one important focus of recent research. Important advances in the search for strategies to establish long-term hematopoetic chimerism without or with minimal cytoreductive conditioning regimen, employing biological or pharmacological agents have been made. Fuchimoto et al. have reported the induction of stable mixed chimerism tolerance using donor peripheral blood progenitor cells and a non-myelosuppressive conditioning protocol involving anti-CD3 immunotoxin T cell depletion, thymic irradiation and cyclosporine A in a miniature swine allogeneic transplantation model across major histocompatibility barriers [86]. While cyclosporine A may actually inhibit tolerogenic effects of donor bone marrow cells by suppression of TGF-ß1-mediated apoptosis of activated T cells [87], initial studies indicate that alternative pharmacologic immunosuppressive agents as part of a preconditioning regimen may be effective: Hale et al. have recently reported successful induction of persistent multilineage chimerism and predominantly peripherally sustained tolerance in a complete mismatch mouse skin transplant model using administration of ALS, donor bone marrow and sirolimus [88]. In addition, in yet another promising advance in the search for strategies to establish long-term hematopoetic chimerism without or with minimal cytoreductive conditioning, the induction of stable mixed chimerism and donor-specific graft tolerance in the majority of treated animals using a protocol involving two injections of anti-CD45 mAb in a fully MHC-mismatched rat skin allograft model has been reported [89].

The perhaps most promising synergistic strategy for potential clinical applicability of the mixed chimerism approach to tolerance induction, however, is concurrent costimulatory blockade. This strategy may have applicability to humans, because it may allow clinical translation of the bone marrow chimerism approach, without myeloablation or T cell depletion of the host [19]. Furthermore, Wekerle et al. have demonstrated in a recent landmark study that in the absence of cytoreductive therapy or any irradiation, induction of high levels of mixed chimerism and donor-specific transplantation tolerance could be achieved by combining high-dose bone marrow transplantation (BMT) with anti-CD154 mAb- and CTLA4Ig-mediated costimulatory blockade in a fully MHC-mismatched mouse skin transplant model [90]. The significance of costimulatory pathway blockade as a synergistic therapy in tolerance induction is underlined further by a recent report by Kawai et al., demonstrating the ameliorating effects of CD154 costimulatory blockade for the induction of mixed chimerism and renal allograft tolerance in a non-human primate model, by improving donor cell engraftment and facilitating long-term allograft survival without the need for splenectomy as part of a non-myeloablative conditioning regimen [91]. Attempts have also been made to arrive at potential clinical strategies that meet the temporal requirements of cadaveric organ transplantation: Wekerle et. al have reported a conditioning regimen consisting of a one-day protocol of bone marrow transplantation with costimulatory blockade, administered less than 24h prior to allogeneic skin transplantation, for the rapid induction of donor-specific graft tolerance [92]. These findings point to a potential applicability of such an approach to cadaveric organ transplantation.

The mechanisms underlying the synergistic tolerogenic effects of mixed chimerism and costimulatory blockade are subject of intensive investigation. Studies in CD28 -/- and CD40L-/- mice have suggested CD28 signal-mediated peripheral donor-reactive T cell deletion as a possible mechanism for CTLA4Ig-facilitated tolerance and inhibition of APC activation as a possible mechanism for anti-CD40L mAb-mediated tolerance [93]. These studies point to the co-existence of both central and peripheral deletional, and also regulatory mechanisms, in a tolerogenic regimen consisting of BMT and costimulatory blockade. Durham et al. have reported durable mixed hematopoetic chimerism and robust transplantation tolerance in a mouse allogeneic skin transplant model induced by donor bone marrow infusion combined with costimulatory blockade using solely anti-CD40L mAb, and found that tolerance in this model was at least in part mediated by the deletion of donor-reactive T cells [94]. Dissecting further the mechanisms underlying the synergistic tolerogenic effects of costimulatory blockade and hematopoetic chimerism, Bingaman et al. have found that CD40 and CD28 costimulatory blockade during adoptive transfer of allogeneic T cells into T cell deficient hematopoetic allochimeric mice facilitated long term acceptance of chimeric T cells and induced donor specific tolerance to skin allografts by specific peripheral deletion of alloreactive T cells [95]. Thus, allochimeric- and costimulatory blockade-mediated tolerogenic synergy likely involves both central and peripheral immune mechanisms.

The demonstration in animal models that allogeneic hematopoetic chimerism can be induced in the absence of toxic preconditioning regimen represents a critical advance towards the potential clinical applicability of such an approach in humans. Indeed, a recent case report directly demonstrates the immediate clinical relevance of the mixed chimerism approach to tolerance induction: Following an earlier observation of inadvertent induction of immunologic tolerance to renal allografts after bone marrow transplants from the same donors [96], Spitzer et al. have now reported tolerance to a renal allograft in a patient upon the deliberate induction of mixed lymphohematopoietic chimerism specifically aimed at treating a hematological malignancy and at providing allotolerance, after a nonmyeloablative preparative regimen [97].

Closest to clinical translation as a tolerogenic strategy, however, is costimulatory blockade. Indeed, preclinical studies in non-human primate islet allograft recipients, using CD80/CD86 – CD28/CTLA4 blockade [98] or CD40-CD40L blockade [99, 100], as well as renal non-human primate transplant recipients (synergistic costimulatory pathway blockade) [101] have indicated the efficacy of costimulatory blockade-based approaches, and provide the rationale to develop such strategies in human organ transplant recipients. In addition, after a decade of laboratory studies, CTLA4Ig now has been used in the clinical arena.

Abrams and others have recently published the results of a phase I clinical trial describing the immunosuppressive effects of CTLA4Ig in the T cell mediated autoimmune disease, psoriasis vulgaris [102]. This timely initial trial serves to underscore the possible application of costimulatory blockade to various clinical diseases, including transplant rejection [22]. Recent studies have therefore focused on developing strategies involving costimulatory pathway blockade in conjunction with conventional immunosuppressive agents that would facilitate initial clinical application of this approach, especially in the light of recent findings that agents such as cyclosporine A, tacrolimus and steroids may exhibit anti-tolerogenic effects.

Kirk et al. have reported synergistic effects of concurrent CD80/CD86 – CD28/CTLA4 and CD40 – CD40L blockade in a MHC disparate rhesus monkey renal transplantation model by inhibition of development of a donor-reactive antibody response which was observed when using CD40-CD40L blockade alone. Furthermore, when MMF, tacrolimus or chronic steroids were added to a CD40 – CD40L costimulatory blockade-based regimen, MMF, as opposed to tacrolimus and chronic steroids, exhibited the lowest degree of unwanted anti-tolerogenic effects, pointing to its potential usefulness as an initial clinical strategy [103]. Topham et al. have reported that addition of sirolimus, but not tacrolimus, to costimulatory blockade in a mouse cardiac allograft model resulted in suppression of induction of chemokine and chemokine receptor mediated signals for host T cell and macrophage recruitment and activation [104]. In addition, sirolimus, but not cyclosporine, when added to costimulatory blockade in a mouse skin allograft model, facilitated tolerance induction [56]. Other authors have found that addition of anti-CD3 immunotoxin to synergistic costimulatory blockade was effective in inducing tolerance in non-human primates [105]. This is particularly interesting as anti-CD3 immunotoxin, in another primate model, has been found tolerogenic in conjunction with DSG even in the absence of costimulatory blockade [106], thus pointing to tolerogenic synergy of these approaches. That costimulatory blockade involving anti-CD40L may not be entirely risk-free, however, was demonstrated by recent reports of potential prothrombotic effects of this agent in non-human primates (107), putting long-awaited clinical trials using CD40L-mediated costimulatory blockade on hold for now. Additional studies will provide us with further critical insights for the rational selection and combination of therapeutic modalities for trials involving costimulatory blockade.

Summary

The major shortcomings of modern transplantation medicine are the consequences of lifelong immunosuppression. Achievement of a state of immunologic tolerance, which would obviate the need for immuno-suppression, is more desirable. Ground-breaking advances in trans-plantation tolerance have been made which promise to facilitate translation of established experimental approaches to tolerance induction to humans in the near future. However, even when the most promising tolerogenic strategies are eventually being applied in clinical trials, we will still need to find ways in which to better assess the clinical tolerant state so that immunosuppressive agents may be withdrawn. Therefore, we must continue the process of defining transplantation tolerance in clinical, immunologic and molecular terms. Once we accomplish this task and develop the "tolerance assay", achievement of transplantation tolerance will become a clinical reality.

References

1. Kahan, B. D. 1989. Cyclosporine [see comments]. *N Engl J Med 321:1725.*
2. Denton, M. D., C. C. Magee, and M. H. Sayegh. 1999. Immunosuppressive strategies in transplantation. *Lancet 353:1083.*
3. Carpenter, C. B. 1995. Long-term failure of renal transplants: adding insult to injury. *Kidney Int Suppl 50:S40.*
4. Suthanthiran, M., and T. B. Strom. 1994. Renal transplantation [see comments]. *N Engl J Med 331:365.*
5. Billingham, R. E., L. Brent, and P. Medawar. 1953. Actively acquired tolerance to foreign cells, twin diagnosis and the Freemartin condition in cattle. *Nature 172:603.*
6. Nickerson, P. W., W. Steurer, J. Steiger, and T. B. Strom. 1994. In pursuit of the "holy grail": allograft tolerance. *Kidney Int Suppl 44:S40.*
7. Suthanthiran, M. 1996. Transplantation tolerance: fooling mother nature [comment]. *Proc Natl Acad Sci U S A 93:12072.*
8. Dong, V. M., K. L. Womer, and M. H. Sayegh. 1999. Transplantation tolerance: the concept and its applicability. *Pediatr Transplant 3:181.*
9. Sayegh, M. H., and C. B. Carpenter. 1997. Tolerance and chronic rejection. *Kidney Int Suppl 58:S11.*
10. Kappler, J. W., N. Roehm, and P. Marrack. 1987. T cell tolerance by clonal elimination in the thymus. *Cell 49:273.*
11. Davis, M. M., and P. J. Bjorkman. 1988. T cell antigen receptor genes and T cell recognition [published erratum appears in Nature 1988 Oct 20;335(6192):744]. *Nature 334:395.*
12. Sprent, J., E. K. Gao, and S. R. Webb. 1990. T cell reactivity to MHC molecules: immunity versus tolerance. *Science 248:1357.*
13. Blackman, M., J. Kappler, and P. Marrack. 1990. The role of the T cell receptor in positive and negative selection of developing T cells. *Science 248:1335.*
14. Anderson, G., N. C. Moore, J. J. Owen, and E. J. Jenkinson. 1996. Cellular interactions in thymocyte development. *Annu Rev Immunol 14:73.*
15. Van Parijs, L., and A. K. Abbas. 1998. Homeostasis and self-tolerance in the immune system: turning lymphocytes off. *Science 280:243.*
16. Charlton, B., H. Auchincloss, Jr., and C. G. Fathman. 1994. Mechanisms of transplantation tolerance. *Annu Rev Immunol 12:707.*
17. Ildstad, S. T., and D. H. Sachs. 1984. Reconstitution with syngeneic plus allogeneic or xenogeneic bone marrow leads to specific acceptance of allografts or xenografts. *Nature 307:168.*
18. Kawai, T., H. Sogawa, M. Koulmada, D. Ko, J. Oneal, S. L. Wee, R. N. Smith, H. Hong, D. Wu, R. B. Colvin, D. H. Sachs, H. Auchincloss, and A. B. Cosimi. 2000. Successful induction of tolerance of pancreatic islets between MHC-mismatched nonhuman primates. *Transplantation 69:A740.*
19. Wekerle, T., M. H. Sayegh, J. Hill, Y. Zhao, A. Chandraker, K. G. Swenson, G. Zhao, and M. Sykes. 1998. Extrathymic T cell deletion and allogeneic stem cell engraftment induced with costimulatory blockade is followed by central T cell tolerance. *J Exp Med 187:2037.*
20. Kawai, T., A. B. Cosimi, R. B. Colvin, J. Powelson, J. Eason, T. Kozlowski, M. Sykes, R. Monroy, M. Tanaka, and D. H. Sachs. 1995. Mixed allogeneic chimerism and renal allograft tolerance in cynomolgus monkeys. *Transplantation 59:256.*
21. Durham, M. M., A. W. Bingaman, A. B. Adams, J. Ha, S. Y. Waitze, T. C. Pearson, and C. P. Larsen. 2000. Cutting edge: administration of anti-CD40 ligand and donor bone marrow leads to hemopoietic chimerism and donor-specific tolerance without cytoreductive conditioning. *J Immunol 165:1.*

22. Sayegh, M. H. 1999. Finally, CTLA4Ig graduates to the clinic. *J Clin Invest 103:1223.*
23. Sayegh, M. H., and L. A. Turka. 1998. The role of T cell costimulatory activation pathways in transplant rejection. *N Engl J Med 338:1813.*
24. Schwartz, R. H. 1992. Costimulation of T lymphocytes: the role of CD28, CTLA-4, and B7/BB1 in interleukin-2 production and immunotherapy. *Cell 71:1065.*
25. Boussiotis, V. A., G. J. Freeman, G. Gray, J. Gribben, and L. M. Nadler. 1993. B7 but not intercellular adhesion molecule-1 costimulation prevents the induction of human alloantigen-specific tolerance. *J Exp Med 178:1753.*
26. Radvanyi, L. G., Y. Shi, H. Vaziri, A. Sharma, R. Dhala, G. B. Mills, and R. G. Miller. 1996. CD28 costimulation inhibits TCR-induced apoptosis during a primary T cell response. *J Immunol 156:1788.*
27. Linsley, P. S., W. Brady, M. Urnes, L. S. Grosmaire, N. K. Damle, and J. A. Ledbetter. 1991. CTLA-4 is a second receptor for the B cell activation antigen B7. *J Exp Med 174:561.*
28. Walunas, T. L., D. J. Lenschow, C. Y. Bakker, P. S. Linsley, G. J. Freeman, J. M. Green, C. B. Thompson, and J. A. Bluestone. 1994. CTLA-4 can function as a negative regulator of T cell activation. *Immunity 1:405.*
29. Walunas, T. L., C. Y. Bakker, and J. A. Bluestone. 1996. CTLA-4 ligation blocks CD28-dependent T cell activation [published erratum appears in J Exp Med 1996 Jul 1;184(1):301]. *J Exp Med 183:2541.*
30. Tivol, E. A., F. Borriello, A. N. Schweitzer, W. P. Lynch, J. A. Bluestone, and A. H. Sharpe. 1995. Loss of CTLA-4 leads to massive lymphoproliferation and fatal multiorgan tissue destruction, revealing a critical negative regulatory role of CTLA-4. *Immunity 3:541.*
31. Karandikar, N. J., C. L. Vanderlugt, T. L. Walunas, S. D. Miller, and J. A. Bluestone. 1996. CTLA-4: a negative regulator of autoimmune disease. *J Exp Med 184:783.*
32. Perez, V. L., L. Van Parijs, A. Biuckians, X. X. Zheng, T. B. Strom, and A. K. Abbas. 1997. Induction of peripheral T cell tolerance in vivo requires CTLA-4 engagement. *Immunity 6:411.*
33. Bluestone, J. A. 1997. Is CTLA-4 a master switch for peripheral T cell tolerance? *J Immunol 158:1989.*
34. Linsley, P. S., P. M. Wallace, J. Johnson, M. G. Gibson, J. L. Greene, J. A. Ledbetter, C. Singh, and M. A. Tepper. 1992. Immunosuppression in vivo by a soluble form of the CTLA-4 T cell activation molecule. *Science 257:792.*
35. Tan, P., C. Anasetti, J. A. Hansen, J. Melrose, M. Brunvand, J. Bradshaw, J. A. Ledbetter, and P. S. Linsley. 1993. Induction of alloantigen-specific hyporesponsiveness in human T lymphocytes by blocking interaction of CD28 with its natural ligand B7/BB1. *J Exp Med 177:165.*
36. Gimmi, C. D., G. J. Freeman, J. G. Gribben, G. Gray, and L. M. Nadler. 1993. Human T cell clonal anergy is induced by antigen presentation in the absence of B7 costimulation. *Proc Natl Acad Sci U S A 90:6586.*
37. Sayegh, M. H. 1999. Finally, CTLA4Ig graduates to the clinic [In Process Citation]. *J Clin Invest 103:1223.*
38. Russell, M. E., W. W. Hancock, E. Akalin, A. F. Wallace, T. Glysing-Jensen, T. A. Willett, and M. H. Sayegh. 1996. Chronic cardiac rejection in the LEW to F344 rat model. Blockade of CD28-B7 costimulation by CTLA4Ig modulates T cell and macrophage activation and attenuates arteriosclerosis. *J Clin Invest 97:833.*
39. Azuma, H., A. Chandraker, K. Nadeau, W. W. Hancock, C. B. Carpenter, N. L. Tilney, and M. H. Sayegh. 1996. Blockade of T cell costimulation prevents development of experimental chronic renal allograft rejection [see comments]. *Proc Natl Acad Sci U S A 93:12439.*

40. Chandraker, A., H. Azuma, K. Nadeau, C. B. Carpenter, N. L. Tilney, W. W. Hancock, and M. H. Sayegh. 1998. Late blockade of T cell costimulation interrupts progression of experimental chronic allograft rejection. *J Clin Invest 101:2309.*
41. Noelle, R. J. 1996. CD40 and its ligand in host defense. *Immunity 4:415.*
42. Marshall, L. S., A. Aruffo, J. A. Ledbetter, and R. J. Noelle. 1993. The molecular basis for T cell help in humoral immunity: CD40 and its ligand, gp39. *J Clin Immunol 13:165.*
43. DiSanto, J. P., J. Y. Bonnefoy, J. F. Gauchat, A. Fischer, and G. de Saint Basile. 1993. CD40 ligand mutations in x-linked immunodeficiency with hyper-IgM [see comments]. *Nature 361:541.*
44. Grewal, I. S., J. Xu, and R. A. Flavell. 1995. Impairment of antigen-specific T cell priming in mice lacking CD40 ligand. *Nature 378:617.*
45. Grewal, I. S., H. G. Foellmer, K. D. Grewal, J. Xu, F. Hardardottir, J. L. Baron, C. A. Janeway, Jr., and R. A. Flavell. 1996. Requirement for CD40 ligand in costimulation induction, T cell activation, and experimental allergic encephalomyelitis. *Science 273:1864.*
46. Ranheim, E. A., and T. J. Kipps. 1993. Activated T cells induce expression of B7/BB1 on normal or leukemic B cells through a CD40-dependent signal. *J Exp Med 177:925.*
47. Klaus, S. J., L. M. Pinchuk, H. D. Ochs, C. L. Law, W. C. Fanslow, R. J. Armitage, and E. A. Clark. 1994. Costimulation through CD28 enhances T cell-dependent B cell activation via CD40-CD40L interaction. *J Immunol 152:5643.*
48. Hancock, W. W., M. H. Sayegh, X. G. Zheng, R. Peach, P. S. Linsley, and L. A. Turka. 1996. Costimulatory function and expression of CD40 ligand, CD80, and CD86 in vascularized murine cardiac allograft rejection. *Proc Natl Acad Sci U S A 93:13967.*
49. Larsen, C. P., D. Z. Alexander, D. Hollenbaugh, E. T. Elwood, S. C. Ritchie, A. Aruffo, R. Hendrix, and T. C. Pearson. 1996. CD40-gp39 interactions play a critical role during allograft rejection. Suppression of allograft rejection by blockade of the CD40-gp39 pathway. *Transplantation 61:4.*
50. Parker, D. C., D. L. Greiner, N. E. Phillips, M. C. Appel, A. W. Steele, F. H. Durie, R. J. Noelle, J. P. Mordes, and A. A. Rossini. 1995. Survival of mouse pancreatic islet allografts in recipients treated with allogeneic small lymphocytes and antibody to CD40 ligand. *Proc Natl Acad Sci U S A 92:9560.*
51. Judge, T. A., A. Tang, L. M. Spain, J. Deans-Gratiot, M. H. Sayegh, and L. A. Turka. 1996. The in vivo mechanism of action of CTLA4Ig. *J Immunol 156:2294.*
52. Judge, T. A., Z. Wu, X. G. Zheng, A. H. Sharpe, M. H. Sayegh, and L. A. Turka. 1999. The role of CD80, CD86, and CTLA4 in alloimmune responses and the induction of long-term allograft survival. *J Immunol 162:1947.*
53. Wells, A. D., X. C. Li, Y. Li, M. C. Walsh, X. X. Zheng, Z. Wu, G. Nunez, A. Tang, M. Sayegh, W. W. Hancock, T. B. Strom, and L. A. Turka. 1999. Requirement for T cell apoptosis in the induction of peripheral transplantation tolerance. *Nat Med 5:1303.*
54. Waldmann, H. 1999. Transplantation tolerance-where do we stand? *Nat Med 5:1245.*
55. Ferguson, T. A., and D. R. Green. 1999. T cells are just dying to accept grafts [news]. *Nat Med 5:1231.*
56. Li, Y., X. C. Li, X. X. Zheng, A. D. Wells, L. A. Turka, and T. B. Strom. 1999. Blocking both signal 1 and signal 2 of T cell activation prevents apoptosis of alloreactive T cells and induction of peripheral allograft tolerance. *Nat Med 5:1298.*
57. Sayegh, M. H., E. Akalin, W. W. Hancock, M. E. Russell, C. B. Carpenter, P. S. Linsley, and L. A. Turka. 1995. CD28-B7 blockade after alloantigenic challenge in vivo inhibits Th1 cytokines but spares Th2. *J Exp Med 181:1869.*

58. Hancock, W. W., R. Buelow, M. H. Sayegh, and L. A. Turka. 1998. Antibody-induced transplant arteriosclerosis is prevented by graft expression of anti-oxidant and anti-apoptotic genes. *Nat Med 4:1392.*

59. Zhou, P., G. L. Szot, Z. Guo, G. He, J. Wang, K. A. Newell, J. R. Thistlethwaite, J. A. Bluestone, and M. Alegre. 2000. Signaling through STAT4 or STAT6 is not required for acute allograft rejection or for the induction of tolerance by CTLA4-Ig treatment in a murine cardiac transplant model. *Tranplantation 69:A1026.*

60. Dong, V. M., K. Kishimoto, A. Exeni, A. Yamada, A. Waaga, D. Briscoe, H. Auchincloss, M. J. Grusby, S. J. Khoury, and M. H. Sayegh. 2000. The differential role of CD28-B7 versus CD40L-CD40 in regulating alloimmune responses in STAT4 versus STAT6 gene knockout mice. *Transplantation 69:A1027.*

61. Dai, Z., B. Konieczny, and F. G. Lakkis. 2000. Generation and maintanance of allospecific CD8+ memory T cells in the absence of interleukin-2. *Transplantation 69:A1024.*

62. Larsen, C. P., E. T. Elwood, D. Z. Alexander, S. C. Ritchie, R. Hendrix, C. Tucker-Burden, H. R. Cho, A. Aruffo, D. Hollenbaugh, P. S. Linsley, K. J. Winn, and T. C. Pearson. 1996. Long-term acceptance of skin and cardiac allografts after blocking CD40 and CD28 pathways. *Nature 381:434.*

63. Lin, H., S. F. Bolling, P. S. Linsley, R. Q. Wei, D. Gordon, C. B. Thompson, and L. A. Turka. 1993. Long-term acceptance of major histocompatibility complex mismatched cardiac allografts induced by CTLA4Ig plus donor-specific transfusion. *J Exp Med 178:1801.*

64. Chandraker, A., M. E. Russell, T. Glysing-Jensen, T. A. Willett, and M. H. Sayegh. 1997. T cell costimulatory blockade in experimental chronic cardiac allograft rejection: effects of cyclosporine and donor antigen. *Transplantation 63:1053.*

65. Sayegh, M. H., X. G. Zheng, C. Magee, W. W. Hancock, and L. A. Turka. 1997. Donor antigen is necessary for the prevention of chronic rejection in CTLA4Ig-treated murine cardiac allograft recipients. *Transplantation 64:1646.*

66. Jones, N. D., A. Van Maurik, M. Hara, B. M. Spriewald, O. Witzke, P. J. Morris, and K. J. Wood. 2000. CD40-CD40L independent activation of CD8+ T cells can trigger allograft rejection. *Transplantation 69:A1152.*

67. Szot, G. L., P. Zhou, J. Wang, Z. Guo, K. A. Newell, J. R. Thistlethwaite, J. A. Bluestone, and M. Alegre. 2000. Role of CD8+ T cells in cardiac allograft rejection in wild-type and CD28-deficient mice. *Transplantation 69:A1054.*

68. Li, Y., X. C. Li, A. Coyle, J. Carlos, A. Ima, X. X. Zheng, and T. B. Strom. 2000. CD8+ dependent allograft rejection is resistant to conventional costimulation blockade: Emerging therapies. *Transplantation 69:A1153.*

69. Hutloff, A., A. M. Dittrich, K. C. Beier, B. Eljaschewitsch, R. Kraft, I. Anagnostopoulos, and R. A. Kroczek. 1999. ICOS is an inducible T cell co-stimulator structurally and functionally related to CD28. *Nature 397:263.*

70. Sayegh, M. H., B. Watschinger, and C. B. Carpenter. 1994. Mechanisms of T cell recognition of alloantigen. The role of peptides. *Transplantation 57:1295.*

71. Shoskes, D. A., and K. J. Wood. 1994. Indirect presentation of MHC antigens in transplantation. *Immunol Today 15:32.*

72. Magee, C. C., and M. H. Sayegh. 1997. Peptide-mediated immunosuppression. *Curr Opin Immunol 9:669.*

73. Sayegh, M. H., and A. M. Krensky. 1996. Novel immunotherapeutic strategies using MHC derived peptides. *Kidney Int Suppl 53:S13.*

74. Boytim, M. L., S. C. Lyu, R. Jung, A. M. Krensky, and C. Clayberger. 1998. Inhibition of cell cycle progression by a synthetic peptide corresponding to residues 65-79 of an HLA class II sequence: functional similarities but mechanistic differences with the immunosuppressive drug rapamycin. *J Immunol 160:2215.*

75. Murphy, B., C. C. Magee, S. I. Alexander, A. M. Waaga, H. W. Snoeck, J. P. Vella, C. B. Carpenter, and M. H. Sayegh. 1999. Inhibition of allorecognition by a

human class II MHC-derived peptide through the induction of apoptosis. *J Clin Invest 103:859.*

76. Sayegh, M. H., S. J. Khoury, W. W. Hancock, H. L. Weiner, and C. B. Carpenter. 1992. Induction of immunity and oral tolerance with polymorphic class II major histocompatibility complex allopeptides in the rat. *Proc Natl Acad Sci U S A 89:7762.*

77. Ciubotariu, R., Z. Liu, A. I. Colovai, E. Ho, S. Itescu, S. Ravalli, M. A. Hardy, R. Cortesini, E. A. Rose, and N. Suciu-Foca. 1998. Persistent allopeptide reactivity and epitope spreading in chronic rejection of organ allografts. *J Clin Invest 101:398.*

78. Vella, J. P., M. Spadafora-Ferreira, B. Murphy, S. I. Alexander, W. Harmon, C. B. Carpenter, and M. H. Sayegh. 1997. Indirect allorecognition of major histocompatibility complex allopeptides in human renal transplant recipients with chronic graft dysfunction. *Transplantation 64:795.*

79. Perez, J., J. Yu, P. Song, S. Stepkowski, and B. D. Kahan. 1999. Class I MHC protein tolerogens for rat cardiac allografts across major histocompatibility barriers. *Transplantation 67:A241.*

80. Behrens, D., K. Lange, M. Krönke, and N. Zavazava. 1999. Soluble, recombinant MHC class I molecules induce indefinite graft survival. *Transplantation 67:A249.*

81. Garrovillo, M., A. Ali, and S. F. Oluwole. 1999. Indirect allorecognition in acquired thymic tolerance: induction of donor-specific tolerance to rat cardiac allografts by allopeptide-pulsed host dendritic cells. *Transplantation 68:1827.*

82. Ali, A., M. Garrovillo, O. O. Oluwole, R. Gopinathan, H. A. DePaz, M. X. Jin, M. A. Hardy, and S. F. Oluwole. 2000. Mechanisms of acquired thymic tolerance: Induction of transplant tolerance by intrathymic injection of in vivo allopeptide primed alloreactive host T cells. *Transplantation 69:A1084.*

83. Shirwan, H., A. Mhoyan, and I. Sherif. 2000. Prevention of chronic rejection with immunoregulatory cells induced by intrathymic immune modulation with class I MHC allopeptides. *Transplantation 69:A129.*

84. Quingsheng, J., J. Yu, C. B. Carpenter, M. H. Sayegh, and B. Murphy. 2000. Induction of apoptosis by a MHC class II derived peptide through a caspase independent pathway. *Transplantation 69:A880.*

85. Li, Y., X. X. Zheng, X. C. Li, M. S. Zand, and T. B. Strom. 1998. Combined costimulation blockade plus rapamycin but not cyclosporine produces permanent engraftment. *Transplantation 66:1387.*

86. Fuchimoto, Y., C. A. Huang, K. Yamada, A. Shimizu, H. Kitamura, R. B. Colvin, V. Ferrara, M. C. Murphy, M. Sykes, M. White-Scharf, D. M. Neville, Jr., and D. H. Sachs. 2000. Mixed chimerism and tolerance without whole body irradiation in a large animal model [see comments]. *J Clin Invest 105:1779.*

87. Asiedu, C. K., W. Wang, and J. M. Thomas. 1999. Cyclosporine A suppresses the tolerogenic effect of donor bone marrow cells by inhibiting TGF-beta1-mediated apoptosis. *Transplantation 67:A1027.*

88. Hale, D. A., A. Umemura, R. Gottschalk, T. Maki, and A. P. Monaco. 1999. Mechanistic characterization of tolerance induced with ALS, donor bone marrow and sirolimus. *Transplantation 67:A272.*

89. Jaeger, M. D., T. Tsui, O. S. Lauth, M. H. Dahlke, A. Deiwick, M. Neipp, K. Wonigeit, and H. J. Schlitt. 2000. A new conditioning protocol for fully MHC-mismatched bone marrow transplantation consisting only of an alloantibody against CD45 as basis for donor-specific tolerance in the rat. *Transplantation 69:A992.*

90. Wekerle, T., J. Kurtz, H. Ito, J. V. Ronquillo, V. Dong, G. Zhao, J. Shaffer, M. H. Sayegh, and M. Sykes. 2000. Allogeneic bone marrow transplantation with co-stimulatory blockade induces macrochimerism and tolerance without cytoreductive host treatment. *Nat Med 6:464.*

91. Kawai, T., G. Abrahamian, H. Sogawa, S. L. Wee, S. Boskovic, O. Nadazdin, D. Andrews, S. Mauiyyedi, H. Hong, D. Wu, J. Phelan, D. Weymouth, D. Ko, R. B. Colvin, D. H. Sachs, and A. B. Cosimi. 2000. Costimulatory blockade for induction of mixed chimerism and renal allograft tolerance in non-human primates. *Transplantation 69:A991.*

92. Wekerle, T., M. H. Sayegh, H. Ito, J. Hill, A. Chandraker, D. A. Pearson, K. G. Swenson, G. Zhao, and M. Sykes. 1999. Anti-CD154 or CTLA4Ig obviates the need for thymic irradiation in a non-myeloablative conditioning regimen for the induction of mixed hematopoietic chimerism and tolerance. *Transplantation 68:1348.*

93. Kurtz, J., T. Wekerle, H. Ito, J. Shaffer, and M. Sykes. 1999. An unexpected role for CD28 and lack of a role for CD40L signaling in peripheral deletion of donor-reactive CD4+ T cells and establishment of mixed chimerism through costimulatory blockade. *Transplantation 67:A453.*

94. Durham, M. M., A. W. Bingaman, A. B. Adams, J. Ha, T. C. Pearson, and C. P. Larsen. 2000. Administration of repeated doses of anti-CD40L and donor bone marrow leads to hematopoietic chimerism and donor specific tolerance without cytoreductive conditioning. *Transplantation 69:A494.*

95. Bingaman, A. W., M. M. Durham, A. B. Adams, J. Ha, T. C. Pearson, and C. P. Larsen. 2000. Hematopoietic chimerism in the presence of CD40 and CD28 blockade leads to peripheral deletion of donor reactive T cells and development of donor specific transplantation tolerance. *Transplantation 69:A495.*

96. Sayegh, M. H., N. A. Fine, J. L. Smith, H. G. Rennke, E. L. Milford, and N. L. Tilney. 1991. Immunologic tolerance to renal allografts after bone marrow transplants from the same donors [see comments]. *Ann Intern Med 114:954.*

97. Spitzer, T. R., F. Delmonico, N. Tolkoff-Rubin, S. McAfee, R. Sackstein, S. Saidman, C. Colby, M. Sykes, D. H. Sachs, and A. B. Cosimi. 1999. Combined histocompatibility leukocyte antigen-matched donor bone marrow and renal transplantation for multiple myeloma with end stage renal disease: the induction of allograft tolerance through mixed lymphohematopoietic chimerism. *Transplantation 68:480.*

98. Levisetti, M. G., P. A. Padrid, G. L. Szot, N. Mittal, S. M. Meehan, C. L. Wardrip, G. S. Gray, D. S. Bruce, J. R. Thistlethwaite, Jr., and J. A. Bluestone. 1997. Immunosuppressive effects of human CTLA4Ig in a non-human primate model of allogeneic pancreatic islet transplantation. *J Immunol 159:5187.*

99. Kenyon, N. S., M. Chatzipetrou, M. Masetti, A. Ranuncoli, M. Oliveira, J. L. Wagner, A. D. Kirk, D. M. Harlan, L. C. Burkly, and C. Ricordi. 1999. Long-term survival and function of intrahepatic islet allografts in rhesus monkeys treated with humanized anti-CD154. *Proc Natl Acad Sci U S A 96:8132.*

100. Kenyon, N. S., L. A. Fernandez, R. Lehmann, M. Masetti, A. Ranuncoli, M. Chatzipetrou, G. Iaria, D. Han, J. L. Wagner, P. Ruiz, M. Berho, L. Inverardi, R. Alejandro, D. H. Mintz, A. D. Kirk, D. M. Harlan, L. C. Burkly, and C. Ricordi. 1999. Long-term survival and function of intrahepatic islet allografts in baboons treated with humanized anti-CD154. *Diabetes 48:1473.*

101. Kirk, A. D., D. M. Harlan, N. N. Armstrong, T. A. Davis, Y. Dong, G. S. Gray, X. Hong, D. Thomas, J. H. Fechner, Jr., and S. J. Knechtle. 1997. CTLA4-Ig and anti-CD40 ligand prevent renal allograft rejection in primates. *Proc Natl Acad Sci U S A 94:8789.*

102. Abrams, J. R., M. G. Lebwohl, C. A. Guzzo, B. V. Jegasothy, M. T. Goldfarb, B. S. Goffe, A. Menter, N. J. Lowe, G. Krueger, M. J. Brown, R. S. Weiner, M. J. Birkhofer, G. L. Warner, K. K. Berry, P. S. Linsley, J. G. Krueger, H. D. Ochs, S. L. Kelley, and S. Kang. 1999. CTLA4Ig-mediated blockade of T cell costimulation in patients with psoriasis vulgaris. *J Clin Invest 103:1243.*

103. Kirk, A. D., L. C. Burkly, D. S. Batty, R. E. Baumgartner, J. D. Berning, K. Buchanan, J. H. Fechner, Jr., R. L. Germond, R. L. Kampen, N. B. Patterson, S. J.

Swanson, D. K. Tadaki, C. N. TenHoor, L. White, S. J. Knechtle, and D. M. Harlan. 1999. Treatment with humanized monoclonal antibody against CD154 prevents acute renal allograft rejection in nonhuman primates [see comments]. *Nat Med 5:686.*

104. Topham, P. S., Y. Li, T. B. Strom, and W. W. Hancock. 1999. Choosing rational combinations of therapeutic agents: Contrasting effects of costimulation blockade plus rapamycin or cyclosporine on intragraft expression of chemokines, chemokine receptors and apoptotic genes. *Transplantation 67:A455.*

105. Knechtle, S. J., A. D. Kirk, J. H. Fechner, Jr., X. Hong, Y. Dong, M. M. Hamawy, and D. M. Harlan. 1999. Inducing unresponsiveness by the use of anti-CD3 immunotoxin, CTLA4-Ig, and anti-CD40 ligand. *Transplant Proc 31:27S.*

106. Thomas, J. M., J. L. Contreras, X. L. Jiang, D. E. Eckhoff, P. X. Wang, W. J. Hubbard, A. L. Lobashevsky, W. Wang, C. Asiedu, S. Stavrou, W. J. Cook, M. L. Robbin, F. T. Thomas, and D. M. Neville, Jr. 1999. Peritransplant tolerance induction in macaques: early events reflecting the unique synergy between immunotoxin and deoxyspergualin. *Transplantation 68:1660.*

107. Kawai, T., D. Andrews, R. B. Colvin, D. H. Sachs, and A. B. Cosimi. 2000. Thromboembolic complications after treatment with monoclonal antibody against CD40 ligand [In Process Citation]. *Nat Med 6:114.*

PART FOUR: GENE THERAPY

MOLECULAR MEDICINE IN ORGAN TRANSPLANTATION: HOW AND WHEN?

Ariela Benigni, Norberto Perico, and Giuseppe Remuzzi

Introduction

Short-term graft survival has been remarkably improved in the past two decades thanks to increased skill coupled with new immuno-suppressants. Although 1 year graft survival is now close to 85-90%, at least for cadaver kidney transplant, long-term results are less impress-sive [1] despite recent data open new hopes. Data from the UNOS registry in more than 93,000 patients who had a renal transplant between the years 1988-1996 showed a projected graft half-life of 21.6 years living and 13.8 years for cadaver donors, respectively [S. Hariharan, personal communication]. The remark-able success is mostly related to the ability of new anti-rejection drugs to limit acute rejections within the first year post surgery. Whether these important findings can be extended also to other transplants is unknown at the present, so that up to now the half-life for most organs other than kidney is only 9.9 years, with no substantial improvement over the past 20 years. Medications moreover have to be given long-life, which invariably impairs systemic immunity translating in more risk of infections and cancers. Tumors of viral origin, including non-Hodgkin's lymphoma, squamous cell-carcinoma of the skin, and Kaposi's sarcoma are 6.5 times more common in transplant recipients than in the general population [2], and their frequency is estimated to increase with time. The future goal of transplant medicine is therefore to induce donor-specific unresponsiveness to alloantigens rather than focus on more potent antirejection molecules as it was done for the past few years. Animals have been rendered tolerant to transplant antigens by various

Mohamed Sayegh and Giuseppe Remuzzi (editors), Current and Future
Immunosuppressive Therapies Following Transplantation, 317-334.
© 2001 Kluwer Academic Publishers. Printed in the Netherlands.

means, and even patients, can occasionally tolerate liver or kidney graft [3], indicating that this is a pursuable goal.

More and more sophisticated knowledge of the basic mechanism of host-immune response to alloantigens paralleled in the recent years technical advances in the development of strategies to transfer genes into mammalian cells. This represents a tremendous opportunity for approaching tolerance induction by gene transfer techniques. Gene therapy can be targeted to recipient's organs involved in modulating immune response or to hematopoietic cell precursors. Systems to insert specific genes into donor organs *ex vivo* before they are actually transplanted have also been developed. All these strategies are currently been explored in animals with the perspective of inducing donor-antigen-specific tolerance or restricting the immune-incompetence locally with no need of systemic immunosuppression.

Targeting the Recipient's Immune Organs or Tissues

To preserve the integrity of the host, the immune system responds to foreign antigens but remains unresponsive to its own molecules. In mammals, tolerance to self-antigens is established perinatally or early after birth, and actively involves the thymus, where maturing thymocytes are exposed to self-proteins before migrating as mature lymphocytes to peripheral lymphoid tissues. In the thymus, antigen recognition occurs after processing and presentation of the protein in the context of molecules of the major histocompatibility complex on the surface of antigen-presenting cells (APCs)/dendritic cells to specific receptor of immature thymocytes termed "T cell receptor" (TCR). Engagement of TCR on immature thymocytes appears to play a critical role, both during the development of those T cells bearing receptors appropriate for foreign antigen and in the deletion of potentially harmful self-reactive T cells.

Of interest intrathymic recognition of alloantigens also prevents maturing T cells from reacting to the same allopeptides in the periphery to the extent that subsequent islet or kidney grafts survived indefinitely when pancreatic islets or isolated glomeruli from the same rodent donor were implanted in the thymus of an incompatible recipients [4,5]. Indefinite survival and antigen-specific unresponsiveness to cardiac, liver, and small bowel allografts in adult rats has been achieved by intrathymic inoculation of donor cells, even in high-responder donor-recipient rat combination [6-9]. Similarly, intrathymic injection of donor cells can prolong survival of skin allografts and xenografts murine models [10,11].

Findings that intrathymic inoculation of cell membrane extracts induced donor-specific tolerance to rat organ allografts as well as islets indicate that the tolerogenic effect of solute antigen is independent of the presence of intact cells [12]. Reports are also available that intrathymic inoculation of synthetic polymorphic class II or class I MHC allopeptides can induce donor-specific unresponsiveness to syngeneic organ transplant when injected into an allogeneic recipient [13,14]. Both donor cells and MHC allopeptides however can sensitize the recipients in case of leakage into the systemic circulation during the maneuver of intrathymic injection. Synthetic peptides, in addition, will never mimic the entire MHC and thus its relative antigenicity would render tolerogenic efforts, based on such strategy, hopeless for future clinical application. Cells made transgenic to express the desired donor antigens would theoretically be preferable to naive donor cells or synthetic allopeptides. Few experiments have been done already in this regards. Thus injecting the thymus of rat recipients with autologous muscle cells genetically modified to express donor-type MHC class I prolonged liver allograft survival, or in some instance even induced tolerance [15]. The specificity of the thymic approach rests on data that transgenic cells never induce tolerance if given intravenously or intraperitoneally. To which extent this method is feasible for clinical application, remains, however, ill defined. One emerging problem with such approach is the nature of the antigen expressed by transgenic cells which may become a critical factor for the success of the entire procedure. Indeed thymic implantation of genetically modified fibroblasts prevents tolerization toward the corresponding soluble fibroblast gene product, which would certainly depend on the level of gene expression but even more on the soluble nature of the product [16].

Direct gene transfer into the recipient thymus of plasmid cDNA encoding donor MHC class I was recently attempted to take advantage of the tolerogenic potential of exposing maturing ï cells to relevant alloantigens while reducing at the same time the rate of non-success and side effects [17]. Plasmid MHC class I DNA injected into the thymus elicited a transient gene expression but sufficient to prolong subsequent liver allograft to induce tolerance in 70% of the rat recipients [17]. While promising, this approach still has specific problems, the antigenic disparity between donor and recipient being a major issue. Dominant alloantigens indeed vary with organs as shown for MHC class I in the liver [18] rather than MHC class II in renal graft rejection [13]. Tolerogenic strategies based on intrathymic cDNA need validation in organs other than liver which by itself has a remarkable tolerogenic potential [19]. In the past years the intrathymic approach has been used to try and induce tolerance to the adenoviral vectors in an attempt to prevent the immune response elicited by the vectors when they are delivered to the periphery [20,21]. Data showed that induction of central tolerance by intrathymic inoculation of adenoviral vector carrying the gene for human bilirubin-UGT-1 (hBUGT), the only enzyme that significantly contributes to bilirubin glucuronidation in human liver, into Gunn rats - an animal model of human Crigler-Najjar syndrome type I - permitted long-term gene expression by repeated administration of the virus [21]. Both the appearance of neutralizing antibodies and cytotoxic lymphocytes against the recombinant adenovirus were markedly inhibited. Whether thymic-dependent strategies will become in the near future a major approach for tolerance induction in human, is still far from clear. An obvious question related to the applicability of acquired thymic tolerance to humans is the best patient population that would benefit for, or for whom the thymic strategy would be technically feasible. Thus it may be that acquired thymic unresponsiveness will prove useful in selected subpopulation like pediatric patients, where the thymus has not been completely involuted yet. Living transplants are also good candidates since sufficient time can be allowed to the necessary DNA manipulations, since donor MHC specificity can easily be determined in advance.

Targeting Hematopoietic Precursor/Dendritic Cells of Donor or Host Origin

It has been proposed that organ transplant implies a migratory flux of donor "passenger " leukocytes out of the graft into the recipient tissues or organ, serving to establish a persistent condition of "microchimerism", and being a tolerogenic precursor of chimeric cells. Although there is evidence that the same migratory mechanism applies to all organ grafts, migration of passenger leukocytes is less in organs other than the liver, such as the kidney and heart. To enhance the acceptance of organs less tolerogenic than the liver, perioperative infusion of donor bone marrow has been attempted to increase the migration of donor leukocytes of bone marrow origin. Such peripheral donor microchimerism not only appears associated with long-term acceptance of the allograft, but it is suggested to play an active role in mitigating host immune-reactivity to graft antigens [3]. The novel modality of gene transfer is currently being used to monitor bone marrow-derived cell engraftment as recently done for multiple myeloma and breast cancer [22]. Beside assessing engraftment by gene transfer techniques, one may try to induce tolerance thanks to the properties of hematopoietic precursor cells to self-renew and remain long-enough in the circulation of the host. Here the ratio between the relatively small number of transfected hematopoietic precursors and the large population of host cell will be a crucial issue to engraftment success. Studies will possibly be designed in the future to confer growth advantage to genetically modified progenitor cells [23]. Gene transfer has used to explore the molecular mechanism by which bone marrow cells injected into immune-incompetent mice can promote tolerance, as shown by transfecting donor bone marrow cells with the Fas ligand gene which appears instrumental to the purpose [24].

Since a decade ago blood transfusion has been the most common source of alloantigens used in clinical transplantation as a means to modulate immune response to allograft. The risk associated with the use of blood products from unrelated subjects provided, however, the rationale for searching alternative strategies for antigen delivery at pre- or peri-transplant period. Among these, an elegant approach implies the use of recipient bone marrow as a vehicle for donor antigen delivery *in vivo*. Sykes and coworkers [25] were the first to report transduction of recipient bone marrow cells to express a donor MHC gene in a protocol in mice designed to induce tolerance to skin allograft. They also found that nonmyeloablative protocols facilitate engraftment of the transduced bone marrow cells [26]. Expression of donor MHC genes in recipient's bone marrow cells may also facilitate the development of tolerance in fully mismatched vascularized organ grafts and strategies have been designed to transfect selective MHC genes into recipient cells that serve as vehicle for alloantigen delivery before transplantation. Combining anti-CD4 monoclonal antibody, an agent that modulates T cell function, with recipient bone marrow cells expressing single donor MHC locus products further promoted the operational tolerance in the above models [27]. Recipient murine bone marrow cells transduced with a replication defective retrovirus encoding a donor MHC class I gene induced indefinite survival of fully allogeneic cardiac grafts in 50% of recipients (28,29), another example of linked unresponsiveness *in vivo*. This approach has also been evaluated in a pig kidney model. Here three out of six miniature swines, whose autologous bone marrow cells were transduced with a single donor MHC class II cDNA, had a markedly prolonged survival of a subsequent kidney allograft mis-matched for multiple alloantigens compared with controls [30]. Transfer of swine MHC II into autologous bone marrow cells of baboons resulted in a prolongation of skin and renal graft survival in baboons, opening new perspectives of gene therapy in the induction of tolerance in xenograft [31].

Beside bone marrow cells, dendritic cells (DC) have also been described to down regulate immune response [32]. This property adds to the more common activity of dendritic cells, a special subset of antigen presenting cells, to highly activate immunologically naive T cells. It has been shown that repeated activation of T cells by DC triggers 'fratricidal' death by a CD95/CD95L-dependent mechanism, a phenomenon known as activation-induced cell death [33]. Interactions of CD95 (Fas) with its ligand CD95L (FasL) are thought to play a major role in the maintenance of immunological homeostasis and peripheral tolerance by leading to T cell apoptosis. CD95 is expressed by many cell types, mainly after stimulation. Immunologically naive T cells express little or no detectable CD95, whereas they acquire its expression rapidly after activation by antigen pulsed DC, becoming susceptible to CD95 / CD95L-induced apoptosis [34]. In contrast CD95L is expressed by selected cell types including immunocompetent leukocytes (such as activated T cells, natural killer cells, macrophages and perhaps certain DC cell subsets). It has been recently reported that DC engineered to over-express CD95L might deliver death signals, instead of activation signal to T cells after antigen-specific interaction, thereby leading to the depletion of antigen-reactive T cells [32]. A recent study has documented that injection of antigen-pulsed autologous skin DC, transfected with CD95 cDNA, into mice before sensitization with the antigen ovoalbumin induced antigen-specific immunosuppression as shown by preventing of delayed-type hypersensitivity responses [32]. These findings suggest that the CD95L-transfected DC technology might be translatable into a new form of immune suppressive therapy designed to reduce the frequency of the alloreactive T cells that recognize given antigens. Whether this approach can be extended to organ transplantation with the aim of inducing tolerance to allograft will be tested soon.

Thus despite encouraging initial results, research in the area of manipulating donor bone marrow-derived cells or dendritic cells to prolong survival of organ transplant is still at a very primitive stage at the moment.

Targeting Syngeneic Genetically Modified Non-Hematopoietic Cells Together with the Graft

Gene transfer strategies offer the possibility of delivering molecules with immunomodulating activity to defined sites in the recipient. Combined transplantation of genetically modified cells with the graft is a way for biologically active molecules to reach their relevant target. These carrier cells, however, should be easy to transfect, allow a rather stable expression of the gene of interest, long-term survival and have not to produce toxic substances that might compromise the function of the combined graft transplant. In this respect myoblasts, unlike many other populations of primary cells, fulfil all these requirements and have been used alongside the pancreatic islets to prevent graft rejection [35,36]. Syngeneic myoblasts transfected with plasmid cDNA encoding the fusion protein CTLA4Ig - an inhibitor of antigen presenting cell / Tcell costimulatory interaction - co-transplanted with islet allograft under the kidney capsule of the recipient mice significantly prolonged mean graft survival up to 31 days [36]. Moreover, expression of FasL by the syngeneic myoblasts to protect allogeneic islets from rejection in a mouse model of diabetes, reversed the diabetes state for an even longer period [35].

Although promising, it appears, however, that this approach would have limited potential application, probably restricted to cellular graft such as the pancreatic islets.

Delivery of Genes to Donor Graft Itself

The need to target and restrict immunosuppression to the isolated organ before transplantation has stimulated approaches based on local delivery of immunomodulating genes whose protein products can limit antigen presenting T cell interaction as an alternative to systemic treatments.

The first studies of this type focussed on transfection of genes encoding TGF-b or interleukin-10 (IL-10), cytokines with immunoregulatory activity that down-regulate immune response. Thus, in a murine cardiac transplantation model, allografts injected with plasmid encoding TGF-b1 under the control of the SV40 promoter, survived 26 days compared with 12 day survival for allografts injected with the control plasmid [37]. Injection of a retroviral vector encoding viral IL-10 further prolonged cardiac graft survival up to 36 days without any toxic effect [37]. A modest effect was also achieved with an adenoviral vector encoding IL-10 on cardiac allograft survival after intracoronary perfusion with the viral vector [38]. Co-transfer of TGF-b and IL-10 genes by adenoviral vector to canine islet cells also served to enhance early islet graft function as well as to prolong graft survival in rats [39]. *Ex vivo* perfusion experiments delivering TGF-b1 to the liver using adenoviral vectors have also been performed in order to down regulate the immune response after transplantation, but the results are too preliminary to reach any solid conclusion [40]. Induction of local production of the p40 subunit of IL-12, that blocks the action of IL-12, suppressed T helper-1-mediated immune responses and prevented allogenic myoblast rejection [41]. Given the ability of TGF-b in some circumstances to promote cell proliferation [42], however, such strategy may have side effects. On the other hand, the use of viral IL-10 to modulate the immune response by direct delivery to the graft may be strictly dependent on the level of viral IL-10 expression achieved to the extent that in human pancreatic islets transfected with adenovirus carrying IL-10 gene *in vitro* proliferative response to T cells was enhanced at low concentration of expression, whereas it was inhibited at high concentration [43].

Acute rejection of the graft is always accompanied by high levels of interstitial leukocyte infiltration. The initial stage of leukocyte migration into tissues at the site of an inflammatory response depends on enhanced expression of adhesion molecules that interact with their ligands on the surface of endothelial and other cells (tubular epithelial cells in the case of kidney) [44]. In addition, antigen-nonspecific adhesion molecules promote the attachment of T cells to their 'professional' APC and transduce regulatory signals to the T cells upon TCR binding to specific MHC peptides [45]. Several adhesion molecule/ligand pairs have been described and characterized, but those involving intercellular adhesion molecule-1 (ICAM-1) and its ligand leukocyte function-associated antigen-1 (LFA-1) and LFA-3/CD3 interaction are probably the most important in the graft rejection process [46]. Antisense oligodeoxynucleotides will soon offer a major investigational tool to clarify the relevance of adhesion molecule in the above setting. Data are already available that an antisense oligodeoxynucleotide, which hybridizes to the 3'-end ICAM-1 mRNA, actually lowers gene expression of ICAM-1 in rat endothelial cells in culture [47] activated by interferon. *In vivo* the same product dose-dependently prolonged heart and kidney allograft survival in rats [47]. Remarkably similar results have been obtained with the human oligodeoxynucleotide antisense ICAM-1 in monkey recipients of a kidney allograft [48]. The above are still systemic approaches that down-regulate expression of ICAM-1 in all vascular beds, more than simply in the transplanted organ.

Possibly more relevant to the future of transplant medicine are findings that pre-transplant exposure of rat kidneys to antisense oligodeoxynucleotide for ICAM-1 inhibited in a rather specific fa-shion intragraft ICAM-1 expression which did prevent delayed graft function, and immune response to MHC class II antigens [49].

Signals generated through the T cell receptor are not sufficient for full activation of T cells. Additional antigen-nonspecific costimulatory signals through particular molecules on the surface of T lymphocytes are required for Il-2 production, cell proliferation and differentiation to effector function, otherwise T cells are anergized [50]. T cells circulating in the graft can therefore be rendered anergic to transplant antigens, at least theoretically, by local transfer of genes whose protein product by inhibiting costimulatory signals would block T cell activation. Rat recipients of livers transduced with an adenovirus vector bearing murine CTLA4-Ig cDNA had an unusually prolonged graft survival accompanied by donor-specific unresponsiveness *in vitro* [51]. Similarly, prolonged survival of rat cardiac [52,53] and murine pancreatic islet allografts [53] as well as of pancreatico-duodenal grafts in rats [54,55] has been achieved by adenoviral CTLA4Ig gene transfer. We recently succeeded in prolonging allograft survival by adenovirus-mediated transduction of cold-preserved rat kidney with sequences encoding CTLA4Ig wish no need of immunosuppression [56]. Organ expression of the transgene was achieved associated with mild infiltration of mononuclear cells in the transfected kidney. Mixed lymphocyte reaction as well as the production of both Th1 and Th2 cytokines were reduced [56]. Very recent data showed that a single *ex vivo* intra-aortic infusion of adenovirus encoding CTLA4Ig gene promoted indefinite survival of cardiac allografts in nonimmunosuppressed hosts. Interestingly, the beneficial effect of local immunosuppression on cardiac allograft survival was not accompanied by donor specific peripheral tolerance, since donor-strain skin graft were rejected by long term recipients of cardiac allografts [57].

With further refinements in gene transfer techniques similar approaches are expected to open exciting possibilities to control post transplant immunity via co-stimulatory molecule/receptor modulations.

Based on data that T cells activated to express Fas - a cell surface molecule belonging to the tumor necrosis factor family - undergo apoptosis on engagement with Fas ligand [58], gene transfer technique has been attempted targeting such system.

Transplantation of FasL expressing islets from transgenic mice resulted in their rapid destruction [59] which may be due to interaction and subsequent self destruction of Fas-expressing islets. However, gene transfer of FasL cDNA into rat renal grafts by a replication-defective adenoviral vector instead clearly prolonged graft survival beyond controls [60]. Similarly, the liver grafts induced to express FasL promoted apoptotic death of infiltrating lymphocytes and were protected from acute rejection [61]. Thus, the complexity of these pathways exposes to unpredictable outcomes. Attempts have been done recently to render pancreatic islets resistant to death, by transfection of adenoviral vector expressing antiapoptotic genes [62].

While most of gene transfer approaches attempted so far appeared somehow promising for reducing acute rejection, results on long term organ survival have been generally modest and the few positive findings rather difficult to reproduce. Gene transfer strategies have been used successfully to prevent chronic organ lesions in aortic and heart transplantation. Transduction of rat aorta with inducible nitric oxide synthase by adenoviral vector technique fully suppressed allograft arteriosclerosis, the key feature of chronic rejection [63]. Moreover, transfecting murine cardiac allografts with antisense cyclin-dependent kinase oligodeoxynucleotides substantially reduced intimal thickening of graft coronary arteries [64]. Additional applications of gene transfer technology to transplantation should consider the area of preventing injury of organs to be grafted. Bovine and porcine aortic endothelial cells in culture transfected with human superoxide dismutase and exposed to cold preservation survive better than unmanipulated cells [65]. Genetic cytoprotection of human endothelial cells during cold preservation has also been attempted with an adenovirus vector encoding the anti-apoptotic genes [66]. *In vivo* studies in mice found reduction of liver ischemia/reperfusion injury by human Bcl-2 gene transfer [67]. Other investigators found high expression of the transgene in rat livers perfused *ex vivo* with adenoviral vector encoding inducible nitric oxide [68]. These data would suggest that in the near future organs can be induced to generate more nitric oxide before transplantation and take advantage of its vasodilator and anti-apoptotic potential. Thus the technology of transferring exogenous genes to organ transplant has theoretically enormous investigational and therapeutic potential which would leave intact the overall competence of the immune system and inhibit the rejection process locally.

Toward Gene Therapy in Human Transplant Medicine

After an initial failure to meet expectations, gene therapy has now settled into a phase of more conservative but rather realistic achievements that appear definitely promising for the future [69]. Already clinical studies found that transferring genetic material to human target cells can exert biological effects [70,71]. However, as animal models have revealed, impediments remain. With current techniques the exogenous genes are transferred in an expression 'cassette', with a promoter that regulates expression of the gene of interest and stops signals to terminate translation [72]. The expression 'cassette' is transfected to target cells, organs or tissues using a 'vector' of viral or non-viral origin. Crucially required is a system that mediates local transfer and expression of the DNA of interest with a reliably high efficiency. Recombinant retroviral or adenoviral vectors to direct ex-pression of a protein product have been largely used so far. Retroviral gene transfer results in efficient, long-term gene expression with inte-gration into genomic DNA; however, this approach requires target cell proliferation which is not always feasible *in vivo*. Recombinant replica-tion-deficient adenovirus vectors instead deliver genes into dividing and nondividing cells, and can carry a large gene fragment and efficiently transfer DNA when high-titre viral stocks are employed as shown in the kidney [73]. Organs that are in any case stored and perfused *ex vivo* before transplantation can indeed be used to address whether adding adenoviral vectors to the perfusion fluid does enhance transfection efficiency. Recent data are available that, by pretransplant perfusion procedure, adenoviral vectors can effectively transmit their cDNA into the kidney better than with direct injection with a clear advantage in transfection efficiency [74]. Such procedure easily can be performed during organ harvesting time without any special needs.

Despite the efficacy of this approach in animals, limitations of DNA size and potential safety issues might limit the application of this gene transfer technology to human tissues and organs. To circumvent var-ious problems associated with viral gene transfer methods, strategies have been developed to allow target gene delivery by receptor-media-ted endocytosis pathway employing molecular conjugate vectors [75]. This delivery system mediates highly efficient gene transfer *in vitro* into primary cells and lines [76]. A preliminary recent report claimed the feasibility of adenovirus-polylysine-DNA complex to deliver expression of a reporter gene in a rat model of renal transplantation [77] and in humans under routine conditions of organ preservation [78], but negative data are also available [79].

Studies have also attempted to clarify whether indeed genes could be delivered to the kidney employing as DNA-complexing agent the cationic polymer polyethylenimine (PEI 25k) to avoid problems related to injecting viral material [80]. When complexes of PEI 25k/DNA were injected into the renal artery they did localize at proximal tubuli, but the transfection efficiency was remarkably low [80]. Moreover the low transfection efficiency of PEI 25k used to deliver genes to the kidney could not be ameliorated by *ex vivo* perfusion of the organ [74]. On the other hand, prolonging exposure of the kidney to the polymer produced microvascular thrombosis which impaired organ reperfusion as to pre-vent any future possibility for this technique to be used in patients.

Novel vector developments including virulence factor-deleted lentiviral vectors capable of gene transfer to non-dividing cells *in vivo* and modified herpes simplex virus vector can be considered as an alternative to enhance efficiency when the organ perfusion is precluded. A totally synthetic vector will eventually be developed that possibly supersedes all the above by combining the optimal properties of each.

Utility of novel vectors, such as adeno-associated virus (AAV) vector for the use in gene therapy has been reviewed recently [81]. Adeno-associated virus 2 (AAV) is a single stranded DNA-containing human parvovirus. Its potential advantages over other viral vectors relate to the safety and to the fact that it can stably integrate into a single site in the genomic DNA of the recipient cells. Indeed between 80-90% of the human population has been exposed to AAV and no symptoms or pathology have been attributed to this infection [82]. The property of stably integrating into the chromosomal DNA in a site-specific manner [83] is of value, since retroviral vectors which integrate into random sites of genomic DNA have potential for mutagenesis and carcinogenesis. One of the major limitations with AAV vectors has been the difficulty in generating large quantities of high-titer vector stocks [84], a problem that, however, is no more insurmontable with the more recent advances in vector technology. AAV vector also does not induce the significant immune response associated with adenoviral vectors.

Indeed, an additional major limitation to gene therapy rests on the immune response elicited by viral proteins, which prevents repeated administrations of the vector. New strategies to limit or eliminate these unwanted effects showed promising preliminary results [85-87] and should be explored in more detail in the next future. They include internal deletions of adenoviral constructs that have led to decreased immunogenicity and increased duration of gene therapy [88], cotransfection of viral IL-10 that inhibits the immune response to adenoviral antigen [89], blockade of co-stimulatory influences, such as the CD28 and CD40 pathways [69]. In the case of organ transplantation, anti-viral immune response may not always be an issue at least for the modulation of early post-transplant events. Actually, over 80% of acute rejection for the kidney as well as for other solid organs manifests within the first 15 days after surgery. Remarkably, studies have found that, albeit transient, expression of exogenous delivered genes by viral vectors does however persist in the transfected organs for up to 2 weeks [90]. Thus in the context of strategies addressed to minimize the consequences of acute rejection, long-term expression of the therapeutic gene product appears definitely less important. This does not apply to chronic rejection that initiates several months post-transplant, which would imply that gene therapy cannot help for the above unless ways to prolong the true expression of the transgene become available. Another issue here is that the inflammatory reaction stimulated by adenoviral-mediated gene transfer might be expected to worsen chronic rejection process and accelerate allograft arteriosclerosis and interstitial scarring. To control the level of protein production induced by gene transfer technique, a fascinating novel approach has been attempted based on pharmacologic control of gene expression by the drug rapamycin [91]. This is based on the fact that eukariotic transcription factors consist of two domains each with a peculiar function, namely DNA binding and transcriptional activation. If the two domains are separated the transcription factor is rendered inactive. In the new proposed system rapamycin is used as a bridge to bring the two domains of a given transcription factor together. Thus the gene controlled by the transcription factor can be turned on. This system has been shown to control circulating level of human growth hormone in mice implanted with engineered human cells [91].

Conclusion

Extensive experimental work has laid a solid scientific basis for gene therapy in organ transplantation and indicated that this is a potentially powerful clinical approach at least to control the acute rejection process. With this promising technology, studies should now focus on the possibility of gene therapy intervention to manipulate the progressive deterioration of graft function - i. e. chronic allograft rejection - that invariably occurs in the most of transplants and is today the most relevant problem for transplant medicine.

Before moving into clinical trials, however, investigators should provide evidence that non-human primates can indeed be transfected safely and efficiently with 'anti-rejection' genes, and, more importantly, effectively enough to control immune response at local organ level. Should studies end with encouraging results, molecular medicine will possibly become instrumental to truly prolong organ graft survival, and contribute to make donor-specific tolerance in human transplantation a reality. The future of transplant medicine will change substantially.

Acknowledgements

The Authors thanks Dr. Susanna Tomasoni for helpful support in preparing the tables.

Laura Arioli helped preparing the manuscript.

References

1. Sayegh MH, Carpenter CB: Tolerance and chronic rejection. Kidney Int 51 (Suppl.58):S-11-S-14, 1997
2. London NJ, Farmery SM, Will EJ, Davison AM, Lodge JPA: Risk of neoplasia in renal transplant patients. Lancet 346:403-406, 1995
3. Starzl TE, Demetris AJ, Murase N, Trucco M, Thomson AW, Rao AS: The lost chord: microchimerism and allograft survival. Immunol Today 17:577-584, 1996
4. Posselt AM, Barker CF, Tomaszewski JE, Markmann JF, Choti MA, Naji A: Induction of donor-specific unresponsiveness by intrathymic islet transplantation. Science 249:1293-1295, 1990
5. Remuzzi G, Rossini M, Imberti O, Perico N: Kidney graft survival in rats without immunosuppressants after intrathymic glomerular transplantation. Lancet 337:750-752, 1991
6. Remuzzi G: Cellular basis of long-term organ transplant acceptance: pivotal role of intrathymic clonal deletion and thymic dependence of bone marrow microchimerism-associated tolerance. Am J Kidney Dis 31:197-212, 1998
7. Perico N, Barbui C, Remuzzi G: Studies of privileged sites and organ transplantation. Exp Nephrol 1:120-127, 1993
8. Remuzzi G, Perico N, Carpenter CB, Sayegh MH: The thymic way to transplantation tolerance. J Am Soc Nephrol 5:1639-1646, 1995
9. Naji A: Induction of tolerance by intrathymic inoculation of alloantigen. Curr Opin Immunol 8:704-709, 1996
10. Ohzato H, Monaco AP: Induction of specific unresponsiveness (tolerance) to skin allografts by intrathymic donor-specific splenocyte injection in antilymphocyte serum-treated mice. Transplantation 54:1090-1095, 1992
11. Dono K, Wood ML, Ohzato H, Otsu I, Gottschalk R, Maki T, Monaco AP: Marked prolongation of rat skin xenografts induced by intrathymic injection of xenogeneic splenocytes and a short course of rapamycin in antilymphocyte serum-treated mice. Transplantation 59:929-932, 1995
12. Oluwole SF, Jin M-X, Chowdhury NC, Ohajekwe OA: Effectiveness of intrathymic inoculation of soluble antigens in the induction of specific unresponsiveness to rat islet allografts without transient recipient immunosuppression. Transplantation 58:1077-1081, 1994
13. Sayegh MH, Perico N, Imberti O, Hancock WW, Carpenter CB, Remuzzi G: Thymic recognition of class II major histocompatibility complex allopeptides induces donor-specific unresponsiveness to renal allografts. Transplantation 56:461-465, 1993
14. Shirwan H, Mhoyan A, Leamer A, Wang C, Makowka L, Cramer DV: The role of donor class I peptides in the induction of allograft tolerance. XVI International Congress of the Transplant Society, Barcelona, Spain, August 25 47, 1996 (abstract)
15. Knechtle SJ, Wang J, Shoushu J, Geissler EK, Sumimoto R, Wolff J: Induction of specific tolerance by intrathymic injection of recipient muscle cells transfected with donor class I major histocompatibility complex. Transplantation 57:990-996, 1994
16. Behara AMP, Westcott AJ, Chang PL: Intrathymic implants of genetically modified fibroblasts. FASEB J 6:2853-2858, 1992
17. Knechtle SJ, Wang J, Graeb C, Zhai Y, Hong X, Fechner Jr,J.H., Geissler EK: Direct MHC class I complementary DNA transfer to thymus induces donor-specific unresponsiveness, which involves multiple immunologic mechanisms. J Immunol 159:152-158, 1997
18. Sumimoto R, Shinomiya T: A role for MHC class I antigens in the protective preoperative blood transfusion effect on liver allograft survival in rats. Transplant Proc 23:2012-2016, 1991

19. Davies HS, Pollard SG, Calne Y: Soluble HLA antigens in the circulation of liver graft recipients. Transplantation 47:524-527, 1989
20. De Matteo R, Rapor S, Ahn M, Fisher K, Burke C, Radu A, Widera G, Claytor B, Barker C, Markmann J: Gene transfer to the thymus. Ann Surg 222:229-242, 1995
21. Ilan Y, Atlavar P, Takahashi M, Davidson A, Horwitz M, Guida J, Chowdhury N, Chowdhury J: Induction of central tolerance by intrathymic inoculation of adenoviral antigens into the host thymus permits long-term gene therapy in Gunn rats. J Clin Invest 98:2640-2647, 1996
22. Dunbar CE, O'Shaughnessy JA, Doren S, Carter C, Berenson R, Brown S, Greenblatt J, Stewart M, Leitman SF, Wilson WH, Cowan K, Young NS, Nienhuis AW: Retrovirally marked CD34-enriched peripheral blood and bone marrow cells contribute to long-term engraftment after autologous transplantation. Blood 85:3048-3057, 1995
23. Brenner MK: Gene transfer to hematopoietic cells. N Engl J Med 335:337-339, 1996
24. George JF, Sweeney SD, Kirklin JK, Simpson EM, Goldstein DR, Thomas JM: An essential role for Fas ligand in transplantation tolerance induced by donor bone marrow. Nature Medicine 4:333-335, 1998
25. Sykes M, Sachs DH, Nienhuis AW, Pearson DA, Moulton AD, Bodine DM: Specific prolongation of skin graft survival following retroviral transduction of bone marrow with an allogeneic major histocompatibility complex gene. Transplantation 55:197-202, 1993
26. Hayashi H, Le Guern C, Sacha D, Sykes M: Long-term engraftment of precultured post-5-fluorouracll allogeneic marrow in mice conditioned with a nonmyeloablative regimen: relevance for a gene therapy approach to tolerance induction. Transplant Immunol 4:86-90, 1996
27. Saitovitch D, Morris P, Wood K: RecipienT cells expressing single donor MHC locus products can substitute for donor specific transfusions in the induction of transplantation tolerance when pretreatment is combined with anti-CD4 monoclonal antibody: evidence for a vital role of CD4+T cells in the induction of tolerance to class I molecules. Transplantation 61:1532-1538, 1996
28. Wong W, Stranford S, Morris P, Wood K: Retroviral gene transfer of a donor class I MHC gene is recipient bone marrow cells induces tolerances to alloantigens *in vivo*. Transplant Proc 29:1130, 1997
29. Wong W, Morris P, Wood K: Pretransplant administration of a single donor class I MHC molecule is sufficient for the indefinite survival of fully allogeneic cardiac allografts: evidence for linked epitope suppression. Transplantation 63:1490-1494, 1997
30. Sonntag K-C, Emery D, Yasumoto A, Sablinski T, Yamada K, Shimada H, Arn S, Sachs DH, LeGuern C: Retrovirus-mediated transfer of MHC class II genes into bone marrow leads to transplantation tolerance. American Society of Gene Therapy 105a, 1998 (abstract)
31. Ierino FL, Gojo S, Banerjee PT, Giovino M, Xu Y, Gere J, Kaynor C, Awwad M, Monroy R, Rembert J, Hatch T, Foley A, Kozlowski T, Yamada K, Neethling FA, Fishman J, Bailin M, Spitzer TR, Cooper DKC, Cosimi AB, LeGuern C, Sachs DH: Transfer of swine major histocompatibility complex class II genes into autologous bone marrow cells of baboons for the induction of tolerance across xenogeneic barriers. Transplantation 67:1119-1128, 1999
32. Matsue H, Matsue K, Walters M, Okumura K, Yagita H, Takashima A: Induction of antigen-specific immunosuppression by CD95L cDNA-transfected 'killer' dendritic cells. Nature Med 5:930-937, 1999
33. Ju S-T, et al. : Fas(CD95)/FasL interactions required for programmed cell death after T cell activation. Nature 373:444-448, 1995

34. Matiba B, Mariani SM, Krammer PH: The CD95 system and the death of a lymphocyte. Semin Immunol 9:59-68, 1997
35. Lau HT, Yu M, Fontana A, Stoeckert Jr,CJ: Prevention of islet allograft rejection with engineered myoblasts expressing fasL in mice. Science 273:109-112, 1996
36. Chahine AA, Yu M, McKernan MM, Stoeckert C, Lau HT: Immunomodulation of pancreatic islet allografts in mice with CTLA4Ig secreting muscle cells. Transplantation 59:1313-1318, 1995
37. Qin L, Chavin KD, Ding Y, Favaro JP, Woodward JE, Lin J, Tahara H, Robbins P, Shaked A, Ho DY, Sapolsky RM, Lotze MT, Bromberg JS: Multiple vectors effectively achieve gene transfer in a murine cardiac transplantation model. Transplantation 59:809-816, 1995
38. Wang CK, Zuo XJ, Carpenter D, Jordan S, Nicolaidou E, Toyoda M, Czer LSC, Wang H, Trento A: Prolongation of cardiac allograft survival with intracoronary viral interleukin-10 gene transfer. Transplant Proc 31:951-952, 1999
39. Deng S, Ketchum RJ, Kucher T, Weber M, Shaked A, Naji A, Brayman KL: Adenoviral transfection of canine islet xenografts with immunosuppressive cytokine genes abrogates primary nonfunction and prolongs graft survival. Transplant Proc 29:770, 1997
40. Drazan KE, Olthoff KM, Wu L, Shen XD, Gelman A, Shaked A: Adenovirus-mediated gene transfer in the transplant setting: early events after orthotopic transplantation of liver allografts expressing TGF-beta1. Transplantation 62:1080-1084, 1996
41. Kato K, Shimozato O, Hoshi K, Wakimoto H, Hamada H, Yagita H, Okumura K: Local production of the p40 subunit of interleukin 12 suppresses T helper-1 mediated immune responses and prevents allogeneic myoblast rejection. Proc Natl Acad Sci USA 93:9086-9089, 1996
42. Lawrence DA: Transforming growth factor-b: An overview. Kidney Int 47 (Suppl.49):S-19-S-23, 1995
43. Benhamou P, Mullen Y, Shaked A, Bahmiller D, Csete M: Decreased alloreactivity to human islets secreting viral interleukin 10. Transplantation 62:1306-1312, 1996
44. Hall B, Bishop G, Farnsworth A, et al.: Identification of the cellular subpopulations infiltrating rejection cadaver renal allografts: preponderance of the T4 subset of T cells. Transplantation 37:564-570, 1984
45. van Seventer G, Shimizu Y, Shaw S: Roles of multiple accessory molecules in T cell activation. Curr Opin Immunol 3:294-303, 1991
46. Springer T: Adhesion receptors of the immune system. Nature 346:425-434, 1990
47. Stepkowski SM, Wang ME, Condon TP, Flournoy S-C, Stecker K, Graham M, Qu X, Tian L, Chen W, Kahan BD, Bennett CF: Protection against allograft rejection with intercellular adhesion molecule-1 antisense oligodeoxynucleotides. Transplantation 66:699-707, 1998
48. Stepkowski S, Wang M, Amante A, et al.: Antisense intracellular adhesion molecule-1 (ICAM-1) oligodeoxynucleotide blocks allograft rejection in rat and monkey models. XVI International Congress of the Transplantation Society, August 25-30, Barcelona 112, 1996 (abstract)
49. Dragun D, Gross V, Lukitsch I, Park JK, Maasch C, Lippoldi A, Tullius SG, Luft FC, Haller H: Inhibition of ICAM-1 expression by antisense oligonucleotides prevents ischemia/reperfusion injury, reduces MHCII expression and enables immediate graft function after renal transplantation. J Am Soc Nephrol 8:655A, 1997 (abstract)
50. Perico N, Remuzzi G: Prevention of transplant rejection. Current treatment guidelines and future developments. Drugs 54 (4):533-570, 1997
51. Olthoff KM, Judge TA, Gelman AE, da Shen X, Hancock WW, Turka LA, Shaked A: Adenovirus-mediated gene transfer into cold-preserved liver allografts: survival

pattern and unresponsiveness following transduction with CTLA4Ig. Nature Medicine 4:194-200, 1998

52. Kita Y, Li X-K, Hayashi S, Funeshima N, Enosawa S, Tamura A, Suzuki K, Kazui T, Amemiya H, Suzuki S: Prolonged rat cardiac allograft survival using adenoviral vector containing the CTLA4Ig gene. Transplant Proc 30:1079-1080, 1998

53. Yang Z, Chen M, Rostami S, Gelman A, Shen X-D, Shaked A, Barker C, Naji A: Induction of prolonged allograft survival by CTLA4Ig gene transfer. American Society of Gene Therapy 108a, 1998 (abstract)

54. Liu C, Deng S, Yang Z, Kucher T, Guo F, Gelman A, Chen H, Naji A, Shaked A, Brayman KL: Local production of CTLA4-Ig by adenoviral-mediated gene transfer to the pancreas induces permanent allograft survival and donor-specific tolerance. Transplant Proc 31:625-626, 1999

55. Uchikoshi F, Yang Z-D, Rostami S, Yokoi Y, Capocci P, Barker CF, Naji A: Prevention of autoimmune recurrence and rejection by adenovirus-mediated CTLA4Ig gene transfer to the pancreatic graft in BB rat. Diabetes 48:652-657, 1999

56. Tomasoni S, Azzollini N, Casiraghi F, Capogrossi M, Remuzzi G, Benigni A: Renal allograft survival is prolonged by CTLA4Ig gene transfer in the absence of systemic immunosuppression. Abstract. J Am Soc Nephrol 1999 (in press)

57. Yang Z, Rostami S, Koeberlein B, Barker CF, Naji A: Cardiac allograft tolerance induced by intra-arterial infusion of recombinant adenoviral CTLA4Ig. Transplantation 67:1517-1523, 1999

58. Nagata S: Fas and Fas ligand: a death factor and its receptor. Adv Immunol 57:129-144, 1994

59. Allison J, Georgiou HM, Strasser A, Vaux DL: Transgenic expression of CD95 ligand on islet B cells induces a granulocytic infiltration but does not confer immune privilege upon islet allografts. Proc Natl Acad Sci USA 94:3943, 1997

60. Swenson KM, Ke B, Wang T, Markowitz JS, Maggard MA, Spear GS, Imagawa DK, Goss JA, Busuttil RW, Seu P: Fas ligand gene transfer to renal allografts in rats. Effects on allograft survival. Transplantation 65:155-160, 1998

61. Li X-K, Tamura A, Funeshima N, Kaneda Y, Kita Y, Enosawa S, Amemiya H, Suzuki S: Prolonged survival of recipient rats with fas-ligand-transfected liver allografts by using HVJ-liposome. Transplant Proc 30:943, 1998

62. Bilbao G, Contreras J, Oliver J, Mikheeva G, Gomez-Navarro J, Eckhoff D, Krasnykh V, Suzuki K, Kasano K, Curiel DT, Thomas JM, Thomas F: *In vitro* cytoprotection of murine pancreatic islets by genetic modification with an adenoviral vector encoding human Bcl-2. American Society of Gene Therapy 11a, 1998 (abstract)

63. Shears II LL, Kawaharada N, Tzeng E, Billiar TR, Watkins SC, Kovesdi I, Lizonova A, Pham SM: Inducible nitric oxide synthase suppresses the development of allograft arteriosclerosis. J Clin Invest 100:2035-2042, 1997

64. Suzuki J-I, Isobe M, Morishita R, Aoki M, Horie S, Okube Y, Kaneda Y, Sawa Y, Matsuda H, Ogihara T, Sekiguchi M: Prevention of graft coronary arterioscelosis by antisense cdk2 kinase oligonucleotide. Nature Medicine 3:900-903, 1997

65. Negita M, Hayashi S, Yokoyama I, et al. : Protective effect of human superoxide dismutase cDNA transfection in the prevention of cold preservation injury. XVI International Congress of the Transplantation Society, August 25-30, Barcelona 496, 1996 (abstract)

66. Bilbao G, Contreras J, Gomez-Navarro J, Mikheeva G, Eckhoff D, Asiedu C, Kasano K, Xing J, Krasnykh V, Thomas F, Thomas JM, Curiel DT: Genetic cytoprotection of human endothelial cells (EC) during cold preservation. The Transplantation Society, XVII World Congress, July 12-17, Montreal 79, 1998

67. Perico N, Amuchastegui S, Bontempelli M, Remuzzi G: CTLA4Ig alone or in combination with low-dose cyclosporine fails to reverse acute rejection of renal allograft in the rat. Transplantation 61:1320-1322, 1996

68. Chia SH, Kibbe M, Tzeng E, Geller DA, Murase N: Adenoviral-mediated delivery of the human iNOS gene to liver isografts: an improved model of ex-vivo gene transfer. American Society of Gene Therapy 12a, 1998 (abstract)
69. Blau H, Khavari P: Gene therapy: progress, problems, prospects. Nature Medicine 3:612-613, 1997
70. Miller AD: Human gene therapy comes of age. Nature 357:455-460, 1992
71. Rosenberg SA, Aebersold P, Cornetta K, Kasid A, Morgan RA, Moen R, Karson EM, Lotze MT, Yang JC, Topalian SL, Merino MJ, Culver K, Miller AD, Blaese RM, Anderson WF: Gene transfer into humans-Immunotherapy of patients with advanced melanoma, using tumor-infiltrating lympocytes modified by retroviral gene transduction. N Engl J Med 323:570-578, 1990
72. Crystal RG: The Gordon Wilson Lecture. *In vivo* gene therapy: a strategy to use human genes as therapeutics. Trans Am Clin Climatol Assoc 106:87-99, 1994
73. Schneider MD, French BA: The advent of adenovirus. Gene therapy for cardiovascular disease. Circulation 88:1937-1942, 1993
74. Tomasoni S, Lutz J, Corna D, Capogrossi M, Remuzzi G, Benigni A: Adenoviral gene transfer in renal transplantation. J Am Soc Nephrol 8:667A, 1997 (abstract)
75. Zeigler ST, Kerby JD, Thompson JA: Molecular conjugated-mediated gene transfer into isolated human and transplanted rat kidneys. Exp Nephrol 5:508-513, 1997
76. Lozier JN, Thompson AR, Hu PC, Read M, Brinkhous KM, High KA, Curiel DT: Efficient transfection of primary cells in a canine hemophilia B model using adenovirus-polylysine-DNA complexes. Hum Gene Ther 5:313-322, 1994
77. Zeigler ST, Kerby JD, Curiel DT, Wehby JN, Diethelm AG, Thompson JA: Molecular conjugate-mediated gene transfer in renal transplantation. Transplant Proc 28:2046-2048, 1996
78. Zeigler ST, Kerby JD, Curiel DT, Diethelm AG, Thompson JA: Molecular conjugate-mediated gene transfer into isolated human kidneys. Transplantation 61:812-817, 1996
79. Wang J, Ma Y, Knechtle SJ: Adenovirus-mediated gene transfer into rat cardiac allografts. Transplantation 61:1726-1729, 1996
80. Boletta A, Benigni A, Lutz J, Remuzzi G, Soria MR, Monaco L: Nonviral gene delivery to the rat kidney with polyethylenimine. Hum Gene Ther 8:1243-1251, 1997
81. Jindal RM, Sidner RA, Bochan MR, Srivastava A: Adeno-associated virus vectors: potential for gene therapy. Graft 1:147-153, 1998
82. Blacklow NR, Hoggan MD, Sereno MS, et al.: A seroepidemiological study of adeno-associated virus infection in infants and children. Am J Epidemiol 94:359-366, 1971
83. Kotin RM, Siniscalco M, Samulski RJ, et al.: Site-specific integration by adeno-associated virus. Proc Natl Acad Sci USA 87:2211-2215, 1990
84. Bromberg JS: A review of adeno-associated virus vectors: potential for gene therapy. Graft 1:135, 1998
85. Fisher KJ, Jooss K, Alston J, Yang Y, Haecker SE, High K, Pathak R, Raper SE, Wilson JM: Recombinant adeno-associated virus for muscle directed gene therapy. Nature Med 3:306-312, 1997
86. Kay MA, Holterman A-X, Meuse L, Gown A, Ochs HD, Linsley PS, Wilson CB: Long-term hepatic adenovirus-mediated gene expression in mice following CTLA4Ig administration. Nature Genetics 11:191-197, 1995
87. Koeberl DD, Alexander IE, Halbert CL, Russell DW, Miller AD: Persistent expression of human clotting factor IX from mouse liver after intravenous injection of adeno-associated virus vectors. Proc Natl Acad Sci USA 94:1426-1431, 1997
88. Ilan Y, Droguett G, Chowdhury NR, Li Y, Sengupta K, Thummala NR, Davidson A, Chowdhury JR, Horwitz MS: Insertion of the adenoviral E3 region into a

L

recombinant viral vector prevents antiviral humoral and cellular immune responses and permits long-term gene expression. Proc Natl Acad Sci USA 94:2587-2592, 1997

89. Qin L, Ding Y, Robson N, Pahud DR, Shaked A, Bromberg JS: Adenovirus-mediated gene transfer of viral interleukin 10 inhibits the immune response to both alloantigen and adenoviral antigen. American Society of Transplant Physicians, 15th Annual Meeting, May 26-30, Dallas (TX) 110, 1996 (abstract)

90. Shaked A, Csete ME, Drazan KE, Bullington KE, Wu L, Busuttil RW, Berk AJ: Adenovirus-mediated gene transfer in the transplant setting. Transplantation 57:1508-1511, 1994

91. Rivera VM, Clackson T, Natesan S, Pollock R, Amara JF, Keenan T, Magari SR, Phillips T, Courage NL, Cerasoli Jr,F., Holt DA, Gilman M: A humanized system for pharmacologic control of gene expression. Nature Medicine 2:1028-1032, 1996

GENE THERAPY IN ORGAN TRANSPLANTATION: APPLICABILITIES AND SHORTCOMINGS

John C. Magee, Randall S. Sung, and Jonathan S. Bromberg

Introduction

Gene therapy holds great promise for the treatment of many conditions but it is currently limited by the inability to effectively introduce the transgene into the tissue of interest, as well as low level and transient transgene expression. Furthermore, once long term transgene expression is achieved, it will need to be responsive to regulation via normal homeostatic mechanisms or via pharmacologic means. These hurdles are significant and limit the current application of gene therapy in many areas, but may pose less of an issue in the context of transplantation. Trans-plantation is a relatively unique setting where one might envision gene therapy being applied *in situ* to the cadaveric donor prior to organ retrieval, or *ex vivo* prior to implantation of the cells or organ into the recipient, allowing for higher doses of vector to be administered without systemic toxicity. Furthermore, this selective perfusion of the organ *ex vivo* provides a functional tissue specificity independent of vector design, a current hurdle for *in vivo* gene therapy in other applications. The transient expression of the transgene, while a shortcoming in applications such as gene replacement therapy, may actually be bene-ficial in the context of transplantation. The limited expression of an immunomodulatory molecule in the microenvironment of the graft may be sufficient to alter the interaction between the donor antigens and the recipient immune system so that a state of donor specific hypores-ponsiveness or functional tolerance is generated. Transient transgene expression may provide a further advantage in that the long-term consequences of prolonged vector expression are not known, and

Mohamed Sayegh and Giuseppe Remuzzi (editors), Current and Future Immunosuppressive Therapies Following Transplantation, 335-356.
© 2001 Kluwer Academic Publishers. Printed in the Netherlands.

regulation of transgene expression is problematic despite the use of tissue specific promoters and regulatable expression elements.

Additional advantages of gene therapy in transplantation include the possibility that introducing immunomodulatory molecules into allografts by gene transfer may allow localized immunosuppression, thus avoiding the side effects associated with conventional systemic immunosuppression such as infection, malignancy, or drug specific toxicities. Gene therapy allows the delivery of peptides which would otherwise be expensive to manufacture and difficult to administer by conventional means. Furthermore, because these immunomodulatory molecules are limited to the microenvironment of the graft, it is possible that some degree of functional antigen specificity will be achieved.

Gene Delivery Approaches

Gene delivery vectors which might be considered for application in transplantation are identical to those being developed for other settings. Gene delivery vectors fall broadly into two categories: viral vectors and nonviral vectors. Viral vectors carry the transgene of interest into the cell by exploiting pre-existing viral receptors and cell surface receptors to gain entry into the cell. Once internalized by receptor mediated endocytosis, the particles escape cellular endosomal degradative pathways and are transported to the nucleus. Such vectors can be very efficient at introducing the transgene of interest but still face many shortcomings. Viral vector approaches are limited by size of cDNA that can be packaged into the viral particle, although this may not pose a particular problem for most molecules relevant to transplantation. The target cells to be transfected must also express the appropriate receptor for the vector. Additionally, many viral based delivery vectors are hampered by specific host humoral and cellular responses as well as components of innate immunity which limit their effectiveness (Bromberg, 1998).

Despite their shortcomings, the development of viral vectors is a promising area of investigation. Many are focusing on integrating viral vectors, including retroviral, lentiviral, and adeno-associated viral vectors. These vectors stably integrate the transgene into genomic DNA. This promotes stable, prolonged transgene expression, but also carries with it the potential risk of mutagenesis and malignant transformation. Of the integrating vectors, retroviral vectors were among the first delivery systems to be used in gene therapy (Eglitis, 1985; Gordon, 1994). These viruses are 10-kb RNA viruses which once inside the cell, use reverse transcriptase to synthesize double stranded DNA, which is then transferred to the nucleus. Host cell replication must occur for the viral DNA sequences to become integrated in the host genome, which may limit the utility of these vectors in organ transplantation. Lentiviral vectors are integrating viruses which can stably infect nondividing cells and thus might be more effective (Naldini, 1996). Adeno-associated viruses are parvoviruses which integrate their DNA at site specific sequences on the long arm of chromosome 19, which could potentially decrease the risk of insertional mutagenesis from random integration (Samulski, 1991).

Concerns for mutagenesis from integrating vectors has provided a stimulus for investigating nonintegrating viral vectors. With these vectors, the viral genome is maintained within the nucleus in an extrachromosomal state as an episome. Because the transgene is extrachromosomal, it is not replicated during cell division. Adenoviral vectors are the prototypic nonintegrating viral vectors (Ghosh-Choudhury, 1987; Rosenfeld, 1991; Kozarsky, 1993). These 36-kb dsDNA viruses are able to infect many non-dividing cells with a high transduction efficiency but are limited by transient expression because there is no stable integration. Additionally, the immune response to adenoviral vectors presents a significant obstacle.

Nonviral vectors are attractive in their simplicity and lack of an antiviral immune response. The simplest nonviral approach is the use of naked plasmid DNA. Plasmid DNA is taken up, albeit at low levels, by cells in culture (Wolff, 1990) and by myocytes *in vivo* (Lin, 1990; Wolff, 1990). Multiple approaches to improve DNA entry into cells have been studied in hopes of improving transduction efficiency. Calcium phosphate coprecipitation is one such *in vitro* approach but it is inefficient compared to viral vectors and relatively impractical for *in vivo* applications. Electroporation is another alternative to improve gene delivery. Although initially described for *in vitro* application, recent work has suggested this approach can be applied *in vivo* to whole organs (Aihara, 1998; Suzuki T, 1998). Other investigators have focused on complexing DNA with other molecules, believing that strategies designed to improve the physical transfer of plasmid DNA into cells might markedly improve the potential of nonviral vectors. Prototypic of work in this area are DNA liposomes complexes. Liposomes form lipid envelopes which complex with DNA and promote cellular uptake (Felgner, 1987; Nicolau, 1987). Dendrimers are synthetic cationic polymers which can complex with DNA and also show promise for significantly increasing transgene delivery (Kukowska-Latallo, 1996). In order to provide some tissue specificity with nonviral vectors, some have investigated synthesizing DNA-protein complexes, which then utilize receptor mediated endocytosis to gain entry into the cell (Wu, 1987).

Improvements in these nonviral approaches have been steady, and are beginning to achieve transfection efficiency approaching levels obtained with viral vectors. Approaches are evolving to modify the limiting steps in the cellular transfer of the foreign DNA so as to either bypass the step or enhance its rate. For example, attaching peptides encoding nuclear localizaton signals to dsDNA is one attractive option to increase the efficiency of gene transfer (Sebestyen, 1998; Zanta, 1999).

While these nonviral techniques are limited largely by low transduction efficiency, such vectors do allow delivery of large DNA sequences or multiple genes. Nonviral vectors also appear less susceptible to immune surveillance, though as discussed later, naked plasmid DNA is capable of generating a host immune response which may also limit transduction efficiency.

Gene Delivery Approaches in Transplantation

Regardless of the vector utilized, gene delivery in the setting of transplantation has some unique advantages and constraints. As mentioned previously, the ability to perfuse an organ or isolated cells *ex vivo* relaxes the need for site directed gene therapy, since much of the nonincorporated vector could be removed prior to placement in the recipient. Obviously such approaches would need to be performed under hypothermic conditions for a relatively short (i.e. hours) time period to prevent ischemic injury to the graft. This approach could be limited by impairment of the cellular functions responsible for uptake and intracellular trafficking of the vector under these conditions. Despite this possible limitation, it does appear that reasonable levels of transduction under these conditions can occur (Csete, 1994; Shaked, 1994; Boasquevisque, 1997). Alternatively, the vector could be administered *in vivo* to the donor following the declaration of brain death, provided agents can be identified which are acceptable to all potential procurement teams.

Effector Molecules

The potential candidate molecules for gene transfer are many and diverse. Effective gene therapy will require a thorough understanding of the respective roles of specific molecules in allorecognition, clonal proliferation, and effector mechanisms responsible for graft rejection. As our understanding of these processes grows, so will potential interventions for gene therapy.

While gene therapy is typically thought of as a way to introduce peptide products, in a broader sense it includes the use of nucleic acids as therapeutic agents. A full discussion of these approaches is beyond the scope of this chapter, but includes the use of antisense oligonucleotides, to bind to specific mRNA sequences and inhibit translation of the mRNA. Alternatively ribozymes, which are catalytically active RNA sequences that cleave and inactivate complementary mRNA sequences, could be delivered. Finally "molecular decoys" encoding specific nucleotide sequences could be introduced which would bind to transcription factors. Any of these approaches could be utilized to decrease cellular expression of immune stimulatory molecules (e.g. IL-2), provided the appropriate cell type could be selectively and efficiently targeted.

Because current gene delivery methods only transduce a subset of the total cells contained within an organ, most approaches have focused on soluble immunomodulatory molecules which could act in a paracrine manner, although systemic levels can be generated in some settings (Olthoff, 1997). As vector delivery systems improve to specifically and effectively target given cell populations, one could envision a role for peptides targeted to nuclear, cytoplasmic, mitochondrial, or trans-membrane compartments to alter cellular function.

With respect to specific effector molecules to be delivered via gene therapy, perhaps the best characterized are the immunomodulatory cytokines, such as TGFβ. TGFβ inhibits Th1 polarization, suppresses a variety of inflammatory cell responses, and inhibits lymphocyte development. Gene transfer of TGFβ has prolonged graft survival in both hepatic and cardiac allograft models (Drazan, 1996; Qin, 1995; Qin, 1996). Another potential cytokine for gene therapy is IL-4. IL-4 inhibits Th1 differentiation and can be used to produce immune deviation to Th2 phenotype. Gene transfer of IL-4 has been successful in prolonging rodent cardiac allograft survival when combined with a donor specific transfusion and cyclosporin based induction protocol (Levy, 1995). IL-10 is another potential immunomodulatory cytokine. While possessing some inhibitory action, it also possesses immunostimulatory properties (Rousset, 1992; Thompson-Snipes, 1991). Subsequently, most have focused on viral IL-10, a homologue of cellular IL-10 which is encoded by the BCRF1 open reading frame of the Epstein-Barr virus (Moore, 1990; Hsu ,1990; de Waal, 1991; Vieira, 1991; Suzuki T, 1995). vIL-10 does not possess the immunostimulatory properties of cellular IL-10 and has been shown to extend allograft survival (Qin, 1997a). Other molecules successfully applied in transplantation using gene therapy approaches include CTLA4Ig (Gainer, 1994; Olthoff, 1997) and Fas ligand (Lau 1996).

The ability to alter the initial steps of allorecognition of MHC with gene therapy has been somewhat limited by the ability to transfect all the cells within an organ. Nonetheless, this is one potential point for intervention. For example, a portion of the adenoviral genome in the E3 region encodes a 19 kD gene product which binds to MHC Class I molecules in the endoplasmic reticulum, preventing the expression of these molecules on the cell surface. Gene transfer of islet allografts with E3-19K prolongs survival (Efrat, 1995b).

More recently gene therapy has been used to investigate the role of viral chemokine agonists vMIP-II (Human herpes virus 8) and MC148 (Molluscum contagiosum). Both prolong allograft survival, and diminish donor specific lymphocyte infiltration into the allograft and inhibits allo-antibody production (DeBruyne, 1999). Gene transfer of antagonists of inflammatory cytokines, such as soluble chemokine receptors, may be another therapeutic approach (McCoy, 1995).

As conventional pharmacologic research discovers peptides with immunosuppressive activity, they may be delivered locally within the graft using gene therapy. One such illustration of this approach is the use of gene therapy to locally deliver MHC derived peptides that seem to act through the induction of heat shock proteins (Magee, 1999; DeBruyne, in press).

Because the introduction of one molecule alone is unlikely to be successful, one might envision combination therapy with several gene products, each focused on a separate phase of the alloresponse, similar to our current conventional multi-drug approaches.

Gene Therapy in Cellular Transplantation

Theoretical advantages of cellular transplantation compared with whole organ transplantation include lower surgical morbidity, the ability for *ex vivo* gene transfer at high efficiency with positive selection of trans- duced cells, and the potential for easy replenishment of cell function through the use of multiple donors or cryopreserved cells from the same donor. Disadvantages include a limit to the number of cells which may be transplanted, the limited functional lifespan of some cultured cell types, and the limited survival of transplanted allogeneic cells due to rejection (Raper, 1995; Hatzoglou, 1990). Most research has been focused on islet cell transplantation for the treatment of diabetes, and on hepatocyte autotransplantation for treatment of single-gene-defect metabolic deficiencies such as hemophilia B, ornithine transcarbamylase deficiency, Crigler- Najjar syndrome, and hereditary tyrosinemia (Armentano, 1990; Kay, 1992; Wilson, 1988; Grossman, 1994; Fabrega, 1996)

Significant attention has focused on the engineering of cells with low intrinsic immunogenicity, and a number of gene therapy strategies have evolved to this end (Docherty, 1997). For example, while immortalized pancreatic β-cell lines are less immunogenic than fresh intact islets, they lose glucose responsiveness with long-term culture; this problem has been circumvented by transfection of β-cell lines with the gene encoding the glucose transporter GLUT-2 (Ferber, 1994). Other transgene constructs have incorporated the use of drug-sensitive promoter elements to either inhibit or induce growth of transplanted transformed β-cells (Deuschle, 1989; Efrat, 1995a). Others have utilized the transfection of genes encoding β-cell transcription factors into islet stem cells or pancreatic α-like cells in order to induce growth and differentiation into a β-cell phenotype (Welsh, 1988; Serup, 1996). This raises the possibility of autotransplantation of engineered α- or islet stem cells to recreate β-cell function.

Some investigators have focused on utilizing gene therapy tech- niques to make cellular allografts less immunogenic. A number of investigators have utilized gene transfer methods to induce local immunosuppression of pancreatic islet allografts. Murine islets transfected with a cDNA encoding CTLA4Ig prolong islet allograft survival compared with nontransduced grafts (Gainer, 1997). Murine myoblasts transfected with plasmid encoding CTLA4Ig, and cotransplanted with islet allografts, also prolong graft survival provided that the myoblasts are syngeneic with the recipient (Chahine, 1995). Syngeneic myoblasts expressing Fas ligand [CD95L] cotransplanted with pancreatic islet allografts under the kidney capsule also successfully prolong graft survival (Lau, 1996).

Gene Therapy in Bone Marrow Transplantation

Hematopoietic progenitor cells are logical targets for gene transfer in that they are cellular transplants that can be readily obtained, cultured, selected and returned to the host following manipulation. Gene transfer to a pluripotent stem cell could in principle allow indefinite repopulation with a wide array of genetically modified cells (Brenner, 1994). Vectors which integrate into genomic DNA, i.e. retroviral, lentiviral, or adeno-associated virus vectors are appropriate for this approach. Other applications to bone marrow transplantation include the local production of cytokines such as TNFα (for anti-leukemic effects) and GM-CSF (for neutrophil recovery following chemotherapy), thereby avoiding the systemic effects of these cytokines (Kuhr, 1994; Rosenthal, 1994). Genes conferring resistance to methotrexate and trimetrexate have also been successfully transferred into bone marrow, providing the potential for *in vivo* selection of donor cells and more effective chemotherapeutic options following allogeneic or autologous bone marrow transplantation (Spencer, 1996; Vinh, 1993).

A novel approach to the control of the allogeneic graft-versus-leukemia response has been developed utilizing gene transfer. Bonini et al. treated eight patients with relapse or EBV-induced lymphoma after T cell depleted bone marrow transplantation with immunocompetent, nondepleted donor lymphocytes retrovirally transduced with the Herpes simplex thymidine kinase as a suicide gene (Bonini, 1997). Such therapy produced antitumor activity in five patients, with lymphocyte survival of up to 12 months. Three patients developed significant graft-versus-host disease as a result of the treatment, which was then abrogated by gangciclovir-induced elimination of the transduced cells in all cases. Such an approach may be an attractive alternative to T cell depletion in allogeneic bone marrow transplantation by restoration of the graft-versus-leukemia effect while providing an effective treatment for potential graft-versus-host disease.

Another strategy utilizes the infusion of autologous bone marrow transfected with genes encoding donor-type MHC molecules prior to organ transplantation. Retroviral transduction of allogeneic class I MHC into syngeneic murine bone marrow cells prolongs survival of skin grafts expressing the introduced MHC antigen (Sykes, 1993), but not of those expressing other alloantigens. These animals display a hyporesponsive state secondary to deficient T cell help (Fraser, 1995).

Expression of allogeneic MHC class II DRβ by cDNA transfected into swine bone marrow has been demonstrated in both long-term cultures and in the peripheral blood of irradiated swine after transplantation (Emery, 1993a,1993b,1994). MHC class II DRβ cDNA has also been successfully transduced into umbilical cord blood and CD34+ cells of cynomolgus monkey *in vitro* (Banerjee, 1996). Treatment with syngeneic bone marrow transduced with donor class II cDNA conferred long-term renal allograft survival in miniature swine fully mismatched at the class I locus (Smith, 1992). This approach may be effective for tolerance induction for xenogeneic organ transplants.

Gene Therapy in Stem Cell Transduction

The stable transduction of human CD34+ bone marrow stem cells with retroviral or lentiviral vectors can produce long-term transgene expression in multiple lineages of hematopoietic cells (Miyoshi, 1999). The ability to transduce marrow progenitor cells may have more far-reaching implications. The finding that endothelial progenitor cells derived from bone marrow can be induced by cytokines or ischemia suggests a method by which stably transfected progenitors are mobilized to populate neovascularized tissue and therefore express transgene at these locations (Takahashi, 1999). This may prove to have beneficial effects in the treatment of ischemic coronary and vascular disease as well as for inhibition of tumorigenesis. Similarly, cardiomyocytes, which have also been generated from adult bone marrow stromal cells *in vitro*, may be transfected to express desirable genes and then subsequently transferred to the hearts of patients with cardiomyopathy (Makino, 1999). Furthermore, the genes which are found to determine specific differentiation of marrow-derived precursor cells could be incorporated into gene transfer vectors, and the vectors utilized to effect specific differentiation (Leiden, 1999).

Gene Therapy in Organ Transplantation

Gene therapy is beginning to show promise for widespread clinical applicability in cellular transplantation. Such approaches may be used to correct single gene defects, or as part of a tolerogenic protocol combined with organ transplantation. At present, a more broad application of gene therapy to organ transplantation is still confined to the laboratory. The current shortcomings of gene therapy still present

significant hurdles which limit any widespread application of this technology. As our understanding of gene therapy grows, and as advantages are made in the arena of cellular transplantation, it is likely
advances will be possible in organ transplantation.

Promoter Selection

In addition to the problems of efficient vector delivery and choice of the
appropriate effector molecules, one of the shortcomings currently
limiting the application of gene therapy is the design of the ideal
promoter. The efficiency and durability of transgene expression by
gene transfer vectors is profoundly influenced by the type of promoter
directing transgene expression. A wide variety of promoter types have
been studied, and the most commonly used are viral promoters such as
MMLV, RSV, SV40 or CMV, but cellular promoters such as the β-actin
promoter have also been utilized. Other promoter characteristics may
have dramatic influences on transgene expression. The efficiency of
the CMVie promoter differs depending on whether the promoter is
derived from human or murine CMV, on the size of the promoter
fragment used in the vector, and on the cell type transfected *in vitro*
(Addison, 1997). The nature of the promoter may determine
interactions with a number of transcription factors or viral gene products which may ultimately determine vector efficacy. For example, the
adenoviral E4 region gene products can activate transgene expression
in cis or in trans directed by an RSV but not a CMV promoter (Brough,
1997).
    Interactions of promoters with components of the immune system
represent an important means by which transgene expression is attenuated. Interferons and TNFα are known to have a variety of antiviral
activity. Interferon-γ regulates MCMV infection and inhibits reactivation
of MCMV from latency (Presti, 1998). Such inhibition may occur by
blockade of replication (Lucin, 1994), but there is evidence that
interferons inhibit the onset of MCMVie gene transcription as well,
implying a more direct effect on promoter function (Harms, 1995; Qin,
1997b; Gribaudo, 1993). Inhibition of transgene expression by interferons at a post-transcriptional level has been demonstrated in HBV
infection, and in MMLV-based retroviral vectors (Guidotti, 1996;
Ghazizadeh, 1997). In contrast, CMV promoter activity, which increases
following adenovirus vector administration, is stimulated by the transcription factor NF-κB (Looser, 1998). This may explain the early
efficiency of CMV promoter based vectors, as NF-κB activation can be
induced by TNFα, IL-1 and IL-6, all of which are stimulated by vector
administration. Whether an individual cytokine inhibits or augments
transgene expression may also be determined by vector promoter
structure (unpublished observations); for example, the deletion or

mutation of a transcription factor binding site may lead to loss of inhibition by a given cytokine. Precise characterization of the interactions between cytokines and promoter elements may ultimately lead to gene therapy vectors with promoters designed to capitalize on the cytokine milieu of the target tissue, resulting in augmentation of expression rather than attenuation.

Cytokines induced by immune responses to gene transfer vectors may also exert competitive or synergistic effects on transgene expression at the promoter level. We have shown that IFNγ and TNFα in combination are synergistic in inhibition of β-gal expression by adenoviral, retroviral and plasmid vectors *in vitro*, and by adenoviral vectors *in vivo* (Qin, 1997b). In contrast, NF-κB - dependent HIV gene expression is stimulated by TNFα but inhibited by IFNγ by competitive binding of transcription factors induced by these cytokines to the NF-κB coactivator p300 (Hottiger, 1998).

Regulation of Transgene Expression

The physical act of gene transfer gives rise to an array of responses including release of cytokines, initiation of various cell signaling cascades, induction of transcription factors, and production of vector-encoded proteins. Characterization of these responses has spurred approaches designed to exploit these properties so that gene expression can be turned on and off following vector administration (Pan, 1999). Transgene expression by adeno-associated virus vectors utilizing the CMV promoter can be repetitively induced by LPS administration (via an NF-κB–dependent mechanism) even after apparent extinction of gene expression (Loser, 1998). Vectors have been constructed which encode drug-sensitive transcription factors which then regulate the target gene. Genes encoding these transcription factors can be introduced either in the same vector or in an accompanying vector administered simultaneously. In one experiment, an adeno-associated virus vector was given encoding two proteins which reconstitute into a transcription factor complex after administration of the immunosuppressive drug rapamycin (Ye, 1999). This vector was coadministered with an AAV vector expressing the erythropoietin gene under the control of a promoter responsive to this complex. Transcription of the erythropoietin gene was induced 200-fold by rapamycin treatment. In another study, a chimeric transactivating protein was constructed which consisted of a progesterone receptor-ligand binding domain, a DNA binding domain, and an activation domain of the human p65 protein of the NF-κB complex. By including the gene encoding this chimeric protein into the same vector as the reporter transgene, transgene expression could be controlled by the administration of an antiprogestin (Burcin, 1999).

Adaptive Immune Responses to Vector Antigens

Adenoviral vectors are attractive for gene transfer because of their broad host range, capacity for large DNA inserts, and high efficiency of transduction. However, administration of first-generation adeno-virus vectors (those with viral genes E1 and E3 deleted) generates well-characterized adaptive immune responses against viral proteins which appear to be the primary mechanism by which expression is extinguished (Yang, 1994a; Yang, 1994b). The nature of adaptive immunity to gene transfer vectors has been the subject of numerous reports and reviews and will only be briefly reviewed here. Both the cellular and humoral arms of the adaptive immune response are triggered, the former effecting viral clearance, and the latter preventing effective readministration of vector. These responses have been attributed to low levels of viral gene expression by first-generation vectors, or may reflect contamination by wild-type virus. The importance of viral gene expression is supported by a diminution of both Th2 responses and neutralizing antibodies when E4 is deleted from first-generation vectors (Chirmule, 1998), and by the absence of late inflammation in muscle when vectors lacking all viral genes are employed (Chen, 1999). However, cellular responses may not necessarily require viral gene expression, as vectors rendered biologically inactive generate similar infiltration of CD4+ and CD8+ lymphocytes as do untreated vectors (Kafri, 1998). Adeno-associated virus (AAV) vectors incite much less of an immune response in tissues such as muscle fibers and neurons, and expression by these vectors results in a greater persistence of expression (Fisher, 1997). Antigen-presenting cells may be critical to the generation of the immune response to gene therapy vectors. For example, APCs transfected by adenovirus can be adoptively transferred to effect immune mediated elimination of adenovirus or AAV infected cells, but AAV-transfected APCs cannot. This may be due to the inability of AAV to transduce or to effectively activate APCs (Lieber, 1998).

Adaptive Immune Responses to Transgenes

Immune responses to encoded transgenes also limit expression by gene therapy vectors. Indeed much of the literature describing immunity to adenovirus vectors has been generated using vectors expressing the immunogenic reporter β-galactosidase. Human α_1- antitrypsin and human factor IX are two examples of less immunogenic reporter proteins whose duration of expression by adeno-virus vectors exceeds that of β-gal (Wadsworth, 1997; Poller, 1996). Thus, immune responses to adenovirus proteins per se may be less important in limiting expression than originally believed. Long-term expression has also been demonstrated in mice transgenic for hAAT and β-galactosidase, indicating that the anti-adeno-viral immune response does not always limit expression (Wadsworth, 1997; Chen, 1997). Vectors encoding murine erythropoietin demonstrate superior long-term expression in mice compared with identical vectors encoding the human homologue (Tripathy, 1996). Furthermore, the magnitude of immune responses to transgene products may be more strain-dependent than responses to viral antigens, which may account for the strain variation in expression by these vectors (Suzuki M,1998). Regardless of the relative contributions of immune responses to vector antigens and transgene products, it is clear that any gene therapy strategy must account for both in order to achieve long-term expression.

Role of Dendritic Cells

The mechanisms underlying adaptive immune responses to gene therapy vectors include a prominent role for dendritic cells (DC) not only in indirect presentation of soluble antigen, but also directly via vector uptake. Inoculation of plasmid DNA into muscle or skin results in activation of plasmid-containing dendritic cells at the injection site, in draining lymph nodes, and in the systemic circulation (Caseres,1997; Chattergoon,1998). These cells function as APC, can induce specific proliferation of CD4+ T cells and generation of CD8+ CTLs, and can induce both primary and secondary adaptive immune responses (Bouloc, 1998; Porgador, 1998). Much of the transgene product can be presented directly by transfected DC, since antigen-bearing DC in draining lymph nodes can be depleted by antibodies to a surface protein encoded by cotransfected DNA (Porgador, 1998). This direct pathway appears to be the primary mode of antigen presentation in this model, rather than cross- or indirect presentation of antigen by untransfected DC that have taken up soluble antigen.

Adenovirus vector-transfected dendritic cells also are important in the development of anti-vector immune responses. Adenovirus vectors efficiently transfect both mature and immature DC without altering maturation or function (Zhong, 1999). Adoptively transferred dendritic cells transfected with adenovirus encoding LacZ can mediate the immune elimination of muscle fibers stably transfected with an adeno-associated virus containing LacZ (Jooss, 1998). Dendritic cells infected *in vitro* with adenovirus encoding an antigenic peptide can subsequently induce strong specific CTL responses that can be augmented with repeated administration of transfected DC (Brossart,1997). Low titers of neutralizing antibody are generated with this method; in contrast, direct immunization generates high titers of neutralizing antibody, which limits the efficacy of repeated administration. Such an approach may have advantages in designing vaccination therapies or in tumor immunization.

Innate Immunity

In addition to antigen specific immune responses generated by vector proteins and transgenes, the importance of innate immune responses in limiting vector efficiency and persistence independent of, and in advance of, adaptive immune responses has recently received increasing attention. Resident macrophages, such as alveolar macrophages in the lung and Kupffer cells in the liver, clear a vast majority of adeno-virus vector genomes within 24 hours of administration (Worgall, 1997a; Worgall, 1997b). Kupffer cell depletion by gadolinium chloride treatment substantially reduces this vector clearance (Lieber, 1997). These cells, in addition to directly clearing vector, release cytokines such as TNFα, IL-6, IFNγ and IL-1β. While some of these cytokines such as TNFα and IFNγ possess intrinsic antiviral properties, they also induce a profound inflammatory response mediated by neutrophils, NK cells, and monocytes (Muruve, 1999; Lieber, 1997; Yei, 1994; Adesanya, 1996). This response is not dependent on viral gene expression, as such responses occur early after infection (Otake, 1998), and vectors progressively deleted of viral genes incite similar inflammatory responses and vector persistence (Lusky, 1998). Furthermore, viral antigen recognition may not be required, as inflammation can occur in mice bearing irrelevant transgenic TCR (Gangappa, 1998).

The cytokines induced following virus or viral vector administration are potent inducers of proinflammatory chemokines such as RANTES, MCP-1, MIP-1α, MIP-1β, and MIP-2 (Muruve, 1999; Otake, 1998; Thomas, 1998; Olszewska-Pazdrak, 1998). Specific inhibition of TNFα or MIP-2 can attenuate virus-induced inflammation (Otake, 1998; Elkon, 1997). Many of these effects are mediated through NF-κB activation, as inhibition of NF-κB activation either by overexpression of its inhibitor IkB or by expression of a mutant of the p65/RelA subunit of NF-kB leads to inhibition of cytokine expression, chemokine expression, and leukocyte infiltration (Soares, 1998; Thomas, 1998; Lieber, 1998). However, NF-κB also appears to exert a protective effect on vector-induced hepatic injury; NF-κB inhibition by introduction of an expression vector encoding IκB results in greater susceptibility to TNFα- mediated apoptosis, although antagonism of p65/RelA binding does not. Such protection may be due to feedback inhibition of TNFα production by the p50 subunit of NF-κB (Bohuslav, 1998). Vector persistence during NF-κB inhibition by IκB overexpression is enhanced only by simultaneous overexpression of the anti-apoptotic gene bcl-2 (Lieber, 1998).

Immune Responses to Nucleic Acids

Immune responses to nucleic acids in gene therapy vectors also contribute to limitation of expression. Bacterial DNA is a powerful stimulator of polyclonal proliferation in B cells and cytokine production by monocytes and lymphocytes (Ballas, 1996; Klinman 1996). The immunostimulatory properties of bacterial DNA are attributed to un-methylated CpG motifs, which may be present in plasmid DNA or synthetic oligonucleotides. These responses are sensitive to inhibitors of endosomal acidification such as bafilomycin A or chloroquine (Yi, 1998a; Macfarlane, 1998). This acidification is coupled to the generation of intracellular reactive oxygen species, which in turn is linked to the degradation of IκB (Yi, 1998a), and inhibition of IkB degradation suppresses the immunostimulatory effects of CpG DNA (Yi, 1998b). CpG DNA also induces the activation of c-Jun N-terminal kinase and p38 which leads ultimately to activation of the transcription factor AP-1 (Yi, 1998c; Hacker, 1998). The actions of CpG motifs stimulate innate immune responses via TNFα and IL-6 secretion, monocyte activation, and increased NK cell activity (Yamamoto, 1988; Yi, 1996;Yi, 1998a). In addition, type I interferons, IFNγ, IL-12, and IL-18 are also induced, and subsequently stimulate Th1 responses and enhance adaptive immunity (Sun, 1998; Roman, 1997; Chu, 1997; Weiner, 1997). While the ability of these motifs to function as immune adjuvants to coad-ministered antigens are advantageous for vaccination, they are potentially deleterious to gene therapy applications which require sustained expression of transgene product.

Conclusions

Gene therapy for the treatment of diseases is still an evolving field, very much in its infancy. This brief review delineates a number of distinct areas in which further significant development will be required before gene therapy in organ transplantation can become a clinical reality. First and foremost, the selection of a vector (viral or nonviral) which provides high transduction efficiency, stable cellular incorporation, and high-level regulated gene expression will be the sine qua non of a clinically successful delivery vehicle. The advances necessary to achieve these goals will require major efforts to understand vector entry and transport in the cell; nucleic acid structure and stability within the nucleus; and diverse determinants of gene expression including chromatin structure, promoter and enhancer function, and the inter-action of transcriptional and recombinational complexes with vector DNA. Further advances in the understanding of the interactions of the immune system and vectors will also be required to enhance vector stability and avoid activation of deleterious adaptive and innate immune responses. Lastly, the choice of an appropriate immunosuppressive effector molecule is not certain and the large catalogue of potential choices currently makes the selection difficult.

References

1. Addison CL, Hitt M, Kunsken D, Graham FL. Comparison of the human versus murine cytomegalovirus immediate early gene promoters for transgene expression by adenoviral vectors. *J Gen Virol.* 78 (Pt 7):1653-61, 1997.
2. Adesanya MR, Redman RS, Baum BJ, O'Connell BC. Immediate inflammatory responses to adenovirus-mediated gene transfer in rat salivary glands. *Hum Gene Ther.* 7(9):1085-93, 1996.
3. Aihara H, Miyazaki J. Gene transfer into muscle by electroporation in vivo. *Nat Biotech* 16(9):867-870, 1998.
4. Armentano D, Thompson AR, Darlington G, Woo SL. Expression of human factor IX in rabbit hepatocytes by retrovirus-mediated gene transfer: Potential for gene therapy of human hemophilia B. *Proc Natl Acad Sci USA* 87(16):6141-6145, 1990.
5. Ballas ZK, Rasmussen WL,. Krieg AM. Induction of NK activity in murine and human cells by CpG motifs in oligodeoxynucleotides and bacterial DNA. *J. Immunol.* 157(5):1840-5, 1996.
6. Banerjee PT, Ierino F, Kaynor GC, Giovino M, Sablinski T, Emery DW, Rosa MD, LeGuern C, Sachs DH, Monroy RL. Retrovirus-mediated gene transfer and expression of swine MHC Class II genes in CD34+ monkey stem cells. *Transplant Proc* 28(2):747-748, 1996.
7. Boasquevisque CHR, Mora BN, Schmid RA, Lee TC, Nagahiro I, Cooper JD, Patterson GA. Ex vivo adenoviral-mediated gene transfer to lung isografts during cold preservation. *Ann Thorac Surg* 63(6):1556-1561, 1997.
8. Bohuslav J, Kravchenko VV, Parry GC, Erlich JH., Gerondakis S, Mackman N, Ulevitch RJ. Regulation of an essential innate immune response by the p50 subunit of NF-kappaB. *J. Clin Invest.* 102(9):1645-52, 1998.
9. Bonini C, Ferrari G, Verzeletti S, Servida P, Zappone E, Ruggieri L, Ponzoni M, Rossini S, Mavilio F, Traversari C et al. HSV-TK gene transfer into donor lymphocytes for control of allogeneic graft-versus-leukemia. *Science* 276(5319):1719-1724, 1997.
10. Bouloc A, Walker P, Grivel JC, Vogel JC, Katz SI. Immunization through dermal delivery of protein-encoding DNA: a role for migratory dendritic cells. *Eur. J. Immunol.* 29(2):446-54, 1999.
11. Brenner MK, Heslop HE, Rill D, Li C, Nilson T, Roberts M, Smith C, Krance R, Rooney C. Gene transfer and bone marrow transplantation. *Cold Spring Harb Symp Quant Biol* 59:691-697, 1994.
12. Bromberg JS, DeBruyne LA, Qin L. Interactions between the immune system and gene therapy vectors: Bidirectional regulation of response and expression. *Adv Immunol.* 69:353-409, 1998.
13. Brossart P, Goldrath AW, Butz EA, Martin S, Bevan MJ. Virus-mediated delivery of antigenic epitopes into dendritic cells as a means to induce CTL. *J. Immunol.* 158(7):3270-6, 1997.
14. Brough DE, Hsu C, Kulesa VA, Lee GM, Cantolupo LJ, Lizonova A, Kovesdi I. Activation of transgene expression by early region 4 is responsible for a high level of persistent transgene expression from adenovirus vectors in vivo. *J. Virol.* 71(12):9206-13, 1997.
15. Burcin MM, Schiedner G, Kochanek S, Tsai SY, O'Malley BW. Adenovirus-mediated regulable target gene expression in vivo. *Proc. Natl. Acad Sci USA.* 96(2):355-60, 1999.
16. Casares S, Inaba K, Brumeanu TD, Steinman RM, Bona CA. Antigen presentation by dendritic cells after immunization with DNA encoding a major histocompatibility complex class II-restricted viral epitope. *J. Exp Med.* 186(9):1481-6, 1997.

17. Chahine AA, Yu M, McKernan MM, Stoeckert C, Lau HT. Immunomodulation of pancreatic islet allografts in mice with CTLA4Ig secreting muscle cells. *Transplantation*. 59(9):1313-8, 1995.

18. Chattergoon MA, Robinson TM, Boyer JD, Weiner DB. Specific immune induction following DNA-based immunization through in vivo transfection and activation of macrophages/antigen-presenting cells. *J. Immunol.* 160(12):5707-18, 1998.

19. Chen HH, Mack LM, Choi SY, Ontell M, Kochanek S, Clemens PR. DNA from both high-capacity and first-generation adenoviral vectors remains intact in skeletal muscle. *Hum Gene Ther.* 10(3):365-73, 1999.

20. Chirmule N, Hughes JV, Gao GP, Raper SE, Wilson JM. Role of E4 in eliciting CD4 T-cell and B-cell responses to adenovirus vectors delivered to murine and nonhuman primate lungs. *J. Virol.* 72(7):6138-45, 1998.

21. Chu RS, Targoni OS, Krieg AM, Lehmann PV, Harding CV. CpG oligodeoxynucleotides act as adjuvants that switch on T helper 1 (Th1) immunity. *J. Exp Med.* 186(10):1623-31, 1997.

22. Csete ME, Drazan KE, Van Bree M, McIntee DF, McBride WH, Bett A, Graham FL, Busuttil RW, Berk AJ, Shaked A. Adenovirus-mediated gene transfer in the transplant setting. I. Conditions for expression of transferred genes in cold-preserved hepatocytes. *Transplantation* 57:(10)1502-1507, 1994.

23. DeBruyne LA, Kewang L, Bishop K, Bromberg JS. Gene transfer of virally encoded chemokine agonists, vMIP-II and MC148, prolongs cardiac allograft survival. *Transplantation* 67(9):S571, 1999.

24. DeBruyne LA, Magee JC, Buelow R, and Bromberg JS: Gene transfer of immunomodulatory peptides correlates with heme oxygenase-I induction and enhanced allograft survival. *Transplantation* (in press).

25. Deuschle U, Pepperkok R, Wang F, Giordano TJ, McAllister WT, Ansorge W, Bujard H. Regulated expression of foreign genes in mammalian cells under the control of coliphage T3 RNA polymerase and lac repressor. *Proc Natl Acad Sci USA* 86(14): 5600-5604, 1989.

26. De Waal Malefyt R, Haanen J, Spits H, Roncarlol MG, te Velde A, Figdor C, Johnson C, Kastelein R, Yssel H, de Vries JE. Interleulin-10 (IL-10) and viral IL-10 strongly reduce antigen-specific human T cell proliferation by diminishing the antigen-presenting capacity of monocytes via down-regulation of class II major histocompatibility complex expression. *J Exp Med* 174(4):915-924, 1991.

27. Docherty K. Gene therapy for diabetes mellitus. *Clinical Science* 92(4):321-330, 1997.

28. Drazan KE, Olthoff KM, Wu L, Shen X, Gelman A, Shaked, A. Adenovirus-mediated gene transfer in the transplant setting: early events after orthotopic transplantation of liver allografts expressing TGF-□1. *Transplantation* 62(8):1080-1084, 1996.

29. Efrat S, Fusco-Demane D, Lemberg H, Erman OA, Wang X. Conditional transformation of a pancreatic □-cell line derived from transgenic mice expressing a tetracycline-regulated oncogene. *Proc Natl Acad Sci USA* 92(8): 3576-3580, 1995a.

30. Efrat S, Fejer , Brownlee M, Horwitz MS. Prolonged survival of pancreatic islet allografts mediated by adenovirus immunoregulatory transgenes. *Proc Natl Acad Sci USA* 92(15):6947-6951, 1995b.

31. Eglitis MA, Kantoff P, Gilboa E, Anderson WF. Gene expression in mice after high efficiency retroviral-mediated gene transfer. *Science* 230(4732):1395-1398, 1985.

32. Elkon KB, Liu CC, Gall JG, Trevejo J, Marino MW, Abrahamsen KA, Song X, Zhou JL, Old LJ, Crystal RG, Falck-Pedersen E. Tumor necrosis factor alpha plays a central role in immune-mediated clearance of adenoviral vectors. *Proc Natl Acad Sci USA*. 94(18):9814-9, 1997.

33. Emery DW, Shafer GE, Karson EM, Sachs DH, LeGuern C. Retrovirus-mediated transfer and expression of an allogeneic major histocompatibility complex class II DRB cDNA in swine bone marrow cultures. *Blood.* 81(9):2460-5, 1993a.

34. Emery DW, Smith CV, Shafer GE, Karson EM, Sachs DH, LeGuern C. Expression of allogeneic class II cDNA in swine peripheral blood mononuclear cells following retroviral-mediated gene transfer into bone marrow. *Transplantation Proc.* 25(1 Pt 1):140-1, 1993b.

35. Emery DW, Sablinski T, Arn JS, LeGuern C, Sachs DH. Bone marrow culture and transduction of stem cells in a miniature swine model. *Blood Cells.* 20(2-3):498-502, 1994.

36. Fabrega AJ, Fasbender AJ, Struble S, Zabner J. Cationic lipid-mediated transfer of the hIL-10 gene prolongs survival of allogeneic hepatocytes in Nagase analbuminemic rats. *Transplantation* 62(12):1866-1871, 1996.

37. Felgner PL, Gadek TR, Holm M, Roman R, Chan HW, Wenz M, Northrop JP, Ringold GM, Danielsen M. Lipofection: a highly efficient, lipid-mediated DNA-transfection procedure. *Proc Natl Acad Sci USA.* 84 (21):7413-7, 1987.

38. Ferber S, Beltrande I, Rio H, Johnson JH, Noel RJ, Cassidy LE, Clark S, Becker TC, Hughes SD, Newgard CB. GLUT-2 gene transfer into insulinoma cells confers both low and high affinity glucose-stimulated insulin release. *J Biol Chem* 269(15):11523-11529, 1994.

39. Fisher KJ, Jooss K, Alston J, Yang Y, Haecker SE, High K, Pathak R, Raper SE, Wilson JM. Recombinant adeno-associated virus for muscle directed gene therapy. *Nat Med.* 3(3):306-12, 1997.

40. Fraser CC, Sykes M, Lee RS, Sachs DH, LeGuern C. Specific unresponsiveness to a retrovirally-transferred class I antigen is controlled through the helper pathway. *J. Immunol.* 154(4):1587-1595, 1995.

41. Gainer AL, Korbutt GS, Rajotte RV, Warnock GL, Elliott JF. Expression of CTLA4-Ig by biolistically transfected mouse islets promotes islet allograft survival. *Transplantation.* 63(7):1017-21, 1997.

42. Gangappa S, Babu JS, Thomas J, Daheshia M, Rouse BT. Virus-induced immunoinflammatory lesions in the absence of viral antigen recognition. *J. Immunol.* 161(8):4289-300, 1998.

43. Ghazizadeh S, Carroll JM, Taichman LB. Repression of retrovirus-mediated transgene expression by interferons: implications for gene therapy. *J. Virol.* 71(12):9163-9, 1997.

44. Ghosh-Choudhury G, Graham FL. Stable transfer of a mouse dihydrofolate reductase gene into a deficient cell line using human adenovirus vector. *Biochem Biophys Res Comm.* 147(3):964-73, 1987.

45. Gordon EM, Anderson WF. Gene therapy using retroviral vectors. *Curr Opin Biotech* 5(6):611-616, 1994.

46. Gribaudo G, Ravaglia S, Caliendo A, Cavallo R, Gariglio M, Martinotti MG, Landolfo S. Interferons inhibit onset of murine cytomegalovirus immediate-early gene transcription. *Virol.* 197(1):303-11, 1993.

47. Grossman M, Raper SE, Kozarsky K, Stein EA, Engelhardt JF, Muller D, Lupien PJ, Wilson JM. Successful *ex vivo* gene therapy directed to liver in a patient with familial hypercholesterolemia. *Nat Genetics* 6(4):335-341, 1994.

48. Guidotti LG, Ishikawa T, Hobbs MV, Matzke B, Schreiber R, Chisari FV. Intracellular inactivation of the hepatitis B virus by cytotoxic T lymphocytes. *Immunity.* 4(1):25-36, 1996.

49. Hacker H, Mischak H, Miethke T, Liptay S, Schmid R, Sparwasser T, Heeg K, Lipford GB, Wagner H. CpG-DNA-specific activation of antigen-presenting cells requires stress kinase activity and is preceded by non-specific endocytosis and endosomal maturation. *EMBO J.* 17(21):6230-40, 1998.

50. Harms JS, Splitter GA. Interferon-gamma inhibits transgene expression driven by SV40 or CMV promoters but augments expression driven by the mammalian MHC I promoter. *Hum Gene Ther*. 6(10):1291-7, 1995.
51. Hatzoglou M, Lamers W, Bosch F, et al. Hepatic gene transfer in animals using retroviruses containing the promoter from the gene for phosphoenolpyruvate carboxykinase. *J. Biol Chem* 265(28):17285-17293, 1990.
52. Hottiger MO, Felzien LK, Nabel GJ. Modulation of cytokine-induced HIV gene expression by competitive binding of transcription factors to the coactivator p300. *EMBO J*. 17(11):3124-34, 1998.
53. Hsu DH, De Waal Malefyt R, Fiorentino DF, Dang MN, Vieira P, DeVries J, Spits H, Mosmann TR, Moore KW. Expression of interleukin-10 activity by Epstein-Barr virus protein BCRF1. *Science* 250(4982):830-832, 1990.
54. Jooss K, Yang Y, Fisher KJ, Wilson JM. Transduction of dendritic cells by DNA viral vectors directs the immune response to transgene products in muscle fibers. *J. Virol*. 72(5):4212-23, 1998.
55. Kafri T, Morgan D, Krahl T, Sarvetnick N, Sherman L, Verma I. Cellular immune response to adenoviral vector infected cells does not require de novo viral gene expression: implications for gene therapy. *Proc Natl Acad Sci USA*. 95(19):11377-82, 1998.
56. Kay MA, Baley P, Rothenberg S, Leland F, Fleming L, Parker Ponder K, Liu T-J, Finegold M, Darlington G, Pokorny W. et al. Expression of human □1-antitrypsin in dogs after autologous transplantation of retroviral transduced hepatocytes. *Proc Natl Acad Sci USA* 89(4982):89-93, 1992.
57. Klinman DM, Yi AK, Beaucage SL, Conover J, Krieg AM. CpG motifs present in bacteria DNA rapidly induce lymphocytes to secrete interleukin 6, interleukin 12, and interferon gamma. *Proc Natl Acad Sci USA*. 93(7):2879-83, 1996.
58. Kozarsky KF, Wilson JM. Gene therapy: adenovirus vectors. *Curr Opin Genet Dev*. 3(3):499-503, 1993.
59. Kuhr T, Dougherty GJ, Klingermann H-G. Transfer of the tumor necrosis factor a gene into hematopoietic progenitor cells as a model for site-specific cytokine delivery after marrow transplantation. *Blood* 84(9):2966-2970, 1994.
60. Kukowska-Latallo JF, Bielinska AU, Johnson J, Spindler R, Tomalia DA, Baker JR Jr. Efficient transfer of genetic material into mammalian cells using Starburst polyamidoamine dendrimers. *Proc Natl Acad Sci, USA*. 93(10):4897-902, 1996.
61. Lau HT, Yu M, Fontana A, Stoeckert CJ Jr. Prevention of islet allograft rejection with engineered myoblasts expressing FasL in mice. *Science*. 273(5271):109-12, 1996.
62. Leiden JM. Beating the odds: a cardiomyocyte cell line at last. *J. Clin Invest*. 103(5):591-2, 1999.
63. Levy AE, Alexander JW. Administration of intragraft interleukin-4 prolongs cardiac allograft survival in rats treated with donor-specific transfusion/cyclosporine. *Transplantation*. 60(5):405-6, 1995.
64. Lieber A, He CY, Meuse L, Schowalter D, Kirillova I, Winther B, Kay MA. The role of Kupffer cell activation and viral gene expression in early liver toxicity after infusion of recombinant adenovirus vectors. *J. Virol*. 71(11):8798-807, 1997.
65. Lieber A, He CY, Meuse L, Himeda C, Wilson C, Kay MA. Inhibition of NF-kappaB activation in combination with bcl-2 expression allows for persistence of first-generation adenovirus vectors in the mouse liver. *J. Virol*. 72(11):9267-77, 1998.
66. Lin H, Parmacek MS, Morle G, Bolling S, Leiden JM. Expression of recombinant genes in myocardium in vivo after direct injection of DNA. *Circulation* 82(6):2217-2221, 1990.
67. Loser P, Jennings GS, Strauss M, Sandig V. Reactivation of the previously silenced cytomegalovirus major immediate-early promoter in the mouse liver: involvement of NF-kappaB. *J. Virol*. 72(1):180-90, 1998.

68. Lucin P, Jonjic S, Messerle M, Polic B, Hengel H, Koszinowski UH. Late phase inhibition of murine cytomegalovirus replication by synergistic action of interferon-gamma and tumour necrosis factor. *J. Gen. Virol.*. 75 (Pt 1):101-10, 1994.

69. Lusky M, Christ M, Rittner K, Dieterle A, Dreyer D, Mourot B, Schultz H, Stoeckel F, Pavirani A, Mehtali M. In vitro and in vivo biology of recombinant adenovirus vectors with E1, E1/E2A, or E1/E4 deleted. *J. Virol.* 72(3):2022-32, 1998.

70. Macfarlane DE, Manzel L. Antagonism of immunostimulatory CpG-oligodeoxynucleotides by quinacrine, chloroquine, and structurally related compounds. *J. Immunol.* 160(3):1122-31, 1998.

71. Magee JC, DeBruyne LA, Buelow R, Bromberg JS. Gene transfer of immunosuppressive peptides B2702 and RDP1257 prolongs allograft survival: evidence suggesting a role for heme oxygenase-I. *Transplant Proc.* 31(1-2):1194, 1999.

72. Makino S, Fukuda K, Miyoshi S, Konishi F, Kodama H, Pan J, Sano M, Takahashi T, Hori S, Abe H, Hata J, Umezawa A, Ogawa S. Cardiomyocytes can be generated from marrow stromal cells in vitro. *J. Clin Invest.* 103(5):697-705, 1999.

73. McCoy RD, Davidson BL, Roessler BJ, Huffnagle GB, Simon RH. Expression of human interleukin-1 receptor antagonist in mouse lungs using a recombinant adenovirus: effects on vector-induced inflammation. *Gene Ther* 2(7):437-442, 1995.

74. Miyoshi H, Smith KA, Mosier DE, Verma IM, Torbett BE. Transduction of human CD34+ cells that mediate long-term engraftment of NOD/SCID mice by HIV vectors. *Science.* 283(5402):682-6, 1999.

75. Moore KW, Vieira P, Fiorentino DF, Trounstine ML, Khan TA, Mosmann TR. Homology of cytokine synthesis inhibitory factor (IL-10) to the Epstein-Barr virus gene BCRFI. *Science* 248(4960):1230-1234, 1990.

76. Muruve DA, Barnes MJ, Stillman IE, Liebermann TA. Adenoviral genetherapy leads to rapid induction of multiple chemokines and actue neutrophil-dependent hepatic injury in vivo. *Hum Gene Ther.* 10(6):965-976, 1999.

77. Naldini L, Blomer U, Fallay P, Ory D Muligan R, Gage FH, Verma IM, and Trono D. In vivo delivery and stable transduction of nondividing cells by a lentiviral vector. *Science* 272(5259):263-267, 1996.

78. Nicolau C, Legrand A, Grosse E.. Liposomes as carriers for in vivo gene transfer and expression. *Methods Enzymol.* 149:157-76, 1987.

79. Olszewska-Pazdrak B, Casola A, Saito T, Alam R, Crowe SE, Mei F, Ogra PL, Garofalo RP. Cell-specific expression of RANTES, MCP-1, and MIP-1alpha by lower airway epithelial cells and eosinophils infected with respiratory syncytial virus. *J. Virol.* 72(6):4756-64, 1998.

80. Olthoff KM, Da Chen X, Gelman A, Turka L, Shaked A. Adenovirus-mediated gene transfer of CTLA4Ig to liver allografts results in prolonged survival and local T cell anergy. *Transplant Proc* 29(1-2):1030-1031, 1997.

81. Otake K, Ennist DL, Harrod K, Trapnell BC. Nonspecific inflammation inhibits adenovirus-mediated pulmonary gene transfer and expression independent of specific acquired immune responses. *Hum Gene Ther.* 9(15):2207-22, 1998.

82. Pan R-Y, Xiao X, Chen S-L, Li J, Lin L-C, Wang H-J, Tsao Y-P. Disease-inducible transgene expression from a recombinant adeno-associated virus vector in a rat arthritis model. *J. Virol.* 73(4):3410-3417, 1999.

83. Poller W, Schneider-Rasp S, Liebert U, Merklein F, Thalheimer P, Haack A,. Schwaab R, Schmitt C, Brackmann HH. Stabilization of transgene expression by incorporation of E3 region genes into an adenoviral factor IX vector and by transient anti-CD4 treatment of the host. *Gene Ther.* 3(6):521-30, 1996.

84. Porgador A, Irvine KR, Iwasaki A, Barber BH, Restifo NP, Germain RN. Predominant role for directly transfected dendritic cells in antigen presentation to CD8+ T cells after gene gun immunization. *J. Expl Med.* 188(6):1075-82, 1998.
85. Presti RM, Pollock JL, Dal Canto AJ, O'Guin AK, Virgin HW 4th. Interferon gamma regulates acute and latent murine cytomegalovirus infection and chronic disease of the great vessels. *J. Expl Med.* 188(3):577-88, 1998.
86. Qin L, Chavin KD, Ding Y, Favarro JP, Woodward JE, Lin J, Tahara H, Robbins P, Shaked A, et al. Multiple vectors effectively achieve gene transfer in a murine cardiac transplantation model: Immunosuppression with TGF-β1 or vIL-10. *Transplantation* 59(6): 809-816, 1995.
87. Qin L, Ding Y, Bromberg JS. Gene transfer of transforming growth factor-β1 prolongs murine cardiac allograft survival by inhibiting cell mediated immunity. *Hum Gene Ther* 7(16):1981-1988, 1996.
88. Qin L, Ding Y, Pahud DR, Robson ND, Shaked A, Bromberg JS. Adenovirus-mediated gene transfer of viral interleukin-10 inhibits the immune response to both alloantigen and adenoviral antigen. *Hum Gen Ther* 8(11):1365-1374, 1997a.
89. Qin L, Ding Y, Pahud DR, Chang E, Imperiale MJ, Bromberg JS. Promoter attenuation in gene therapy: interferon-gamma and tumor necrosis factor-alpha inhibit transgene expression. *Hum Gene Ther.* 8(17):2019-29, 1997b.
90. Raper SE. Hepatocyte transplantation and gene therapy. *Clin Transplantation.* 9(3 Pt2):249-254, 1995.
91. Roman M, Martin-Orozco E, Goodman JS, Nguyen MD, Sato Y, Ronaghy A, Kornbluth RS, Richman DD, Carson DA, Raz E. Immunostimulatory DNA sequences function as T helper-1-promoting adjuvants [see comments]. *Nat Med.* 3(8):849-54, 1997.
92. Rosenfeld MA, Siegfried W, Yoshimura K, Yoneyama K, Fukayama M, Stier LE, Paakko PK, Gilardi P, Stratford-Perricaudet LD, Perricaudet M, et al. Adenovirus-mediated transfer of a recombinant alpha 1-antitrypsin gene to the lung epithelium in vivo. *Science.* 252(5004):431-4, 1991.
93. Rosenthal FM, Fruh R, Henschler R, Veelken H, Kulmburg P, Mackensen A, Gansbacher B, Mertelsmann R, Lindemannn A. Cytokine therapy with gene-transfected cells: Single injection of irradiated granulocyte-macrophage colony-stimulating factor-transduced cells accelerates hematopoietic recovery after cytotoxic chemotherapy in mice. *Blood* 84(9):2960-2965, 1994.
94. Rousset F, Garcia E, Defrance T, Peronne C, Vezzio N, Hsu DH, Kastelein R, Moore KW, Banchereau J. Interleukin-10 is a potent growth hand differentiation factor for activated human B lymphocytes. *Proc Natl Acad Sci USA* 89(5):1890-1893, 1992.
95. (12), Zhu X,. Xiao X,. Brook JD, Housman DE, Epstein N, Hunter LA. Targeted integration of adeno-associated virus (AAV) into human chromosome 19 [published erratum appears in *EMBO J* 11:1228, 1992] *EMBO J.* 10(12):3941-50, 1991.
96. Sebestyen MG, Ludtke JJ, Bassik MC, Zhang G, Budker V, Lukhtanov EA,. Hagstrom JE,. Wolff JA. DNA vector chemistry: the covalent attachment of signal peptides to plasmid DNA. *Nat Biotech.* 16(1):80-5, 1998.
97. Serup P, Jensen J, Andersen FG, Jaergensen MC, Blume N, Holst JJ, Madsen OD. Induction of insulin and islet amyloid polypeptide production in pancreatic islet glucagonoma cells by insulin promoter factor I. *Proc Natl Acad Sci USA* 93(17):9015-9020, 1996.
98. Shaked A, Csete ME, Drazan KE, Bullington D, WU L, Busuttil RW, Berk AJ. Adenovirus-mediated gene transfer in the transplant setting. . II. Successful expression of transferred cDNA in syngeneic liver grafts. *Transplantation* 57(10):1508-1511, 1994.

99. Smith CV, Nakajima K, Mixon A, Guzetta PC, Rosengard BR, Fishbein JM, Sachs DH. Successful induction of long-term specific tolerance to fully allogeneic renal allografts in miniature swine. *Transplantation* 53(2):438-444. 1992.

100. Soares MP, Muniappan A, Kaczmarek E, Koziak K, Wrighton CJ, Steinhauslin F, Ferran C, Winkler H, Bach FH, Anrather J. Adenovirus-mediated expression of a dominant negative mutant of p65/RelA inhibits proinflammatory gene expression in endothelial cells without sensitizing to apoptosis. *J. Immunol.* 161(9):4572-82, 1998.

101. Spencer HT, Sleep SE, Rehg JE, Blakley RL, Sorrentino BP. A gene transfer strategy for making bone marrow cells resistant to trimetrexate. *Blood* 87(6):2579-2587, 1996.

102. Sun S, Zhang X, Tough DF, Sprent J. Type I interferon-mediated stimulation of T cells by CpG DNA. *J. Expl Med.* 188(12):2335-42, 1998.

103. Suzuki M, Singh R, Moore MA, Song WR, Crystal RG. Similarity of strain- and route-dependent murine responses to an adenovirus vector using the homologous thrombopoietin cDNA as the reporter genes. *Hum Gene Ther.* 9(8):1223-31, 1998.

104. Suzuki T, Tahara H, Narula S, Moore KW, Robbins PD, Lotze MT. Viral interleukin-10 (IL-10), the human herpes virus 4 cellular IL-10 homologue, induces local anergy to allogeneic and syngeneic tumors. *J Exp Med* 182(2):477-486, 1995.

105. Suzuki T, Shin BC, Fujikura K, Matsuzaki T, Takata K. Direct gene transfer into rat liver cells by in vivo electroporation. *FEBS Letters* 425(3):436-440, 1998.

106. Sykes M, Sachs DH, Nienhuis AW, Pearson DA, Moulton AD, Bodine DM. Specific prolongation of skin graft survival following retroviral transduction of bone marrow with an allogeneic major histocompatibility complex gene. *Transplantation.* 55(1):197-202, 1993.

107. Takahashi T, Kalka C, Masuda H, Chen D, Silver M, Kearney M, Magner M, Isner JM, Asahara T. Ischemia- and cytokine-induced mobilization of bone marrow-derived endothelial progenitor cells for neovascularization. *Nat Med.* 5(4):434-8, 1999.

108. Thomas LH, Friedland JS, Sharland M, Becker S. Respiratory syncytial virus-induced RANTES production from human bronchial epithelial cells is dependent on nuclear factor-kappa B nuclear binding and is inhibited by adenovirus-mediated expression of inhibitor of kappa B alpha. *J. Immunol.* 161(2):1007-16, 1998.

109. Thompson-Snipes L, Dhar V, Bond MW, Mosmann TR, Moore KW, Rennick DM. Interleukin-10: a novel stimulatory factor for mast cells and their progenitors. *J Exp Med* 173(2):507-510, 1991.

110. Tripathy SK, Black HB, Goldwasser E, Leiden JM. Immune responses to transgene-encoded proteins limit the stability of gene expression after injection of replication-defective adenovirus vectors. *Nat Med.* 2(5):545-50, 1996.

111. Vieira P, de Waal Malefyt R, Dang MN, Johnson KE, Kastelein R, Fiorentino DF, de Vries JE, Roncarolo MG, Mosmann TR, and Moore KW. Isolation and expression of human cytokine synthesis inhibitory factor cDNA clones: homology to Epstein-Barr virus open reading frame BCRFI. *Proc Natl Acad Sci USA* 88(4):1172-1176, 1991.

112. Vinh DB, McIvor RS. Selective expression of methotrexate-resistant dihydrofolate reductase (DHFR) activity in mice transduced with DHFR retrovirus and administered methotrexate. *J Pharmacol Exp Ther* 267(2):989-996, 1993.

113. Wadsworth SC, Zhou H, Smith AE, Kaplan JM. Adenovirus vector-infected cells can escape adenovirus antigen-specific cytotoxic T-lymphocyte killing in vivo. *J. Virol.* 71(7):5189-96, 1997.

114. Weiner GJ,. Liu HM, Wooldridge JE, Dahle CE, Krieg AM. Immunostimulatory oligodeoxynucleotides containing the CpG motif are effective as immune

adjuvants in tumor antigen immunization. *Proc Nal Acad Sci USA*. 94(20):10833-7, 1997.

115.Welsh M, Welsh N, Nilsson T, Arkhammar P, Pepinsky RB, Steiner DF, Berggren P-O. Stimulation of pancreatic islet beta-cell replication by oncogenes. *Proc Natl Acad Sci USA* 85(1):116-120, 1988.

116.Wilson JM, Johnston DE, Jefferson DM, Mulligan RC. Correction of the genetic defect in hepatocytes from the Watanabe heritable hyperlipidemic rabbit. *Proc Natl Acad Sci USA*. 85:4421-4425, 1988.

117.Wolff JA, Malone RW, Williams P, Chang W, Ascadi G, Jani A, Felgner PL. Direct gene transfer into mouse muscle *in vivo. Science* 247(4949 Pt 1):1465-1468, 1990.

118.Worgall S, Leopold PL, Wolff G, Ferris B, Van Roijen N, Crystal RG. Role of alveolar macrophages in rapid elimination of adenovirus vectors administered to the epithelial surface of the respiratory tract. *Hum Gene Ther.* 8(14):1675-84, 1997a.

119.Worgall S, Wolff G, Falck-Pedersen E, Crystal RG. Innate immune mechanisms dominate elimination of adenoviral vectors following in vivo administration. *Hum Gene Ther.* 8(1):37-44, 1997b.

120.Wu GY, Wu CH. Receptor-mediated in vitro gene transformation by a soluble DNA carrier system. [published erratum appears in *J Biol Chem.* 263:588, 1988]. *J Biol Chem.* 262(10):4429-32, 1987.

121.Yamamoto S, Kuramoto E, Shimada S, Tokunaga T. In vitro augmentation of natural killer cell activity and production of interferon-alpha/beta and -gamma with deoxyribonucleic acid fraction from Mycobacterium bovis BCG. *Japanese J. Can Res.* 79(7):866-73, 1988.

122.Yang Y, Ertl HC, Wilson JM. MHC class I-restricted cytotoxic T lymphocytes to viral antigens destroy hepatocytes in mice infected with E1-deleted recombinant adenoviruses. *Immunity.* 1(5):433-42, 1994a.

123.Yang Y, Nunes FA, Berencsi K, Furth EE, Gonczol E, Wilson JM. Cellular immunity to viral antigens limits E1-deleted adenoviruses for gene therapy. *Proc. Natl Acad Sci USA.* 91(10):4407-11, 1994b.

124.Ye X, Rivera VM, Zoltick P, et al. Regulated delivery of therapeutic proteins after in vivo somatic cell gene transfer. *Science.* 283(5398):88-91, 1999.

125.Yei S, Mittereder N, Wert S, Whitsett JA, Wilmott RW, Trapnell BC. In vivo evaluation of the safety of adenovirus-mediated transfer of the human cystic fibrosis transmembrane conductance regulator cDNA to the lung. *Hum Gene Ther.* 5(6):731-44, 1994.

126.Yi AK, Chace JH, Cowdery JS, Krieg AM. IFN-gamma promotes IL-6 and IgM secretion in response to CpG motifs in bacterial DNA and oligodeoxynucleotides. *J. Immunol.* 156(2):558-64, 1996.

127.Yi AK, Tuetken R, Redford T, Waldschmidt M, Kirsch J, Krieg AM. CpG motifs in bacterial DNA activate leukocytes through the pH-dependent generation of reactive oxygen species. *J. Immunol.* 160(10):4755-61, 1998a.

128.Yi AK, Krieg AM. CpG DNA rescue from anti-IgM-induced WEHI-231 B lymphoma apoptosis via modulation of I kappa B alpha and I kappa B beta and sustained activation of nuclear factor-kappa B/c-Rel. *J. Immunol.* 160(3):1240-5, 1998b.

129.Yi AK, Krieg AM. Rapid induction of mitogen-activated protein kinases by immune stimulatory CpG DNA. *J. Immunol.* 161(9):4493-7, 1998c.

130.Zanta MA,. Belguise-Valladier P, Behr JP. Gene delivery: a single nuclear localization signal peptide is sufficient to carry DNA to the cell nucleus. *Proc Natl Acad Sci USA.* 96(1):91-6, 1999.

131.Zhong L, Granelli-Piperno A, Choi Y, Steinman RM. Recombinant adenovirus is an efficient and non-perturbing genetic vector for human dendritic cells. *Eur J Immunol.* 29(3):964-72, 1999.

IMMUNOMODULATION STRATEGIES IN XENOTRANSPLANTATION

Ian P.J. Alwayn, Leo Bühler, Murali Basker, and David K.C. Cooper

Abstract

Many believe that xenotransplantation – i.e., the transplantation of tissues and/or organs between different species – holds the future of transplantation. Clinical application, however, is currently hampered by many barriers, of which rejection is the most formidable. This chapter focuses on the immunopathological background of xenograft rejection and the therapeutic modalities being explored to prevent it. The pig-to-nonhuman primate experimental model is emphasized, as the pig is the animal most likely to be the organ-source for organ xenotransplantation in humans.

Introduction

The outcome of clinical organ transplantation has dramatically improved since the introduction of cyclosporine (CyA) in 1979 and of other immunosuppressive agents (introduced more recently) as well as refinements of surgical techniques and perioperative management. Due to its relative success, the inclusion criteria for potential organ transplant recipients have been broadened, resulting in an even greater shortage of donor organs. The number of patients with end-stage organ failure that die awaiting organ transplantation is steadily increasing, mainly because of the shortage of appropriate donor organs [1-3]. Many clinicians and investigators believe that strategies directed at expanding the allogeneic donor pool will not be sufficient to resolve this

Mohamed Sayegh and Giuseppe Remuzzi (editors), Current and Future Immunosuppressive Therapies Following Transplantation, 357-388.

problem of organ shortage. In contrast, successful xenotransplantation - the transplantation of tissues and/or organs between two different species - has the potential of providing an unlimited supply of donor organs that would be available when required [4]. However, major immunological barriers, as well as other important issues, at present prevent the implementation of xenotransplantation clinically [5].

Concordant xenografts - tissues/organs transplanted between phylogenetically close species, i.e., mouse and rat, monkey and baboon, or nonhuman primate and human - reject more vigorously than allografts. The mechanism of rejection is thought to be mediated by a combination of humoral and cellular factors. Conventional immunosuppressive therapy cannot guarantee long-term graft survival because of the potent induced antibody response in concordant xenotransplantation. However, with judicious pharmacological immunosuppressive therapy, the reported survival of concordant heart grafts in nonhuman primates exceeds 500 days [6].

Discordant xenotransplantation - xenotransplantation between phylogenetically widely disparate species, i.e., guinea pig and rat, pig and baboon, or pig and human - is characterized by the occurrence of hyperacute rejection (HAR) [7,8]. This type of rejection, mediated in primates by preformed (natural) antibodies (directed against the Galα1-3Gal (α-Gal) epitopes) (**Table 1**) [9], which activate complement, takes place within minutes to hours after transplantation [10]. Histological examination of these rejected grafts reveals intravascular thrombosis and interstitial hemorrhage [11,12].

It has recently become possible to overcome HAR through antibody and/or complement depletion or by utilizing organs from pigs transgenic for human complement regulatory protein [8,13-15]. If HAR is successfully prevented, a delayed type of rejection termed acute

Table 1. Structures of the main carbohydrate epitopes present at the surface of human and porcin vascular endothelium[*]

Human	Pig
Galβ1-4GlcNAcβ1-R[(a)]	Galβ1-4GlcNAcβ1-R[(a)]
ABH-Galβ1-4GlcNAcβ1-R[(b)]	**Galα1-3**Galβ1-4GlcNAcβ1-R[(c)]
NeuAcα2-3Galβ1-4GlcNAcβ1-R[(d)]	NeuAcα2-3Galβ1-4GlcNAcβ1-R[(d)]

Only the underlined epitopes in bold are different between the two species.
R are glycolipid or glycoprotein carrier molecules anchored in the cell membrane.
(a) N acetyllactosamine
(b) The A, B, H, or AB blood group antigen
(c) The α-galactosyl antigen
(d) N-acetylneuraminic acid

 * Modified from Oriol R, et al 1993 [23].

vascular rejection (AVR) occurs within days. Cellular infiltrates are invariably found throughout the xenograft, consisting of macrophages, NK cells, and monocytes [16,17]. Data suggest that this type of rejection is most probably antibody-mediated but complement-independent. It has thus far not been possible to overcome AVR in the pig-to-primate model. Survival of xenografts to date has generally been less than 30 days [18,19], and has not exceeded 99 days (White DJG, personal communication).

These major immunological differences notwithstanding, it is widely thought that the pig will be the most appropriate organ source [20,21], as pigs have a number of advantages over nonhuman primates as a potential source of organs for humans (**Table 2**). Furthermore, pigs can be bred in specific pathogen-free environments, thus eliminating to a large extent the risk of transfer of disease from pig to human. Certain herds of miniature swine have fully documented MHC antigens, which may facilitate certain manipulations aimed at the induction of

Table 2. Relative advantages and disadvantages of pigs and baboons as potential sources of organs and tissues.

		Baboon	**Pig**
Availability		Restricted	Unlimited
Breeding		Poor	Good
Potential	Reproductive age	3-5 years	4-8 months
	Length of pregnancy	173-193 days	114 +/- 2 days
	Number of offspring	1-2	5-12
	Rate of growth	Slow	Rapid
Size of adult organs		Inadequate	Adequate
Maintenance cost		High	Low
Similarity	Anatomical	Similar	Similar
	Physiological	Very similar	Less similar
	Immunological	Close	Distant
Knowledge of tissue typing		Limited	Considerable (in selected herds)
Experience with genetic engineering		None	Considerable
Risk of transfer of infection (xenozoonosis)		High	Low
Availability of specific pathogen-free animals		No	Yes
Public opinion		Mixed	More favorable

tolerance in the recipient, and pigs may be genetically modified to become less immunogenic to humans. Finally, since pigs are currently being bred for human consumption, it is likely that the general public will be amenable to using pigs for human organ xenotransplantation.

Many studies have been directed at attempting to understand the mechanisms of pig-to-nonhuman primate xenograft rejection. Much progress in this field has been made in the last decade, although the pathophysiology of xenograft rejection has not yet been fully eluci- dated. This chapter will briefly summarize our current knowledge of the mechanisms involved in discordant xenograft rejection and describe the techniques being explored to prevent rejection from occurring. Em- phasis will be placed on our experience in the pig-to-nonhuman primate preclinical model. Various methods of immunomodulation will be dis- cussed, including i) those aimed at depleting/inhibiting and/or preven- ting production of antibody, ii) those that deplete or inhibit comple- ment, iii) pharmacological immunosuppressive therapy aimed at sup- pression of both T and B cell function, iv) induction of tolerance and/or accommodation, and v) genetic engineering of the donor animal.

Rejection of Xenografts

Hyperacute Rejection

HAR is an antibody-dependant, complement-mediated process that occurs within minutes to hours after revascularization of the trans- planted discordant xenograft. Perper and Najarian were among the first to describe this process in 1966 in the pig-to-dog model [7]. All nonprimate mammals, including the pig, express terminal $Gal\alpha1$-3Gal oligosaccharides (αGal) as surface antigens on many cells, including the vascular endothelium [22,23]. In 1984 Galili et al. reported that humans possess natural antibodies with anti-αGal specificity [24], but it was not until 7 years later that Good et al. demonstrated that these antibodies (anti-αGal) play a major role in the HAR of pig xenografts in primates [9]. Anti-αGal are of IgG, IgM, and IgA subclasses and account for more than 85% of circulating natural anti-pig antibody in humans and 100% in baboons [24-28]. IgM is thought to be the major contributor to HAR [29]. Binding of these antibodies to the αGal epitopes on porcine tissue results in activation of complement through the classical pathway. This initiates a chain-reaction involving multiple complement components and leads to the formation of complexes, known as the membrane attack complex of complement, which causes lysis and opsonisation of cell membranes, resulting in rapid graft destruction.

Acute Vascular Rejection

Several methods have been developed to successfully prevent HAR, including extracorporeal immunoadsorption (EIA) of anti-αGal antibody, complement depletion or inhibition, and/or the use of pigs transgenic for human complement regulatory proteins. These approaches are discussed below. Once HAR has been averted, however, acute vascular rejection (AVR) develops, most probably as a result of the development of high levels of high-affinity antibody directed against αGal and other pig epitopes [30]. IgG seems to be the antibody subclass mostly responsible as increases in anti-αGal IgG of 100-300-fold have been documented after experimental pig organ and bone marrow transplantation in humans and nonhuman primates [31,32]. These induced antibodies initiate AVR by mechanisms that appear to be independent of complement, although complement fractions may play a role [17,30].

Cells, such as macrophages, NK cells, and monocytes are present in the rejected xenografts at the time of AVR, suggesting that they may be important to the rejection process [33,16,34]. Macrophages, in particular, play an important role in production, mobilization, activation, and regulation of immune effector cells. They participate in the activation of B and T cells. They process and present antigens, secrete various cytokines and chemokines, and phagocytose apoptotic and necrotic cells as well as various pathogens. It is not clear, however, if these cells, as well as NK cells, play a direct role in mediating or effecting AVR, or if they migrate to the graft as a result of presence of antibody.

Whatever the mechanism of AVR, there is growing evidence that it is associated with a state of disseminated intravascular coagulation in the recipient, which may develop before histopathological evidence of AVR is advanced [32,35].

Immunological Events following Antibody-Mediated Rejection

Since it has to date not been possible to routinely avert AVR, discussion of the immunological processes following AVR is mostly hypothetical. However, *in vitro* and *in vivo* studies involving discordant xenogeneic cells or grafts have shown that pig tissues are also rejected by cellular (antibody-independent) mechanisms [36-40]. The transplantation of pig pancreatic islets may be a useful model in that these are transplanted in the absence of a vascular endothelium, and therefore do not express αGal. Ingrowth of recipient vascular endothelium occurs. Nevertheless, porcine islets are rejected by a cellular mechanism in which macrophages and NK cells play a significant role. Although this model cannot be fully extrapolated to the transplantation of a vascularized organ, it seems likely that, if AVR is prevented, a cellular form of rejection will take place in the vascularized organ. Furthermore, chronic rejection, e.g. graft atherosclerosis, is likely to develop early.

Modulation of the Xenogeneic Immune Response

HAR can be prevented by i) depletion/inhibition of anti-αGal, ii) depletion or inhibition of components of complement, or iii) the use of organs from pigs transgenic for human complement regulatory proteins. To date, it has not been possible to prevent AVR in the pig-to-nonhuman primate model. Several methods, largely aimed at depletion/inhibition of anti-αGal combined with prevention of production of induced antibody, are currently being studied. Since non-specific cells, such as macrophages and NK cells, appear to be important in the pathogenesis of AVR, agents targeting these cells may also be essential in preventing AVR.

Present progress with these various therapeutic modalities will be presented and discussed.

Depletion of Anti-Pig (Anti-αGal) Antibody

The first reported attempts at removing preformed xenoreactive antibodies date from the 1960s and 1970s. The recipient's blood or plasma was perfused through a donor-specific organ, such as a pig kidney or liver [41-43]. The anti-species antibodies were thus adsorbed by the perfused organ's vascular endothelium and temporarily depleted from the recipient. This resulted in modestly prolonged survival of a subsequently transplanted organ from the same donor. The pig liver has been shown to be a better immunoadsorbent than the kidney in the pig-to-non-human primate model [8,44,45], and the lung may also be a good immunoadsorbent [46].

Other methods for depleting anti-pig antibody include (i) plasma exchange, (ii) plasma perfusion through non-specific immunoadsorbents (e.g., protein columns), and (iii) plasma perfusion through specific antibody sorbents (e.g., synthetic αGal immunoaffinity columns).

Plasma exchange - the removal of the subject's plasma (with replacement of volume by other fluids) - is utilized as a treatment for numerous conditions, such as myasthenia gravis, thrombotic microangiopathies, and cryoglobulinemias [47-49]. All or most circulating antibodies, including anti-αGal, are temporarily removed, which places the patient at some risk for infection. Furthermore, the patient may be depleted of plasma proteins important to the coagulation cascade. In clinical allotransplantation, Alexandre's group successfully removed circulating anti-A and/or anti-B blood group antibodies from potential kidney transplant recipients utilizing repeated plasma exchanges [50] allowing successful ABO-incompatible kidney transplantation through the development of accommodation (see below). This technique was also moderately successful in depleting xenoreactive natural antibodies in a pig-to-baboon kidney transplant model [51] with graft survival up to 22 days before eventually undergoing AVR.

Nonspecific antibody sorbents. The patient's plasma is passed through an immunoaffinity column containing proteins – such as staphylococcal protein A and protein G - that remove most immunoglobulins. The proteins are efficiently bound to the Fc portion of the antibody but, as they are non-specific, all antibodies are removed, resulting again in temporary hypogamma-globulinemia [52]. After adsorption, the remaining plasma is returned to the patient, which reduces the need for replacement fluids. Palmer et al. [53] and others have reported success using protein A columns to deplete anti-HLA antibodies in potential renal transplant recipients, and this technique has been used in a number of allotransplantation studies [54-56]. Nonspecific immunoadsorbants have also been used in xenotransplantation studies [57].

Specific antibody sorbents. Specific antibody sorbents, consisting of immunoaffinity columns of αGal oligosaccharides, successfully remove anti-αGal from plasma by binding the antibody to the αGal oligosaccharides. Significant hypogammaglobulinemia does not occur. Ye et al. demonstrated that extracorporeal immunoadsorption (EIA) of baboon plasma, utilizing immunoaffinity columns of the relatively non-specific melibiose on 4 consecutive days, could reduce serum cytotoxicity to pig kidney (PK15) cells by 80% [58]. With the availability of more specific synthetic αGal oligosaccharides, such as those consisting of an αGal trisaccharide [59], a course of EIA can result in successful depletion of anti-αGal for 4-5 days, after which anti-αGal returns and leads to AVR of a transplanted porcine organ [60-63]. To enable equilibration of anti-αGal between the intra- and extravascular spaces, Kozlowski et al. provided evidence indicating that EIAs should be carried out approximately 24 – 48 hours apart and that 4 consecutive EIAs were optimal [64]. Our own experience with over 300 EIAs in baboons indicates that a course of 3 EIAs results in 99% and 97% reductions in IgG and IgM, respectively [65].

Although all of the methods mentioned above are efficient in depleting anti-αGal and preventing HAR, antibody production continues and the depletion is only transient. If AVR is to be prevented, other therapeutic modalities are needed to inhibit the production of anti-αGal. To date this has proved extremely difficult to achieve.

Inhibition of Anti-αGal Antibody

Several methods have been devised in an attempt to inhibit anti-αGal *in vivo*.

Oligosaccharide infusion. Extensive *in vitro* studies, largely by Neethling and her collegues, demonstrated that many oligosaccharides, terminating in Galα1-X, can inhibit the action of anti-αGal [26,59, 66,67]. Some have been tested *in vivo* [58,68,69]. The infusion of very high concentrations of melibiose and/or arabinogalactan was found to be partially effective in eliminating cytotoxicity of baboon serum to PK15 cells (which are cultured pig kidney epithelial cells that express considerable Gal) [58]. However, when these di/polysaccharides were infused in such high concentrations, toxic effects were seen. More recently the intravenous administration of more specific saccharides has proven non-toxic, but only partially successful in inhibiting anti-αGal activity [68,69]. HAR of a transplanted pig organ was delayed, but not prevented.

Antiidiotypic antibody infusion.   An alternative approach to using synthetic oligosaccharide columns or intravenous oligosaccharides to bind anti-αGal is to use antiidiotypic antibodies (AIAs) directed against idiotypes expressed on anti-αGal antibodies. AIAs recognize specific idiotypes (antigenic determinants) within the variable regions of immunoglobulins, and are also directed against the B lymphocyte subpopulations that bear the same idiotypes as surface receptors. Koren et al. produced AIAs directed against human anti-pig antibodies in mice [70]. Several of these AIAs, when incubated with human serum, had a major inhibitory effect on serum cytotoxicity towards pig PK15 cells *in vitro.* When infused into baboons, serum cytotoxicity was markedly reduced (to approximately 10%).

We have recently produced a pig polyclonal AIA by immunizing a pig with human anti-αGal antibodies. After repeated administration to a baboon (following repeated EIA of anti-αGal), the purified final preparation (1-2 % AIAs) was able to effect a delayed return of anti-αGal and also to reduce the cytotoxicity of the serum to pig cells [71].

Suppression of Production of Anti-Pig (Anti-αGal) Antibody

Once depletion of anti-αGal has been achieved, unless accommodation develops (see below), it would seem essential to prevent the return of production of anti-αGal. As these (and all) antibodies are produced by B and plasma cells, techniques aimed at targeting these cells would be required. Non-specific methods, such as irradiation and pharmacological immunosuppressive drugs, are the mainstays of several xenotransplantation models, but to date have not resulted in either significantly diminished anti-αGal production or in long-term survival of a transplanted pig organ [5]. More specific therapies, consisting of specific monoclonal antibodies or immunotoxins directed at B cell- or plasma cell-specific surface antigens, might be able to achieve lasting suppression of production of anti-αGal. These various methods are outlined below.

Whole body irradiation.   Irradiation causes cell death, primarily of rapidly dividing cells, such as malignant cells and cells involved in hematopoiesis. Its current use is as an element of the conditioning regimen for bone marrow transplantation [72]. Several protocols aimed at achieving mixed hematopoietic chimerism and the induction of tolerance have therefore incorporated whole body irradiation (WBI)

[32,73,74]. WBI of 300 cGy - a non-lethal dose from which the bone marrow can spontaneously recover - leads to the temporary ablation of B cells in peripheral blood, bone marrow, and lymph nodes (**Figures 1A, B & C**), but results only in a small and temporary reduction in the production of antibody, including anti-αGal [31,32]. WBI, therefore, although creating "space" in the bone marrow to facilitate engraftment of transplanted hematopoietic cells, has only a minimal and transient effect on antibody production. The lack of effect on antibody production suggests that B cells themselves do not produce the majority of anti-αGal. Production is presumably by plasma cells, which are notably radiation-resistant [75].

Pharmacological agents. The effect on anti-αGal production of various conventional immunosuppressive drugs, as well as of several novel drugs, has been studied in baboons by Lambrigts et al [76]. Various combinations of these drugs (along with cyclosporine (CyA)) were used with EIA to deplete and suppress production of anti-αGal. In the absence of immunosuppression, anti-αGal returned to pre-EIA levels within 48 hours after the last of 3 consecutive EIA procedures. The rate of return of anti-αGal could be decreased with several combinations of drugs after EIA, but return could not be completely abolished. Rebound of anti-αGal to levels greater than or equal to pre-treatment levels was, however, successfully prevented.

Mycophenolate mofetil (MMF), an inhibitor of T and B cell proliferation and antibody production through purine synthesis inhibition, was judged to provide most suppression of antibody production in the absence of toxic side effects. It reduced anti-αGal levels to approximately 40% (IgM) and 20% (IgG) of pretreatment levels 48 hours following EIA and also reduced the rate of return of anti-αGal thereafter [76]. Ten days after the last EIA the anti-αGal IgM and IgG were 75 % and 25 % of pretreatment levels.

Cyclophosphamide (CPP), an alkylating metabolite, has also been associated with suppression of both T and B lymphocytes. Two doses of 20 mg/kg iv reduced both T and B cells to approximately 50% of baseline levels (Buhler L, unpublished data). When administered in moderate doses (1 – 20 mg/kg/day) it can significantly reduce the rate of return of anti-αGal after EIA [76]. White and coworkers have used CPP extensively in their hDAF transgenic pig-to-primate heart and kidney transplant models [18,19,77]. Their current CPP dosing regimen consists mainly of induction therapy, with an initial dose of 40 mg/kg iv on day −1 before transplant, followed by 3 doses of 20 mg/kg iv on days 0, 1, and 2, to reach a total of 100 mg/kg. This induction therapy is combined with cyclosporine, steroids, and other agents, such as MMF or a rapamycin derivative. Significant prolongation of xenograft function to a mean of approximately one month can be achieved [19,77], but ultimately the grafts are lost to AVR.

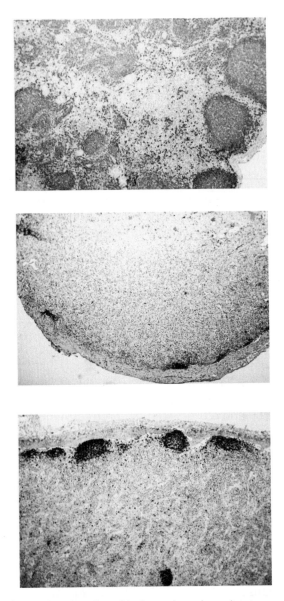

Figure 1. Photomicrographs of baboon lymph nodes immunohistochemically labeled with the B cell-specific anti-CD20 mAb.

A. Lymph node before whole body irradiation (WBI) (300 cGy) showing normal number and distribution of B cells in the follicles.

B. Lymph node 9 days after WBI (300 cGy). Note the complete depletion of B cells.

C. Lymph node 15 days after WBI (300 cGy). Recovery of B cells can be seen, beginning at the periphery of the follicles.

An agent investigated at our center is *zidovudine (AZT),* a purine analogue used in the treatment of HIV infection [78]. Apart from inhibiting viral reverse transcriptase, it also inhibits the mammalian DNA-polymerase that is responsible for DNA synthesis of mitochondria. We hypothesized that, since antibody production is a highly energy-dependant process, depletion of cellular mitochondria might prevent antibody from being produced by B and plasma cells. When AZT was administered to baboons, and anti-αGal was depleted by EIA, a significant reduction of anti-αGal, particularly of IgG, was documented in a previously sensitized baboon, but the drug was less successful in a baboon expressing only natural anti-Gal antibody but not induced antibody. Further studies are needed to fully assess this drug.

The novel antineoplastic drug, *cladribine*, is presently used to treat lymphoproliferative malignancies [79]. Cladribine, unlike other chemotherapeutic agents, is not only toxic to actively dividing lymphocytes but also to quiescent lymphocytes and monocytes, in which it induces apoptosis. It is therefore currently being explored in several transplantation studies [80]. In our own studies in baboons, its efficacy as a suppressor of antibody production is at least equal to that of most of the other agents tested. Baboons receiving cladribine maintained a decrease in anti-αGal levels to approximately 20% - 50% of baseline values for approximately 2 weeks following a course of EIA.

Other drugs, such as melphalan and brequinar sodium, are rather less effective in maintaining depletion of anti-αGal following EIA than are CPP or MMF [76]. Furthermore, methotrexate appears to have no effect on T or B cells in baboons, even when administered at doses that would be considered very high or even lethal in humans (Treter S, personal observation). Leflunomide has been found to be less successful than anticipated (White DJG, personal communication).

Anti-B cell monoclonal antibodies.   Several monoclonal antibodies (mAbs) directed against B cell-specific surface antigens have proven successful in reducing the mass of B cell lymphomas in in vitro, preclinical, and clinical studies [81-84]. Such mAbs, effective through a complement-mediated mechanism and/or antibody-dependant cellular cytotoxicity (ADCC), may be useful in depleting normal B cells and thus perhaps lead to reduced antibody production. This method, although not specific for anti-αGal, might provide a window for the induction of tolerance or accommodation.

The human-mouse chimeric antibody IDEC-C2B8 targets CD20 that is expressed on the surface of normal B cells. This mAb can effectively deplete malignant B cells in the blood of patients with B cell lymphoma [81-84]. We have confirmed the effectiveness of this mAb in our laboratory, where we have treated baboons with a 4 week course (x1 weekly) of anti-CD20 mAb, after which no B cells could be detected in the blood or bone marrow for up to 3 months (**Figure 2**). Lymph nodes, however, could not be fully depleted of B cells; a decrease in B

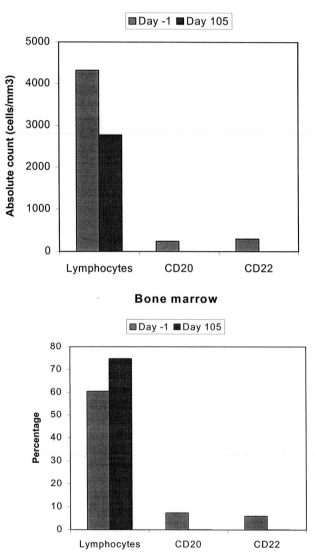

Figure 2. Bar chart demonstrating the depletion of (i) lymphocytes, (ii) CD20- and (iii) CD22-positive cells in blood (as absolute cell count) and bone marrow (as percentage of total cells) before (at −1 day) and after (at 105 days) four doses of the anti-CD20 chimeric mAb, IDEC-C2B8, at weekly intervals. Almost total depletion of B cells (CD20- and CD22-positive) was seen immediately after the course of anti-CD20 mAb therapy, and this depletion persisted for approximately 3 months.

cells to 20% of the initial level was found 5 weeks after the first dose, with recovery beginning by week 6. The addition of 150cGy WBI could effectively eradicate the remaining B cells in these experiments, with recovery not occurring for 3 months. After a course of EIAs, anti-αGal levels remained reduced for 2 – 3 weeks but the reduction was relatively modest and disappointing when compared with the extent of B cell deletion (**Figure 3**).

Immunotoxins. CD22 is a surface molecule involved with the generation of mature B cells within the bone marrow, blood, and marginal zones of lymphoid tissues. An anti-CD22 mAb has been successful in the treatment of non-Hodgkin lymphoma [85]. It has been demonstrated that the conjugation of mAbs to toxins, such as ricin A or sapporin, can significantly increase the efficiency of the antibody in depleting the targeted cells [86]. For this purpose, a murine anti-CD22 mAb was conjugated to the ricin A chain (in the laboratory of Ellen Vitetta) and administered to a baboon. After 4 doses, a rapid reduction of B cells in the blood and bone marrow was observed. However, there was little immediate depletion of B cells in lymph nodes. Further studies involving this immunotoxin are ongoing.

It can be concluded from these data that WBI, pharmacological agents, anti-B cell monoclonal antibodies, and immunotoxins, alone or in combination, can potentially deplete B cells from blood, bone marrow, and lymph nodes for as long as 3 months. After specific immunoadsorption of anti-αGal the levels of anti-αGal, however, recover, suggesting that cells other than B cells (probably plasma cells) are the major source of anti-αGal production.

Prevention of the induced antibody response. Induced anti-αGal IgG, and possibly antibody directed against new porcine (non-αGal) antigenic determinants, are considered to play a major role in AVR. It is believed that these newly-synthesized antibodies are produced in a T cell-dependent fashion. Prevention of this response may therefore prove to be a major step in the prevention of AVR. The costimulatory pathway of CD40 and the T cell ligand, CD40L (or CD154), is crucial for effective activation of T cells to antigen [87] and plays an important role in establishing T cell-dependent B cell activity [88]. Costimulatory blockade may therefore prevent the production of induced antibodies. Blockade of this pathway alone or in combination with blockade of the B7/CD28 pathway has been effective in prolonging survival of skin and organ allografts in rodents [89] and of kidney allografts in monkeys [90,91]. At our center, when combined with a nonmyeloablative regimen, costimulatory blockade has been shown to facilitate the establishment of mixed chimerism and tolerance to skin allografts in rodents [92]. Furthermore, in xenotransplantation, costimulatory blockade has allowed prolonged survival of rat-to-mouse skin and heart grafts, as well as pig-to-mouse skin grafts [93]. We have recently included an anti-CD40L mAb in our tolerance induction regimen in a

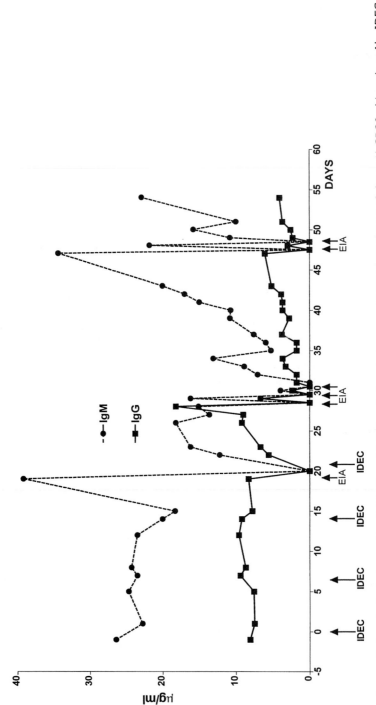

Figure 3. Graph depicting anti-αGal IgG and IgM levels in a baboon receiving four doses of the anti-CD20 chimeric mAb, IDEC-C2B8, at weekly intervals (long arrows). Extracorporeal immunoadsorption (EIA) was performed on the days indicated by short arrows. Following successful removal of anti-αGal antibodies by repeated EIA, the rate of return of antibody was slow. Anti-αGal IgM had returned to pre-treatment level within 2 weeks, but IgG remained at a low level for at least 4 weeks.

pig-to-baboon model (as discussed below). We demonstrated that the anti-CD40L mAb is effective in preventing the induced antibody response (both to αGal and other pig determinants) after the infusion of high doses of mobilized porcine peripheral blood mobilized progenitor cells into baboons [94] (**Figures 4A & B**). We believe that the prevention of an induced response to pig antigens marks a major advance in overcoming the barriers to xenotransplantation.

Depletion or Inhibition of Complement

In the 1960s, cobra venom was important in elucidating the activation of the complement pathway [95]. Cobra venom factor (CVF) was purified and was found to activate the complement system as a functional analogue of C3b [96,97]. Similar to C3b, CVF can bind to factor B, but is approximately 5 times more stable than C3bBb and is resistant to decay acceleration and proteolytic inactivation [98]. The administration of CVF therefore leads to continuous complement activation, resulting in depletion of one or more complement components. Complement depletion by CVF can prolong discordant xenograft survival from minutes to days, but AVR eventually develops by complement-independent mechanisms [14, 99-101].

Inhibition of complement activation can be achieved successfully by administering human soluble complement receptor 1 (sCR1). This leads to acceleration of the proteolytic cleavage of C3/C5-convertases, thus preventing development of MAC and proinflammatory cytokines. sCR1 does not activate and deplete complement components and may therefore be less toxic than CVF. Administered alone, sCR1 can also prolong discordant cardiac xenograft survival in the guinea pig-to-rat model to 32 hours [102] and in the pig-to-primate model to 7 days [103]. When combined with CPP, cyclosporine and steroids, survival of pig cardiac xenografts was further prolonged to a maximum of 6 weeks [104, 105].

Induction of Tolerance

Many investigators believe that the ideal method for avoiding both HAR and AVR is to induce B cell tolerance. Additionally, if T cell tolerance were also induced, the subsequent cellular response would be avoided. This would prevent the complications associated with long-term pharmacological immunosuppressive therapy. Since tolerance can be defined as a state of permanent specific unresponsiveness to donor antigens (but not to other antigens) by the recipient in the absence of maintenance immunosuppressive therapy, immune responses to pathogens would be normal. Sachs and Sykes have developed tolerance in small and large animal allotransplantation models [31,32,73,92,106, 107].

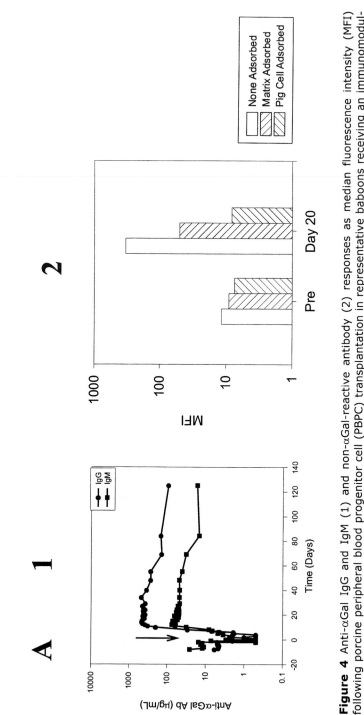

Figure 4 Anti-αGal IgG and IgM (1) and non-αGal-reactive antibody (2) responses as median fluorescence intensity (MFI) following porcine peripheral blood progenitor cell (PBPC) transplantation in representative baboons receiving an immunomodulatory regimen (aimed at inducing mixed chimerism and tolerance) (see Figure 5) **without** (**A**) and **with** an anti-CD40L mAb (**B**). The arrows in (1) indicate the first day of porcine PBPC transplantation, which was administered after the third (cont.)

A1. A rise in both anti-αGal IgG and IgM to above pre-PBPC level occurred by day 10, indicating sensitization to the Gal determinants on the PBPC.

A2. Antibody directed to both αGal and porcine nonαGal determinants on the PBPC developed within 20 days.

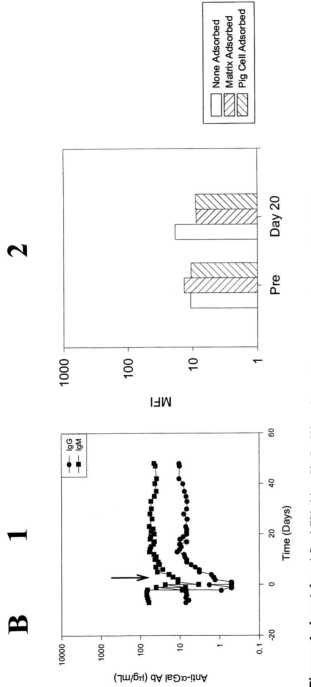

Figure 4. (cont.) and final EIA (day 0). In (2), column 1 represents the serum level of anti-pig antibody, column 2 represents the same serum after immunoadsorption of anti-αGal antibody, and column 3 represents this serum depleted of both αGal-reactive and non-αGal-reactive antibodies. The difference between columns 1 and 2 therefore indicates the amount of anti-αGal antibody, and the difference between columns 2 and 3 indicates the amount of anti-nonαGal antibody.

B1. No rise in αGal-reactive IgG or IgM above pre-PBPC levels occurred, indicating that sensitization to αGal did not develop when anti-CD40L mAb was administered.

B2. No antibody against porcine nonαGal determinants developed.

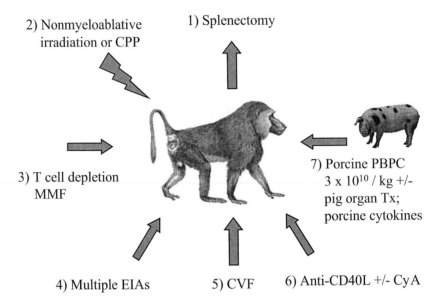

2) Nonmyeloablative irradiation or CPP

1) Splenectomy

3) T cell depletion MMF

7) Porcine PBPC 3 x 10^{10} / kg +/- pig organ Tx; porcine cytokines

4) Multiple EIAs   5) CVF   6) Anti-CD40L +/- CyA

Figure 5. Schematic representation of our immunomodulatory regimen (aimed at obtaining mixed hematopoietic chimerism and inducing tolerance) in baboons. A splenectomy is performed, followed by 300 cGy WBI or induc-tion therapy with cyclophosphamide (CPP). A continuous iv infusion of MMF is commenced. The baboon undergoes multiple EIAs. Anti-complement therapy is initiated with cobra venom factor, dosed according to the results of the measurement of CH50 (EZ-complement, Diamedix Corp., Miami, FL). Anti-CD40L mAb and pig cytokines are started prior to the first infusion of porcine mobilized peripheral blood progenitor cells (PBPC) +/- a pig organ transplant. A total of 3 x 10^{10} cells / kg is infused over 3 days. In some cases, cyclosporine (CyA) has been added to the protocol.

Hematopoietic cell chimerism. One approach to inducing tolerance to a transplanted xenogeneic organ would be to first induce mixed hema-topoietic cell chimerism between pig and primate [32,60]. To induce this state in the pig-to-primate model, a combination of (at least temporary) (i) depletion or inhibition of anti-αGal, (ii) depletion or inhibition of complement, (iii) T cell depletion (and/or costimulatory blockade), and (iv) pig hematopoietic cell engraftment, would appear to be necessary. Our laboratory is involved in studies aimed at inducing mixed hematopoietic chimerism and thus a state of both B and T cell tolerance in this model. We infuse large quantities of cytokine-mobil-ized peripheral blood progenitor cells (approximately 3 x 10^{10} cells/kg) obtained from our MHC-inbred herd of miniature swine into a pre-conditioned recipient baboon. Our current conditioning regimen consists of splenectomy, WBI, thymic irradiation, anti-thymocyte globulin, MMF, CyA, CVF, anti-CD40L mAb, and multiple EIAs [94] (**Figure 5**). With this regimen, we are able to detect porcine cells by flow cytometry until day 6 following infusion, and by polymerase chain reaction consistently

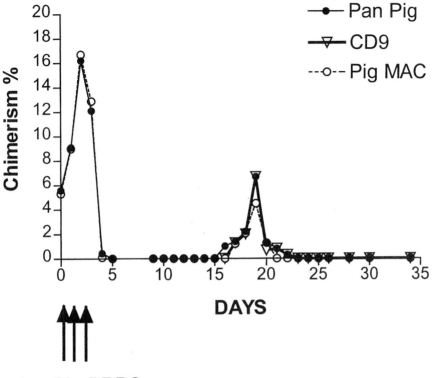

Figure 6. Pig cell chimerism detected by flow cytometry in the blood of a baboon treated with our immunomodulatory regimen (see Figure 5) . Porcine PBPC were infused on days 0 – 2, during which up to 16% of the white blood cells in the baboon were of pig origin. From days 5 through 15 no pig cells could be detected, but on days 16 through 21 a pig monocyte population (stained with markers for pig (pan pig), pig CD9 (platelets, early B cells, activated T cells, and basophils), and pig MAC (monocytes and granulocytes)) could again be detected, indicative of transient pig cell engraftment in the baboon.

through day 30 and intermittently up to 140 days. Although engraftment of porcine cells, measurable by flow cytometry, has been definitively documented only once (**Figure 6**), a state of donor-specific hyporesponsiveness, detected by mixed lymphocyte reaction from day 40-80, has been observed in several cases, indicating that the induction of tolerance through mixed hematopoietic chimerism seems feasible if anti-Gal can be removed for sufficient period of time.

<u>Molecular chimerism.</u>   A second approach to the induction of tolerance is by gene therapy in an attempt to induce what has been termed molecular chimerism. For example, B cell tolerance might be achieved if the primate recipient could be induced to express the Gal epitope on

its tissues, which might lead to the suppression of production of anti-Gal antibody. Autologous transplantation of bone marrow from αGal-knockout mice transduced *ex vivo* with the gene for αgalacto-syltransferase (αGT, the enzyme that leads to the production of the Gal epitopes) resulted in suppression of production of anti-αGal and the achievement of B cell tolerance to αGal [108]. Preliminary studies in baboons, however, demonstrated only transient expression of αGal following the infusion of transduced autologous bone marrow cells. The transduction efficiency of baboon bone marrow cells is currently being optimized with the use of improved vectors and culture parameters.

T cell tolerance might be achieved by the introduction into the recipient of a gene encoding a swine MHC (SLA) class II antigen. The presence of a donor-specific class II antigen in the recipient (following gene transduction of bone marrow cells) has been demonstrated to lead to tolerance to a kidney allograft in miniature swine [109], and its importance has been tested in the pig-to-baboon model [110]. *Ex vivo* transduction of baboon bone marrow cells with an SLA class II gene of a specific MHC-inbred miniature swine genotype was performed. Auto-logous transplantation of these transduced cells led to detection of the transgene in blood and bone marrow, but the transcription was tran-sient. Subsequent pig skin or organ grafts (from a pig matched to the transgene) were rejected within 8 to 22 days from an antibody-mediated mechanism. In contrast to control baboons, however, the induction of IgG against non-αGal antigens was prevented, suggesting prevention of a T cell response.

<u>Thymic transplantation</u>. Zhao et al. demonstrated that the transplantation of fetal pig thymus and liver tissue (as a source of hematopoietic cells) under the kidney capsule of thymectomized and T/NK cell-depleted mouse recipients can induce donor-specific tolerance and restore immune competence [111]. Furthermore, when donor-matched pig skin grafts were transplanted to these mice, permanent graft survival was achieved, whereas allogeneic skin grafts rejected within 26 days [112]. These studies were expanded by Wu et al., who demonstrated in vitro unresponsiveness following fetal porcine thymic tissue grafting in thymectomized, T cell-depleted baboons [113]. Fur-ther studies are underway in this model.

Our center is also involved with the induction of T cell tolerance by the transplantation of a vascularized thymic graft from the donor. Yamada et al. have demonstrated in our MHC-inbred herd of pigs that autologous thymic tissue, when transplanted under the renal capsule, becomes vascularized, regenerates, and functions normally [114] **(Figures 7A & 7B)**. When these "thymo-kidney" composite grafts are transplanted across a fully-mismatched allogeneic barrier, in a T cell depleted and thymectomized recipient, they are able to induce T cell tolerance [115, Yamada, manuscript in preparation]. If anti-αGal could

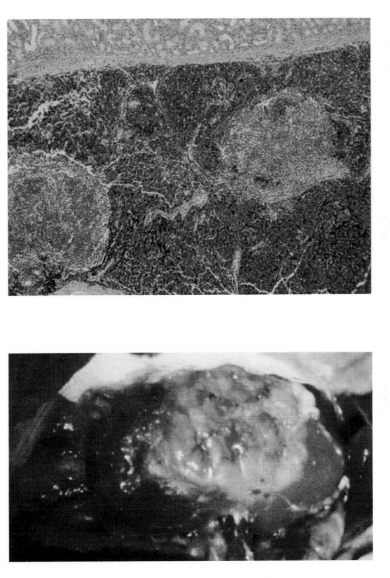

Figure 7. Macroscopic (left) and microscopic (right) appearances of pig thymic tissue 3 months after transplantation under the capsule of an autologous kidney. In (right), kidney tissue can be seen at the right margin of the figure; note the complete reorganization of the thymic tissue, which allowed normal thymopoiesis.

be successfully depleted for a limited period of time, the transplantation of a pig thymokidney could potentially induce T cell tolerance in the pig-to-primate model. The problem of providing an anti-Gal-free environment that would allow T cell tolerance to develop, however, remains unresolved at the present time.

Accommodation

Under certain circumstances, ABO-incompatible allografts or allografts in HLA-sensitized recipients are able to survive despite the presence of circulating antibodies directed against determinants on the grafted organ [50,53,116]. This process has been termed accommodation, and can be summarized as the absence of antibody-mediated rejection of a primary vascularized organ despite the presence of circulating antibodies that are potentially reactive with antigens on the vascular endothelium of that graft [117]. The phenomenon has not yet been documented to conclusively occur in Gal-incompatible large animal models. Possible explanations for the phenomenon of accommodation have been proposed by Bach et al. [117] and are briefly reviewed. Firstly, the returning antibodies may be different in isotype, affinity, and/or specificity, and are thus unable to initiate rejection. Secondly, the surface antigens on the vascular endothelium may show subtle changes during the absence of natural antibodies, thus preventing recognition by the returning antibodies. Finally, during the return of antibodies, the endothelial cells may adapt and either respond differently to these antibodies or become 'desensitized'. It has been proposed that, during accommodation, 'beneficial' genes are upregulated and 'detrimental' genes are downregulated [118].

Genetic Engineering of the Organ-Source Pig

To date, it has proven rather difficult to maintain depletion of anti-αGal antibodies in the recipient primate. A different approach would be to prevent expression of the αGal epitope on the vascular endothelial cells of the pig by genetic manipulation. It is currently not possible to create an αGal-knockout pig (i.e., to disrupt the α1,3galactosyl-transferase gene (αGT) by homologous recombination, thereby preventing αGal expression) because pig embryonic stem cells are not yet available. Furthermore, studies in αGal-knockout mice indicate that the absence of αGal may induce expression of underlying 'cryptic' oliogosaccharide epitopes to which humans may have antibodies [119]. However, several advances have been made in the field of genetic engineering and are discussed below.

    <u>Transgenesis for human complement regulatory proteins.</u> Since complement activation in humans is regulated by membrane bound complement regulatory proteins, such as CD46 (membrane cofactor protein, MCP), CD55 (decay accelerating factor, DAF), and CD59, inducing expression of these human proteins in pigs to inhibit comple-

ment activation seems to be a logical approach. Complement regulatory proteins are largely species-specific, i.e., complement regulatory proteins expressed on porcine tissue do not modulate human complement and vice-versa. The creation of pigs transgenic for human complement regulatory proteins therefore seems desirable. White's group in Cambridge has successfully created pigs transgenic for hDAF. When organs from these pigs are transplanted into nonhuman primates, they are protected from HAR and, in association with intensive immunosuppressive therapy, graft survival of up to 99 days has been reported (White, personal communication). Median graft survival of life-supporting pig kidneys transplanted into cynomolgus monkeys is approximately 30 days and of pig hearts transplanted orthotopically into baboons about 15 days [18,19]. Other groups have created pigs transgenic for more than one human complement regulatory protein but with less prolonged graft survival [120], probably due to differences in the immunosuppressive protocol administered.

Competitive glycosylation As it is not yet possible to create an αGal-knockout pig, alternatives have been proposed to decrease the αGal expression on donor pig organs. The introduction of a gene that would compete with αGT for its substrate, N-acetyllactosamine, is one such approach [121] (**Figure 8**). *In vitro* studies by Sandrin et al. [122,123]

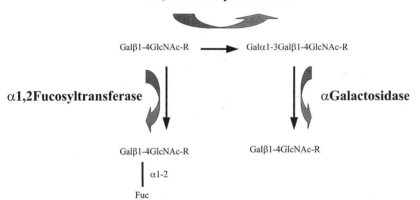

α**1,3Galactosyltransferase**

Galβ1-4GlcNAc-R ⟶ Galα1-3Galβ1-4GlcNAc-R

α**1,2Fucosyltransferase** α**Galactosidase**

Galβ1-4GlcNAc-R   Galβ1-4GlcNAc-R

| α1-2

Fuc

Figure 8. Natural biosynthetic pathway for synthesis of the Gal epitope (Galα1-3Gal), and methods by which this can be modified by transgenic techniques. Galactose is added to the N-acetyllactosamine (Galβ1-4GlcNAc) substrate by the α1,3 galactosyltransferase enzyme to form Galα1-3Gal. Galβ1-4GlcNAc can also form the substrate for the H (O) histo-blood group epitope when the gene for the α1,2 fucosyltransferase enzyme is transgenically introduced. Furthermore, cleavage of Galα1-3Gal occurs when the gene for the α-galactosidase enzyme is introduced. Modification of the natural pathway has been demonstrated in cells in culture and in αGal-knockout (αGal-negative) mice by transgenic techniques, but has not yet been successfully achieved in pigs. (Modified from [123]).

in COS cells demonstrated that competition takes place between αGT and α1,2fucosyltransferase (αFT) in the Golgi apparatus for this substrate, and that αFT takes precedence, thereby resulting in a cell that expresses more H blood group antigen than Gal. COS cells simultaneously transfected with cDNA clones encoding for either αGT or αFT showed greater expression of the αFT-product (the H epitope) than the αGT-product (αGal) [123]. Mice transgenic for αFT demonstrated a major decrease in αGal expression and reduction of reactivity of these cells when challenged with human serum [124]. More recently, evidence has been presented that high-level expression of H antigen on porcine cells reduces human monocyte adhesion and activation [125].

It would be necessary, however, to ensure that <u>all</u> the αGal epitopes are replaced by the H epitopes, or the transplanted organ may still be susceptible to HAR or AVR. It has therefore been proposed to add another gene, namely α-galactosidase, to the donor pig in addition to that for αFT [126]. αGalactosidase removes terminal αGal rather than adding it, and would ensure that those αGal epitopes that are not competitively replaced with H epitopes by αFT are removed by α-galactosidase. Sandrin's group has provided data demonstrating a complete absence of αGal expression in cell cultures containing the genes for both αFT and α-galactosidase [127].

<u>Nuclear transfer.</u> Our knowledge of and ability to genetically manipulate embryonic and adult cells of large mammals has greatly increased in the last few years [128]. In the not too distant future, it may be possible to genetically modify a pig cell in culture by adding or deleting specific genes. The resulting cell can then be selectively cloned, making multiple copies, after which the nuclear material of these cells may be transferred into embryonic cells from which the nucleus has been removed. These embryonic cells would be implanted into surrogate sows, thus enabling the production of an almost "instant" herd of genetically-modified pigs. This technique may therefore prove of great benefit to xenotransplantation.

Comment

Xenotransplantation has potential to change transplantation medicine as it is currently known. No longer will patients with organ failure need to wait weeks, months or years for an organ as a limitless number of animal organs will be readily available. The surgical procedure can be planned electively, during normal working hours, while the patient is still in reasonable health. The use of animals as a source of organs also presents us with new opportunities to manipulate and/or modify a "donor" using techniques such as genetic engineering and nuclear transfer. Manipulation of donor has not been possible in allotransplantation.

The rejection processes that take place following the transplantation of a vascularized organ from a pig to a primate present formidable barriers. Much progress has been made in the last decade in elucidating the pathophysiology of these phenomena. Although major immunological hurdles (such as the prevention of HAR) have been overcome, many remain. It is unlikely that any of the therapeutic modalities discussed in this chapter will be successful in preventing rejection when used alone. A combination of therapies will almost certainly be necessary.

Our own experience, and that of others, would suggest that, using the agents that are available today, pharmacological suppression of the T and B cell responses to the transplanted organ may be insufficient to allow long-term graft survival. It would seem essential to find a means of depleting plasma cells, or inhibiting their activity, as our evidence is that they are the major source of anti-αGal antibody production.

We would suggest that a successful therapeutic regimen is likely to require anti-αGal depletion, and maintenance of depletion for a significant period of time, possibly several weeks. During this period, newly-developing αGal-reactive B cells could be tolerized by, for example, successful porcine hematopoietic cell transplantation. In this respect, the ability of anti-CD40L mAb to prevent the induced antibody response to pig cells represents a significant step in overcoming the immunologic barriers to xenotransplantation, and will undoubtedly facilitate the survival of transplanted pig organs in primates and the induction of tolerance.

However, despite our current preoccupation with the humoral response to a xenograft, antibody is unlikely to be the sole hurdle to overcome. Several non-specific immune cells have been implicated in various stages of rejection. Macrophages and NK cells are consistently found in xenografts undergoing AVR, and may play a role in the onset of this form of rejection [16-129]. Recent studies at our center have been directed at depleting or inhibiting these cells, which it is hoped will contribute to prolonged survival of xenografts. The additional induction of T cell tolerance would ensure prolonged graft survival without the need for further immunosuppressive therapy.

Acknowledgements

We thank our many colleagues at the Transplantation Biology Research Center and at BioTransplant, Inc., who have contributed to the studies outlined in this review and, in particular, Kazu Yamada MD, and David Sachs MD for their constructive comments on the preparation of this chapter.

References

1. Harper AM, Rosendale JD. The UNOS OPTN waiting list and donor registry. Clin Transpl 1997: 61
2. Delmonico FL, Harmon WE, Lorber MI, et al. A new allocation plan for renal transplantation. Transplantation 1999; 67:303
3. Aaronson KD, Mancini DM. Mortality remains high for outpatient transplant candidates with prolonged (>6 months) waiting list time. J Am Coll Cardiol 1999; 33(5): 1189
4. Cooper DKC. Xenografting: how great is the clinical need? Xeno 1993; 1: 25
5. Lambrigts D, Sachs DH, Cooper DKC. Discordant organ xenotransplantation in primates. World experience and current status. Tranplantation 1998; 66: 547
6. Bailey LL, Gundry SR. Survival following orthotopic cardiac xenotransplantation between juvenile baboon recipients and concordant and discordant donor species: foundation for clinical trials. World J Surg 1997; 21:943
7. Perper RJ, Najarian JS. Experimental renal heterotransplantation. I. In widely divergent species. Transplantation 1966; 4: 377
8. Cooper DKC, Human PA, Lexer G, et al. Effects of cyclosporine and antibody adsorption on pig cardiac xenograft survival in the baboon. J Heart Lung Transplant 1988; 7: 238
9. Good AH, Cooper DKC, Malcolm AJ, et al. Identification of carbohydrate structures that bind human anti-porcine antibodies: implications for discordant xenografting in humans. Transplant Proc 1992; 24: 559
10. Platt JL, Fischel RJ, Matas AJ, et al. Immunopathology of hyperacute xenograft rejection in a swine-to-primate model. Transplantation 1991; 52: 514
11. Rose AG, Cooper DKC, Human PA, et al. Histopathology of hyperacute rejection of the heart: experimental and clinical observations in allografts and xenografts. J Heart Lung Transplant 1991; 10: 223
12. Rose AG, Cooper DK. A histopathologic grading system of hyperacute (humoral, antibody-mediated) cardiac xenograft and allograft rejection. J Heart Lung Transplant 1996; 15:804
13. Alexandre GPJ, Gianello P, Latinne D, et al. Plasmapheresis and splenectomy in experimental renal xenotransplantation. In: Hardy MA (ed). Xenograft 25. New York, Elsevier, 1989. p 28.
14. Leventhal JR, Dalmasso AP, Cromwell JW, et al. Prolongation of cardiac xenograft survival by depletion of complement. Transplantation. 1993; 55: 857
15. Cozzi E, White DJG. The generation of transgenic pigs as potential organ donors or humans. Nat Med 1995; 1: 964
16. Fryer JP, Leventhal JR, Dalmasso AP, et al. Cellular rejection in discordant xenografts when hyperacute rejection is prevented: analysis using adoptive and passive transfer. Transpl Immunol 1994; 2:87
17. Bach FH, Robson SC, Winkler H, et al. Barriers to xenotransplantation. Nat Med 1995; 1: 869
18. Schmoeckel M, Bhatti FN, Zaidi A, et al. Orthotopic heart transplantation in a transgenic pig-to-primate model. Transplantation 1998; 65: 1570
19. Zaidi A, Schmoeckel M, Bhatti F, et al. Life-supporting pig-to-primate renal xenotransplantation using genetically modified donors. Transplantation 1998; 65: 1584
20. Cooper DKC, Ye Y, Rolf LL Jr, et al. The pig as a potential organ donor for man. In: Cooper DKC, Kemp E, Reemtsma K, et al. (eds.). Xenotranplantation. Heidelberg, Springer 1991. p481
21. Sachs DH. The pig as a potential xenograft donor. Vet Imm Immunopath 1994; 43: 185

22. Galili U, Shohet SB, Kobrin E, et al. Man, apes, and Old World monkeys differ from other mammals in the expression of α-galactosyl epitopes on nucleated cells. J Biol Chem 1988; 263: 17755

23. Oriol R, Ye Y, Koren E, et al. Carbohydrate antigens of pig tissues reacting with human natural antibodies as potential targets for hyperacute vascular rejection in pig-to-man organ xenotransplantation. Transplantation 1993; 56: 1433

24. Galili U, Rachmilewitz EA, Peleg A, et al. A unique natural human IgG antibody with anti-α-galactosyl specificity. J Exp Med 1984; 260: 1519

25. Cooper DKC, Good AH, Koren E, et al. Identification of α-galatosyl and other carbohydrate epitopes that are bound by human anti-pig antibodies: relevance to discordant xenografting in man. Transplant Immunol 1993; 1: 198

26. Cooper DKC, Koren E, Oriol R. Oligosaccharides and discordant xenotransplantation. Immunol Rev 1994; 141: 31

27. Kujundzic M, Koren E, Neethling FA, et al. Variability of anti-αGal antibodies in human serum and their relation to serum cytotoxicity against pig cells. Xenotransplantation 1994; 1: 58

28. McMorrow IM, Comrack CA, Nazarey PP, et al. Relationship between ABO bloodgroup and levels of Gal alpha,3galactose-reactive human immunoglobulin G. Transplantation 1997; 64: 546

29. Sandrin MS, Vaughan HA, Dabkowski PL, et al. Anti-pig IgM antibodies in human serum react predominantly with Galα(1-3)Gal epitopes. Proc Natl Acad Sci USA 1993; 90: 11391

30. Galili U. Anti-αgalactosyl (anti-Gal) antibody damage beyond hyperacute rejection. In: Cooper DKC, Kemp E, Platt JL, et al. (eds). Xenotransplantation, 2nd edition. Heidelberg, Springer 1997. p 95

31. Kozlowski T, Monroy R, Xu, Y, et al. Anti-Galα1-3Gal antibody response to porcine bone marrow in unmodified baboons and baboons conditioned for tolerance induction. Transplantation 1998; 66: 176

32. Kozlowski T, Shimuzu A, Lambrigts D, et al. Porcine kidney and heart transplantation in baboons undergoing a tolerance induction regimen and antibody adsorption. Transplantation 1999; 67:18

33. Candinas D, Belliveau S, Koyamada N, et al. T cell independence of macrophage and natural killer cell infiltration, cytokine production, and endothelial activation during delayed xenograft rejection. Transplantation 1996; 62:1920

34. Marquet RL, van Overdam K, Boudesteijn EA, et al. Immunobiology of delayed xenograft rejection. Transplant Proc 1997; 29:955

35. Ierino FL, Kozlowski T, Siegel JB, et al. Disseminated intravascular coagulation in association with the delayed rejection of pig-to-baboon renal xenografts. Transplantation 1998; 66:1439

36. Moses RD, Auchincloss H. Mechanism of cellular xenograft rejection. In: Cooper DKC, Kemp E, Platt JL, et al. (ed.), Xenotransplantation 2nd edition. Heidelberg, Springer 1997. p140

37. Vallee I, Guillaumin JM, Thibault G, et al. Human T lymphocyte proliferative response to resting porcine endothelial cells results from an HLA-restricted, IL-10 sensitive, indirect presentation pathway but also depends on endothelial-specific costimulatory factors. J Immunol 1998; 161:1652

38. Simeonovic CJ, Townsend MJ, Morris CF, et al. Immune mechanisms associated with the rejection of fetal murine proislets allografts and pig proislet xenografts: comparison of intragraft cytokine mRNA profiles. Transplantation 1999; 67:963

39. Soderlund J, Wennberg L, Castanos-Velez E, et al. Fetal porcine islet-like cell clusters transplanted to cynomolgus monkeys: an immunohistochemical study. Transplantation 1999; 67:784

40. Siebers U, Horcher A, Brandhorst H, et al. Analysis of the cellular reaction towards microencapsulated xenogeneic islets after intraperitoneal transplantation. J Mol Med 1999; 77:215

41. Moberg AW, Shons AR, Gerwurz H, et al. Prolongation of renal xenografts by the simultaneous sequestration of preformed antibody, inhibition of complement, coagulation, and antibody synthesis. Transplant Proc 1971; 3: 538
42. Slapak M, Greenbaum M, Bardawil W, et al. Effect of heparin, arvin, liver perfusion, and heterologous antiplatelet serum on rejection of pig kidney to dog. Transplant Proc 1971; 3: 558
43. Shons AR, Beir M, Jetzer J, et al. Techniques of *in vivo* plasma modification for the treatment of hyperacute rejection. Surgery 1973; 73: 28
44. Lexer G, Cooper DKC, Rose AG, et al. Hyperacute rejection in a discordant (pig-to-baboon) cardiac xenograft model. J Heart Transplant 1986; 5: 411
45. Azimzadeh A, Meyer C, Watier H, et al. Removal of primate xenoreactive natural antibodies by extracorporeal perfusion of pig kidneys and livers. Transpl Immunol 1998; 1: 13
46. Macchiarini P, Oriol R, Azimzadeh A, et al. Evidence of human non-alpha-galactosyl antibodies involved in the hyperacute rejection of pig lungs and their removal by pig organ perfusion. J Thorac Cardiovasc Surg 1998; 5: 831
47. Siami GA, Siami FS. Plasmapheresis and paraproteinemia: cryoprotein-induced diseases, monoclonal gammopathy, Waldenstrom's macroglobulinemia, hyperviscosity syndrome, multiple myeloma, light chain disease, and amyloidosis. Ther Apher 1999; 3:8
48. Malahati K, Dawson RB, Collins JO, et al. Predictable recovery from myesthenia gravis crisis with plasma exchange: thirty-six cases and review of current management. J Clin Apheresis 1999; 14:1
49. Bosch T, Buhmann R, Lennertz A, et al. Therapeutic plasma exchange in patients suffering from thrombotic microangiopathy after bone marrow transplantation. Ther Apher 1999; 3:252
50. Alexandre GPJ, Squifflet JP, De Bruyere M, et al. Present experiences in a series of 26 ABO-incompatible living donor renal allografts. Transplant Proc 1987; 19: 4538
51. Alexandre GPJ, Gianello P, Latinne D, et al. Plasmapheresis and splenectomy in experimental renal xenotransplantation. In: Hardy MA (ed). Xenograft 25. New York, Elsevier, 1989. p 28.
52. Benny WB, Sutton DM, Oger J, et al. Clinical evaluation of a staphylococcal protein A immunoadsorption system in the treatment of myasthenia gravis patients. Transfuion 1999; 39:682
53. Palmer A, Welsh K, Gjorstrup P, et al. Removal of HLA antibodies by extracorporeal immunoadsorption to enable renal transplantation. Lancet 1989; 1: 10
54. Dantal J, Testa A, Bigot E, et al. Effects of plasma-protein A immunoadsorption on idiopathic nephrotic syndrome recurring after renal transplantation. Ann Med Interne (Paris) 1992; 143:48
55. Pretagostini R, Berloco P, Poli L, et al. Immunoadsorption with proetein A in humoral rejection of kidney transplants. ASAIO J 1996; 42:M645
56. Hickstein H, Korten G, Bast R, et al. Protein A immunoadsorption (i.a.) in renal transplantation patients with vascular rejection. Transfus Sci 1998; Mar:53
57. Leventhal JR, John R, Fryer JP, et al. Removal of baboon and human antiporcine IgG and IgM natural antibodies by immunoadsorption. Results of in vitro and in vivo studies. Transplantation 1995; 59:294
58. Ye Y, Neethling FA, Niekrasz M, et al. Evidence that intravenously administered alpha-galactosyl carbohydrates reduce baboon serum cytotoxicity to pig kidney cells (PK15) and transplanted pig hearts. Transplantation 1994; 58: 330
59. Neethling FA, Cooper DK. Serum cytotoxicity to pig cells and anti-alphaGal antibody level and specificity in humans and baboons. Transplantation 1999; 67:658

60. Sablinski T, Latinne D, Gianello P, et al. Xenotransplantation of pig kidneys to nonhuman primates: I. Development of the model. Xenotransplantation. 1995; 2: 264

61. Cooper DKC, Cairns TDH, Taube DH. Extracorporeal immunoadsorption of anti-pig antibody in pigs using αGal oligosaccharide immunoaffinity columns. Xeno 1996; 4: 27

62. Taniguchi S, Neethling FA, Korchagina EY, et al. *In vivo* immunoadsorption of anti-pig antibodies in baboons using a specific Galα1-3Gal column. Transplantation 1996; 10: 1379

63. Xu Y, Lorf T, Sablinski T, et al. Removal of anti-porcine natural antibodies from human and nonhuman primate plasma *in vitro* and *in vivo* by a Galα1-3Galβ1-Glc-X immunoaffinity column. Transplantation 1998; 65: 172

64. Kozlowski T, Ierino FL, Lambrigts D, et al. Depletion of anti-αGal1-3Gal antibody in baboons by specific immunoaffinity columns. Xenotransplantation 1998; 5: 122

65. Watts A, Foley A, Awwad M, et al. Plasma perfusion by apheresis through a Gal immunoaffinity column successfully depletes anti-Gal antibody – experience with 80 aphereses in baboons. Abstract presented at the 5th International Congress of Xenotransplantation 1999, Nagoya, Japan.

66. Neethling F, Cooper DK, Xu H, et al. Newborn baboon serum anti-alpha galactosyl antibody levels and cytotoxicity to cultured pig kidney (PK15) cells. Transplantation 1995; 60:520

67. Oriol R, Barthod F, Bergemer AM, et al. Monomorphic and polymorphic carbohydrate antigens on pig tissues: implications for organ xenotransplantation in the pig-to-human model. Transpl Int 1994; 7:405

68. Simon PM, Neethling FA, Taniguchi S, et al. Intravenous infusion of Galalpha1-3Gal oligosaccharides in baboons delays hyperacute rejection of porcine heart xenografts. Transplantation 1998; 65:346

69. Romano E, Neethling FA, Nilsson KGI, et al. Intravenous synthetic αGal saccharides delay hyperacute rejection following pig-to-baboon heart transplantation. Xenotransplantation 1999; 6:36

70. Koren E, Milotic F, Neethling FA, et al. Monoclonal antiidiotypic antibodies neutralize cytotoxic effects of anti-αGal antibodies. Transplantation 1996; 62:837

71. Buhler L, Treter S, McMorrow I, et al. Injection of porcine anti-idiotypic antibodies (AIA) to primate anti-Gal antibodies leads to active inhibition of serum cytotoxicity in a baboon. Abstract presented at the 5th International Congress for Xenotransplantation 1999, Nagoya, Japan.

72. Lindsley K, Deeg HJ. Total body irradiation for marrow or stem-cell transplantation. Cancer Invest 1998; 16: 424

73. Sykes M, Sachs DH. Xenogeneic tolerance through hematopoietic cell and thymic transplantation. In: Cooper DKC, Kemp E, Platt JL, et al. (eds). Xenotransplantation, 2nd edition. Heidelberg, Springer 1997. p 496

74. Kimikawa M, Kawai T, Sachs DH, et al. Mixed chimerism and transplantation tolerance induced by a nonlethal preparative regimen in cynomolgus monkeys. Transplant Proc 1997; 29: 1218

75. Clave E, Socie G, Cosset JM. Multicolor flow cytometry analysis of blood cell subsets in patients given total body irradiation before bone marrow transplantation. Int J Radiat Oncol Biol Phys 1995; 34: 881

76. Lambrigts D, Van Calster P, Xu Y, et al. Pharmacologic immunosuppressive therapy and extracorporeal immunoadsorption in the suppression of anti-αGal antibody in the baboon. Xenotransplantation 1998; 5:274

77. Ostlie DJ, Cozzi E, Vial CM, et al. Improved renal function and fewer rejection episodes using SDZ RAD in life-supporting hDAF pig-to-primate renal xenotransplantation. Abstract # 445 at the American Society of Transplantation 1999

78. Lindback S, Vizzard J, Cooper DA, et al. Long-term prognosis following zidovudine monotherapy in primary human immunodeficiency virus type 1 infection. J Infect Dis 1999; 179: 1549

79. Laurencet FM, Zulian GB, Guetty-Alberto M, et al. Cladribine with cyclophosphamide and prednisone in the management of low-grade lymphoproliferative malignancies. Br J Cancer 1999; 79:1215

80. Gorski A, Grieb P, Korczak-Kowalska G, et al. Cladribine (2-chloro-deoxyadenosine, CDA): an inhibitor of human B and T cell activation in vitro. Immunopharmacology 1993; 26: 197

81. Reff ME, Carner K, Chambers KS, et al. Depletion of B cells in vivo by a chimeric mouse human monoclonal antibody to CD20. Blood 1994; 83: 435

82. Maloney DG, Grillo-Lopez AJ, Bodkin DJ, et al. IDEC-C2B8: results of a phase I multiple-dose trial in patients with relapsed non-Hodgkin's lymphoma. J Clin Oncol 1997; 15: 3266

83. Coiffier B, Haioun C, Ketterer N, et al. Rituximab (anti-CD20 monoclonal antibody) for the treatment of patients with relapsing or refractory aggressive lymphoma: a multicenter phase II study. Blood 1998; 92: 1927

84. McLaughlin P, Grillo-Lopez AJ, Link BK, et al. Rituximab chimeric anti-CD20 monoclonal antibody therapy for relapsed indolent lymphoma: half of patients respond to a four dose treatment program. J Clin Oncol 1998; 16: 282

85. Sausville EA, Headlee D, Stetler-Stevenson M, et al. Continuous infusion of the anti-CD22 immunotoxin IgG-RFB4-SMPT-dgA in patients with B cell lymphoma: a phase I study. Blood 1995; 85: 3457

86. Bolognessi A, Tazzari PL, Olivieri F, et al. Evaluation of immunotoxin containing single-chain ribosome-inactivating proteins and an anti-CD22 monoclonal antibody (OM124): in vitro and in vivo studies. Br J Haematol 1998; 101: 179

87. Armitage RJ, Fanslow WC, Strockbine L, et al. Molecular and biological characterization of a murine ligand for CD40. Nature 1992; 357: 80

88. Noelle R, Roy M, Shepherd D, et al. A 39-kDa protein on activated helper T cells binds CD40and transduces the signal for cognate activation of B cells. Proc Natl Acad Sci USA 1992; 89: 6550

89. Larsen CP, Elwood ET, Alexander DZ, et al. Long-term acceptance of skin and cardiac allografts after blocking CD40 ligand. Nature 1996; 381: 434

90. Kirk AD, Harlan DM, Armstrong NN, et al. CTLA4-Ig and anti-CD40 ligand prevent renal allograft rejection in primates. Proc Natl Acad Sci USA 1997; 94: 8789

91. Kirk AD, Burkly LC, Batty DS, et al. Treatment with humanized monoclonal antibody against CD154 prevents acute renal allograft rejection in nonhuman primates. Nature Med 1999; 5:686

92. Wekerle T, Sayegh MH, Hill J, et al. Extrathymic T cell deletion and allogeneic stem cell engraftment induced with costimulatory blockade is followed by central T cell tolerance. J Exp Med 1998; 187:2037

93. Elwood ET, Larsen CP, Cho HR, et al. Prolonged acceptance of concordant and discordant xenografts with combined CD40 and CD28 pathway blockade. Transplantation 1998; 65: 1422

94. Buhler L, Awwad M, Basker M, et al. A nonmyeloablative regimen with CD40L blockade leads to humoral / cellular hyporesponsiveness to pig hematopoietic cells in baboons. Abstract presented at the 5th International Congress for Xenotransplantation 1999, Nagoya, Japan

95. Muller Eberhard HJ, Nilsson UR, Dalmasso AP, et al. A molecular concept of immune cytolysis. Arch Path 1966; 82:205

96. Alper CA, Balatovich D. Cobra venom factor: evidence for its being altered cobra C3 (the third component of complement). Science 1976; 191:1275

97. Vogel CW, Smith CA, Muller Eberhard HJ. Cobra venom factor: structural homology with the third component of human complement. J Immunol 1984; 133:3235
98. Lachmann PJ, Halbwachs L. The influence of C3b inactivator (KAF) concentration on the ability of serum to support complement activation. Clin Exp Immunol 1975; 21:109
99. Adachi H, Rosengard BR, Hutchins GM, et al. Effects of cyclosporine, aspirin, and cobra venom factor on discordant cardiac xenograft survival in rats. Tranplant Proc 1987; 19:1145-1148
100. Scheringa M, Schraa EO, Bouwman E, et al. Prolongation of survival of guinea pig heart grafts in cobra venom factor-treated rats by splenectomy. No additional effect of cyclosporine. Transplantation 1995; 60:1350
101. Kobayashi T, Taniguchi S, Neethling FA, et al. Delayed xenograft rejection of pig-to-baboon cardiac transplants after cobra venom factor therapy. Transplantation 1997; 64: 1255
102. Candinas D, Lesnikoski BA, Robson SC, et al. Effect of repetitive high-dose treatment with soluble complement receptor type 1 and cobra venom factor on discordant xenograft survival. Transplantataion 1996; 62:336
103. Pruitt SK, Bollinger RR, Collins BH, et al. Effect of continuous complement inhibition using soluble complement receptor type 1 on survival of pig-to-primate cardiac xenografts. Transplantation 1997; 63:900
104. Davis EA, Pruitt SK, Greene PS, et al. Inhibition of complement, evoked antibody, and cellular response prevents rejection of pig-to-primate cardiac xenografts. Transplantation 1996; 62:1018
105. Marsh HC Jr, Ryan US. Therapeutic effect of soluble complement receptor type 1 in xenotransplantation. In: Cooper DKC, Kemp E, et al. eds. Xenotransplantation, 2nd edition. Heidelberg, Springer 1997. p 437
106. Yang YG, DeGoma E, Ohdan H, et al. Tolerization of anti-Galα1-3Gal natural antibody-forming B cells by induction of mixed chimerism. J Exp Med 1998; 187:1335-1342
107. Ohdan H, Yang YG, Shimizu A, et al. Mixed chimerism induced without lethal conditioning prevents T cell- and anti-Gal alpha 1,3Gal-mediated graft rejection. J Clin Invest 1999; 104:281
108. Bracy JL, Sachs DH, Iacomini J. Inhibition of xenoreactive natural antibody production by retroviral gene therapy. Science 1998; 281:1845
109. Emery DW, Sablinski T, Shimada H, et al. Expression of an allogeneic MHC DRB transgene, through retroviral transduction of bone marrow, induces specific reduction of alloreactivity. Transplantation 1997; 64:1414
110. Ierino FL, Gojo S, Banerjee PT, et al. Transfer of swine major histocompatibility complex class II genes into autologous bone marrow cells of baboons for the induction of tolerance across xenogeneic barriers. Transplantation 1999; 67:1119
111. Zhao Y, Fishman JA, Sergio JJ, et al. Immune restoration by fetal pig thymus grafts in T cell-depleted, thymectomized mice. J Immunol 1997; 158:1641
112. Zhao Y, Swenson K, Sergio JJ, et al. Skin graft tolerance across a discordant xenogeneic barrier. Nat Med 1996; 2:1211
113. Wu A, Esnaola NF, Yamada K, et al. Xenogeneic thymic transplantation in a pig-to-nonhuman primate model. Transplant Proc 1999; 31:957
114. Yamada K, Shimizu A, Ierino FL, et al. Thymic transplantation in miniature swine: I. Development and function of the "thymokidney". Transplantation 1999, in press
115. Yamada K, Shimizu A, Ierino FL, et al. Allogeneic thymokidney transplants induce stable tolerance in miniature swine. Transplant Proc 1999; 31:1199
116. Chopek MW, Simmons RL, Platt JL. ABO incompatible renal transplantation: initial immunopathologic evaluation. Transplant Proc 1987; 19: 4553

117. Bach FH, Platt JL, Cooper DKC. Accommodation - the role of natural antibody and complement in discordant xenograft rejection. In: Cooper DKC, Kemp E, Reemtsma K, et al. (eds). Xenotransplantation. Heidelberg, Springer 1991. p 81
118. Bach FH, Ferran C, Hechenleitner P, et al. Accommodation of vascularized xenografts: expression of "protective genes" by donor endothelial cells in a host Th2 cytokine environment. Nat Med 1997; 3: 196
119. Shinkel TA, Chen CG, Salvaris E, et al. Changes in cell surface glycosylation in alpha 1,3-galactosyltransferase knockout and alpha 1,2-fucosyltransferase transgenic mice. Transplantation 1997; 64:197
120. Lin SS, Weidner BC, Byrne GW, et al. The role of antibodies in acute vascular rejection of pig-to-primate cardiac transplants. J Clin Invest 1998; 101:1745
121. Cooper DKC, Koren E, Oriol R. Genetically engineerd pigs (Letter). The Lancet 1993; 342:682
122. Sandrin MS, Fodor WL, Mouhtouris E, et al. Enzymatic remodelling of the carbohydrate surface of a xenogenic cell substantially reduces human antibody binding and complement-mediated cytolysis. Nature Med 1995; 1:1261
123. Sandrin MS, Cohney S, Osman N, et al. Overcoming the anti-Galα1-3Gal reaction to avoid hyperacute rejection: molecular genetic approaches. In: Cooper DKC, Kemp E, Platt JL, et al. (eds.) Xenotransplantation, 2nd edition. Heidelberg, Springer 1997. p683
124. Chen CG, Salvaris EJ, Romanella M, et al. Transgenic expression of human alpha1,2-fucosyltransferase (H-transferase) prolongs mouse heart survival in an ex vivo model of xenograft rejection. Transplantation 1998; 65:832
125. Kwiatkowski P, Artrip JH, Edwards NM, et al. High-level porcine endothelial cell expression of alpha(1,2)-fucosyltransferase reduces human monocyte adhesion and activation. Transplantation 1999; 67:219
126. Cooper DKC, Koren E, Oriol R. Manipulation of the anti-αGal antibody-αGal epitope system in experimental discordant xenotransplantation. Xenotransplantation 1996; 3:102
127. Osman N, McKenzie IF, Ostenried K, et al. Combined transgenic expression of alpha-galactosidase and alpha 1,2-fucosyltransferase leads to optimal reduction in the major xenoepitope Galalpha (1,3) Gal. Proc Natl Acad Sci USA 1997; 94:14677
128. Wilmut I, Schnieke AE, McWhir J, et al. Viable offspring derived from fetal and adult mammalian cells. Nature 1997; 385:810
129. Blakely ML, Van der Werff WJ, Berndt MC, et al. Activation of intragraft endothelial and mononuclear cells during discordant xenograft rejection. Transplantation 1994; 58:1059